519

265

303

Ethical Challenges in Managed Care

A CASEBOOK

EDITED BY

Karen G. Gervais
Reinhard Priester
Dorothy E. Vawter
Kimberly K. Otte
Mary M. Solberg

GEORGETOWN UNIVERSITY PRESS / WASHINGTON, D.C.

Georgetown University Press, Washington, D.C.   20007
© 1999 by Minnesota Center for Health Care Ethics. All rights reserved.
Printed in the United States of America.
10 9 8 7 6 5 4 3 2 1 1999
THIS VOLUME IS PRINTED ON ACID-FREE OFFSET BOOKPAPER.

Library of Congress Cataloging-in-Publication Data

Ethical challenges in managed care :   a casebook /   edited by Karen G.
   Gervais . . . [et al.].
      p.   cm.
   Includes index.
      1. Managed care plans (Medical care)—Moral and ethical aspects.
   2. Medical ethics.   I. Gervais, Karen Grandstrand, 1944–   .
   RA413.E876   1999
   362.1'04258—dc21   98-44645
   ISBN 0-87840-718-9 (cloth).—ISBN 0-87840-719-7 (pbk.)

Contents

Acknowledgments   xi

Introduction: Ethical Challenges in Managed Care   1
Karen G. Gervais and Dorothy E. Vawter

Part One: Rationing Shared Resources   15

1   **Balancing a Plan's Obligations to Individual Patients and Its Enrolled Population**
    CASE STUDY   17
    COMMENTARY: *Leonard M. Fleck*   20
    COMMENTARY: *Mitchell Sugarman*   27

2   **Coverage of Emergency Services**
    CASE STUDY   33
    COMMENTARY: *E. Haavi Morreim*   36
    COMMENTARY: *Karen A. Jordan*   41

3   **Coverage of Investigational Interventions for Life-Threatening Conditions**
    CASE STUDY   49
    COMMENTARY: *William T. McGivney*   53
    COMMENTARY: *Gwen Wagstrom Halaas*   58

4   Coverage of Complementary Health Care
CASE STUDY   66
COMMENTARY: *Daniel O. Dugan*   68
COMMENTARY: *Martin Gunderson*   76

5   Coverage Exceptions for Contractually Excluded Benefits
CASE STUDY   83
COMMENTARY: *David Mechanic*   86
COMMENTARY: *Kate T. Christensen*   92

Part Two: Incentives to Contain Costs and Improve Quality   99

6   Referral Practices Under Capitation
CASE STUDY   101
COMMENTARY: *Gail J. Povar*   103
COMMENTARY: *Mark A. Hall*   111

7   Shifting Costs and Care to Public Programs
CASE STUDY   118
COMMENTARY: *Joel E. Frader*   120
COMMENTARY: *Ronald E. Cranford and Karen G. Gervais*   127

8   Choice of Venue and Provider Under Capitation
CASE STUDY   134
COMMENTARY: *Susan B. Rubin and Laurie Zoloth-Dorfman*   138
COMMENTARY: *Arthur L. Caplan*   144

Part Three: Quality Care in a Competitive Market   149

9   Credentialing Standards and Quality Care
CASE STUDY   151
COMMENTARY: *Ruth A. Mickelsen*   153
COMMENTARY: *Matthew K. Wynia and Linda L. Emanuel*   160

10 CEO Salaries in For-Profit and Nonprofit Health Plans
    CASE STUDY   168
    COMMENTARY: *Bradford H. Gray*   169
    COMMENTARY: *David A. Hyman*   176

11 Hospital Staffing Levels   181
    CASE STUDY   181
    COMMENTARY: *Joanne M. Disch*   183
    COMMENTARY: *Judith Shindul-Rothschild*   190

Part Four: Responsibilities to Patients   199

12 Purchaser and Plan Responsibility for Benefit Design
    CASE STUDY   201
    COMMENTARY: *Lisa J. Raiola*   203
    COMMENTARY: *Raymond G. DeVries*   210

13 Advocating for Patients in Managed Care
    CASE STUDY   217
    COMMENTARY: *Susan M. Wolf*   219
    COMMENTARY: *Genevieve Noone Parsons and Peter A. Ubel*   226

14 Similarly-Situated Patients with Different
    Benefits Packages
    CASE STUDY   233
    COMMENTARY: *Larry R. Churchill*   235
    COMMENTARY: *Michael Felder*   241

15 Respecting Patients' Cultural and Religious Beliefs
    CASE STUDY   249
    COMMENTARY: *James Lindemann Nelson*   251
    COMMENTARY: *Kathleen A. Culhane-Pera*   258

Part Five: Managed Care for Vulnerable Populations   265

16 Managing Care for the Seriously Mentally Ill
    CASE STUDY   267
    COMMENTARY: *James E. Sabin*   270
    COMMENTARY: *Mary L. Durham*   276

17 Quality Care for Elderly Nursing Home Patients

CASE STUDY   285
COMMENTARY: *Rosalie A. Kane*   287
COMMENTARY: *Robert M. Veatch*   294

18 Managing Care for Seriously and Chronically Ill Children

CASE STUDY   303
COMMENTARY: *Donald J. Brunnquell*   306
COMMENTARY: *Susan B. Rubin and Laurie Zoloth-Dorfman*   313

Part Six: Responsibilities to the Community 321

19 Health Plan Responsibilities for Public Health Activities

CASE STUDY   323
COMMENTARY: *Mila Ann Aroskar*   325
COMMENTARY: *Gayle Hallin*   332

20 Health Plan Responsibilities for Medical Education and Research

CASE STUDY   340
COMMENTARY: *Howard Brody*   342
COMMENTARY: *Roger J. Bulger*   348

Contributors   357

Index   367

Acknowledgments

The Minnesota Center for Health Care Ethics is an academic, clinical, and policy consortium located in Minneapolis. It is sponsored by the Fairview Health System, HealthEast, and the College of St. Catherine with the Sisters of St. Joseph of Carondelet. The work of the Minnesota Center is inspired by its sponsoring organizations' shared commitments to social justice, to shaping the ethical foundations of our changing health care delivery system, and to providing health care ethics resources for professionals and the community.

Gifted by a planning grant from the Partners in Justice Fund of the Sisters of St. Joseph of Carondelet and the charms of living in Minnesota, a state on the frontier of health system change, we began networking with key individuals and organizations in managed care, developing case materials depicting ethical dilemmas born of the restructuring of the financing and delivery of health care, and laying the groundwork for an ethical framework for managed care practice.

A mandate by the Minnesota State Legislature requiring private health plans to cover a specific investigational intervention (ABMT for breast cancer) galvanized interest in designing a model of an ethically defensible process for making coverage policy decisions. Supported by eleven organizations representing the delivery, financing, and regulation of health care, we convened a multidisciplinary task force that developed a model that now informs the process used by several health plans to decide coverage policy for emerging technologies.

We are exceedingly grateful to our many friends and colleagues in managed care who continue to further our understanding of health system changes, tolerate our probing questions, welcome us into their worlds, and value exploring the ethical issues and developing more adequate ethics resources for managed care. Our work is enriched by our ongoing collaborations with such organizations as the Allina Health System, Blue Cross/Blue Shield of Minnesota, Fairview Health System, HealthEast Care System, HealthPartners, Hennepin Medical Society, the Minnesota Council of Health Plans, the Minnesota Medical Association, UCARE

Minnesota, and the state of Minnesota. It is only through the collaboration of representatives of the cultures of health care delivery, financing, administration, ethics, policy, and law that our health care system will meet the needs of patients and families in the coming years.

This project was made possible by two foundations who share a vision of the contribution ethical reflection can make to our evolving health care system. We owe an exceptional debt of gratitude to the Allina Foundation and the HealthEast Foundation for their generous funding, and we acknowledge the special gifts of encouragement and assistance from Mike Christenson, Dianne Lev, and Linda Smith.

This book offers, in a single volume, the work of forty-seven leading thinkers in their fields on the ethical challenges in managed care. We thank them for their thoughtful and thought-provoking contributions, their enthusiasm for this project, and their responsiveness to a demanding production schedule.

In developing the cases for this book, the authors—Reinhard Priester, Kimberly Otte, Karen Gervais, and Dorothy Vawter—received important and valuable suggestions from many individuals, including Julia Anderson, Robert Beck, David Boyd, Mary Hiber Fenn, Douglas Fenstermaker, Elizabeth Gilles, Lourene Grandstrand, Heidi Groven, Gwen Halaas, Karen Harrison, Cynthia Hart, Ruth Hendrickson, Kathy Hulting, George Isham, Stuart Lancer, Jan Malcolm, Ruth Mickelsen, Gretchen Musicant, Edward Rattner, and unnamed others.

We are especially grateful to Marjorie Noonan for her painstaking attention to the needs of five editors and forty-two commentators, and to the demanding process of readying the final, copyedited manuscript for publication; and we thank Jolee Madl and Kevin Christopherson for their research and technical assistance. In addition, we must extend our deep appreciation to Laura Beaudoin for the care with which she copyedited the manuscript.

Finally, high praise and heartfelt thanks go to the leaders of our sponsoring organizations—Pamela Tibbetts and Gordon Alexander of Fairview Health System, Timothy Hanson of HealthEast, Anita Pampusch and Mary Broderick of the College of St. Catherine, and Sr. Margaret Belanger, Sr. Margaret Kvasnicka, and Sr. Ann Walton of the Sisters of St. Joseph of Carondelet; as well as to our Board members—Charles P. Ceronsky, Joseph R. Clubb, the Rev. Scott W. Hinrichs, Karen Hilgers, CSJ, Daniel A. Johnson, Nancy N. Kari, Robert M. Meiches, and Carol A. Tauer. We could not ask for stronger or more collegial support than they provide.

K.G.G. and D.E.V.

Disclaimer

To the extent the case studies in this book are based on factual situations, identifying characteristics have been changed and facts substituted to protect the identities of the parties involved. The names and geographic information associated with individuals and entities in these case studies are fictitious; any similarity to actual persons, entities, or events is purely coincidental and unintended.

Introduction: Ethical Challenges in Managed Care

Karen G. Gervais and Dorothy E. Vawter

Increasingly, the ethical dilemmas in health care contain unfamiliar elements. For example, financial reimbursement structures appear to play an important role in the quality of patient care, and complicated contractual arrangements among multiple health care providers and payers seem to obstruct rather than facilitate the provision of specific services and continuity of patient care. The organizations that have become the heartbeat of health system change—managed care organizations—are well aware that many of their decisions are value laden and that they lack sufficient ethical resources to guide trade-offs central to their practice, for example, the balancing of individual and population interests, cost and effectiveness, business goals and health care goals, and responsibilities to enrollees and the community. The ethical challenges arising within managed care clearly call for sustained ethical reflection and new ethical guidelines, procedures, and skills.

Since the early 1980s, the prevailing arrangement for financing and delivering health care in the United States has been undergoing a cost-driven and market-based transformation to managed care. "Managed care" is a generic term for the myriad organizational arrangements that integrate the financing and delivery of health care in such a way that the former constrains the latter. It combines the business of insurance with the delivery of professional health care services. Managed care organizations secure enrollees by offering the purchasers of insurance (employers and government) competitively priced enrollment premiums and providing enrollees fair access to quality health care within a finite budget.

The Cases and Commentaries

Because managed care has evolved so rapidly and is still continuing to evolve, the ethical issues it raises have yet to be completely mapped out and adequately explored. This book provides twenty detailed case studies that offer snapshots of managed care arrangements and methods presently used in the United States and the ethical uncertainties they raise for clinicians, health plan administrators, and patients and their families. Each case is accompanied by questions for consideration and a pair of commentaries. The commentaries offer both further clarification of the internal workings of managed care and conceptual and practical guidance in addressing the ethical issues. The commentators bring a breadth of professional expertise to the analyses, representing the fields of bioethics, health policy, clinical practice, health care administration, law, and medical sociology. This book is intended for a broad audience, including clinicians, administrators, and others involved in managed care, as well as students in professional, preprofessional, and continuing education.

Section I examines challenges associated with the central function of managed care—rationing care and allocating shared financial resources. Given that managed care organizations decide what health care interventions will and will not be covered based on trade-offs between the interests of individual enrollees and the enrolled population as a whole, it is important to ask what criteria should be used to make such trade-offs. On what basis, for example, should coverage for emergency services be limited or should coverage of complementary health care be expanded? When, if ever, should managed care make exceptions to coverage policies?

Section II describes situations arising out of some of the incentive arrangements aimed at containing costs and improving quality prevalent in managed care practice in the United States. Capitation, which has been described as "the engine of managed care," is a focal point of the cases in this section.

Section III examines some of the challenges to improving the quality of care raised by managed care operating within a competitive market. Credentialing of providers and staffing levels are important dimensions of quality control but may conflict with other important organizational goals. For-profit managed care organizations pay their administrators more than nonprofits, as well as seek to generate significant financial revenues for shareholders. What effect, if any, do these functions of for-profit managed care organizations have on the quality of service provided their enrollees and the community?

Section IV concerns responsibilities to patients. It explores questions concerning respect for patients and patient advocacy. Whose responsibility is it to advocate for potential enrollees, patients, and enrollees in managed care plans, and what legitimate and illegitimate limits are there on these responsibilities? While coverage denials may be appealed, this process requires a new kind of advocacy by physicians on behalf of their patients, at the same time that managed care organizations may impose barriers on physicians' willingness and ability to advocate for their patients. These changes in the professional role of the physician challenge traditional concepts of patient-centered care.

Section V delves more deeply into the challenges of allocating resources to provide quality care for vulnerable populations, populations that are generally costly to treat, have complex medical and nonmedical needs, and require intensive coordination of services. These patients are often without voice or power and dependent on public programs. We must ask how appropriate structuring of managed care contracts and oversight of managed care operations for these patients will be ensured, and by whom.

Section VI addresses some of the questions concerning managed care's responsibility to the community. As the beneficiary of strong health care education, research, and public health programs, do managed care organizations have a responsibility to support these pursuits? The restructuring of relationships among payers, purchasers, plans, and providers under managed care has left many crucial functions without their historical resource base. We must address the question of who is responsible for supporting these broader system functions. It may be appropriate to ask, Who is currently getting the savings in our restructured health system, and at whose expense?

The strongest message emerging from the contributors to this book is a positive and hopeful one. Each commentator points to strategies for improving managed care policies and practices. They admit that the trade-offs inherent in managed care inevitably allow some harms, but if the trade-offs are based on an ethically justified balancing of interests, they are properly viewed as misfortunes rather than injustices. Some commentators stress that we must attend not only to ethical challenges within managed care organizations but also to the societal challenge to create and maintain a good health care system.

The History of Managed Care in the United States

Since before World War II, the prevailing mode of health care delivery and financing in the United States was fee-for-service indemnity insurance. This traditional fee-for-service arrangement encouraged, and did little to constrain, the delivery of health care services. In that era, insurers paid for the health care services physicians ordered for their patients. The physician and the insured patient bore little if any of the costs and had little need to factor the costs of care into decisions to offer or receive care. Significant overutilization of health care services, inconsistent quality of services, a substantial and growing proportion of uninsured persons in our population, and hyperinflation in societal health care spending are the negative legacies of the fee-for-service era.

In the 1940s, the precursors of modern health maintenance organizations (HMOs) developed in the form of prepaid group health care cooperatives. These were health care delivery arrangements between an enrolled population and a group of physicians who agreed to work on a salaried rather than a fee-for-service basis. Enrollees' prepaid monthly premiums were pooled to cover all the health care services they were predicted to need during the coverage period. Thirty years later, a government-led reform effort resulted in the federal passage of the 1973 HMO Act, which created a favorable economic environment for the creation of "federally qualified" HMOs that would compete with fee-for-service systems on cost and quality by pursuing a "health maintenance" strategy.

Early in the 1980s, the government succeeded in introducing cost controls into the Medicare program in the form of Medicare diagnosis-related groups, creating set payments for the treatment of hospital patients with particular diagnoses. This required hospitals to manage a patient's care within the budget allowed by the diagnosis-related group, or incur financial loss. This cost constraint had indirect impacts on the cost of private insurance, since hospitals, accustomed to cost-shifting, raised the price of services for privately insured patients to offset losses associated with treating Medicare patients. This drove premium costs higher for employers purchasing indemnity coverage for their employees.

Employers were relatively powerless to manage cost until 1983, when the state of California passed legislation that enabled "selective contracting" between private insurers and hospitals for a fixed price per service. Such direct negotiating with hospitals soon spread throughout the United States and began to extend to physicians and clinics as well. Providers were thereby brought into the unfamiliar territory of the marketplace, where negotiation around price could occur.

Throughout the 1980s and 1990s, in response to runaway inflation in health care expenditures, both employers and government, the two primary purchasers of health care insurance in the United States, responded to the financial crisis by seeking lower-cost health insurance for their enrollees. They increasingly turned to managed care organizations. By 1994, nearly two-thirds of insured employees were covered under some form of managed care. However, massive systemic issues remained. The turn to managed care was a response to the cost-containment interests of purchasers. It was a change neither inspired by, nor organized to attain, crucial societal health care goals. In 1994, the Clinton administration made a concerted effort at government-led reform to address the issues of universal access and quality, in addition to cost containment. When this effort failed, managed care organizations stepped up their response to purchasers' demands for cost containment.

The Goals of Managed Care

Our societal embracing of managed care has focused primarily on cost containment, secondarily on quality improvement, and has essentially avoided the issue of expanding access to health care coverage for the uninsured and underinsured. To the extent that containing costs and improving the quality of care are jointly viable goals within a market-based health system, managed care holds great promise for those who have health care coverage. For them, it has the potential to bring costs under control; eliminate the harms and costs associated with overtreatment; reinvigorate primary care; and improve quality of care and the coordination of care across the continuum of services. However, several factors impede managed care organizations from fully attending to improving the quality of care. On the one hand, there is a lack of relevant empirical information about patient outcomes. More seriously, however, the market provides no incentives to managed care organizations to support research and health care education, activities arguably crucial to improving quality. In an environment that pares cost through competition, new funding mechanisms for these activities will have to be developed and the role of managed care organizations clarified. There is a similar absence of incentives to expand access to health care and to attend to the needs of those in our community without health care coverage.

The market may give rise to "healthy" competition, but it is unclear that it can give rise to healthy cooperation in relation to a communal good such as health care. Government-sponsored activity or regulation may be necessary to address and correct the unhealthy outcomes of market competition where the provision of this communal good is either not promoted or perhaps even undermined.

The Methods of Managed Care

Many of the ethical challenges posed by managed care lie in the details of the rationing methods used to achieve cost containment, including: definitions of medical necessity; coverage policies; practice guidelines; and risk-sharing arrangements (such as capitation and other payment arrangements).

DEFINITIONS OF MEDICAL NECESSITY

Managed care organizations are required by law, and in their contracts with enrollees they pledge, to cover medically necessary services. However, medically necessary services do not include all services that could, or even would, benefit an individual. Within the finite resource pool generated from enrollee premiums, a determination of whether an intervention is medically necessary and will be covered for an enrollee depends on the "richness" of the managed care organization's definition of medical necessity. Which definition of medical necessity ought managed care organizations adopt? One that focuses on restoring patients to their premorbid condition, on promising patients normal species function, or on enhancing health status beyond that of normal function? Should there be a single definition that applies to all, or should the definition sometimes be adjusted to meet the needs of different groups of enrollees? The answers to these questions are value-laden and directly affect patient access to health care services.

COVERAGE POLICIES

To control costs and manage the finite budget generated from enrollees' premiums, enrollee contracts list certain categories of interventions that are excluded from coverage, such as investigational interventions. Since contracts cannot list every possible intervention that may ever be desired, managed care plans also develop internal coverage policies that define what interventions will and will not be covered for the enrolled population as a whole. These rationing decisions, for example, about whether to cover an emerging technology, ideally rest on a number of factors, including technology-assessment reports, medical necessity criteria, number of enrollees needing the intervention, costs per individual and population, impact on premium costs and coverage of other interventions, and cost-effectiveness relative to other interventions. Making coverage policies is a complex value-laden task requiring careful attention to the appropriate prioritizing and balancing of individual health care needs and population health care goals.

PRACTICE GUIDELINES

Individual decisions about whether a particular intervention will be covered for a particular patient with a particular condition are further governed by practice guidelines. Managed care organizations increasingly require not simply the physician's belief that an intervention might be medically necessary, but they require that the intervention be consistent with practice guidelines that define care plans for patients with the patient's condition.

Ideally, practice guidelines are formulated against the background of significant scientific and medical research and are based on population studies that measure patient-centered health outcomes and costs of alternative treatments in order to determine the most cost-effective intervention. Consistent with the goal of cost containment, cost-effectiveness—rather than effectiveness alone—becomes the basis for including an intervention in practice guidelines.

In practice, many such guidelines simply reflect the standard of care that has developed over time. There is still a great deal of data gathering to do to improve practice guidelines. Managed care organizations are ideally suited to gather the sort of patient-outcomes data essential to developing good practice guidelines. But once again, it is important that guidelines be based on an ethically defensible balancing of the considerations of benefit and cost.

Managed care organizations' pursuit of evidence-driven practice based on health outcomes and technology-assessment studies stands to benefit enrollees and the enrolled population as a whole by eliminating the risks and harms of overtreatment, inappropriate treatment, and unsafe treatment, and by distributing the pooled resources in ways that maximize the health of the enrollees. Such a basis for rationing health care to enrolled populations has potential drawbacks, however. Since the needs of vulnerable populations have been historically neglected in health care research and in our health care system, there is relatively little data to support conclusions about the efficacy of interventions aimed at their improvement. Those who need interventions lacking good evidentiary bases (for example, mental and physical rehabilitation) may increasingly be denied coverage for interventions that offer them their only chance at a functional life. Hence, one of the ethical challenges managed care organizations now face is to ensure that these historically underserved groups are fairly treated and provided appropriate care. Moreover, it is important that practice guidelines never be allowed to completely replace the judgment of the physician, just as rules of law should never displace the roles of the jury and the judge. Clearly, managed care organizations have a choice to make concerning how wide a berth to give clinicians to exercise professional judgment or whether to give rigid deference to practice guidelines.

RISK-SHARING ARRANGEMENTS

Managed care organizations use a number of strategies to promote provider compliance with coverage policies, definitions of medical necessity, and practice guidelines, most notably by arrangements that spread the financial risks associated with ordering health care interventions to providers. "Risk-sharing" refers to the practice of distributing the financial costs and risks of providing care between insurer and physician, clinic, and/or hospital. By contrast, under indemnity fee-for-service plans, the health insurance companies and patients bear all of the costs and financial risk, while providers bear none (unless they provide uncompensated care).

Most risk-sharing arrangements currently used by managed care organizations place both individual and institutional providers at financial risk whenever they order or provide health care services. Capitation is a common risk-sharing arrangement; providers receive a prepaid per-member per-month amount and must themselves cover the costs of all the care that patients require. Risk-sharing arrangements between a provider and a managed care organization may also include salary withholds and bonuses for provider performance relative to specific financial targets.

The financial risk to providers may range from insignificant to oppressive, depending on such factors as the extent of risk-sharing between the provider and the managed care organization, the number of enrollees in the risk pool, risk-adjustment calculations, and the frequency with which the provider's performance is assessed. Whether the financial arrangements between providers and managed care organizations are described as financial incentives or disincentives, they may function ethically or unethically to influence provider behavior. They may raise the cost-consciousness of health care professionals, inclining them toward caution in the ordering of services; or they may interfere with health care professionals' ordering of services. In general, the more a reimbursement arrangement places a provider at risk, the stronger the provider's disincentive to order at least some types of health services. Whether under fee-for-service or managed care, direct connections between a physician's treatment recommendations and reimbursement can be hazardous to patients; but they are potentially more hazardous if the physician has incentives to undertreat and to withhold from patients information about the full range of treatment options.

Three Ethics Projects

It is sometimes said that managed care poses no new ethical challenges, and that in and of itself, managed care is neutral. What is meant by this is that managed care is not inherently unethical, that it can be part of an ethically defensible health care system. It seems correct to say that the concept of managed care, understood as the endeavor to balance cost and quality concerns in ethically justified ways, is essential to an ethically defensible health care system.

However, the environment within which managed care American-style operates makes our managed care arrangements less than neutral. Managed care organizations currently pursue the goals of cost containment and quality under the profit-oriented aegis of the marketplace, with no necessary commitment to health care as a special need or service that should be available to all without regard to ability to pay.

Health care, the largest human service endeavor in the United States, is a creature of investment and political power. It is guided by a social ethic that permits the claim that the ethical obligations of managed care organizations extend to those entities and individuals with whom they have contractual relationships and no further. Are the ethical obligations of managed care organizations confined to their business relationships, or does the control over societal health care resources they hold in the United States generate ethical obligations that extend to the promotion of societal health care goals? Is the relationship of managed care organization to enrollee simply a contractual one or also a fiduciary one, given the services it covers?

The cases and commentaries in this book suggest at least three major ethics projects: (1) developing procedures and criteria for balancing individual and population health care interests, so that rationing decisions are fair; (2) clarifying the responsibilities and accountability of the multiple players in the health system and strengthening resources and capacities in health care ethics; and (3) reconsidering our social ethic concerning health care and articulating the community responsibilities of managed care organizations.

BALANCING INDIVIDUAL AND POPULATION INTERESTS

Consistent with the American political ethos of individualism, the traditional principles of bioethics (autonomy, beneficence, and justice), developed and implemented over the last thirty-five years, have assigned priority to respect for patient autonomy. This has resulted in the elaboration of the rights of patients in health care and research settings and the duties of health care professionals to defer to patients' autonomous choices. Whenever resources are pooled, however, by or for a defined population to ensure the availability of coverage for health care, an ethical framework and/or procedure is needed to assist with decisions that affect patient care and the overall health status of the population. The ethical quandaries inherent in the balancing of individual and population health care interests have yet to be adequately addressed.

For all but the very wealthy, access to adequate, lifelong, affordable health care can only be secured by individuals pooling their resources to cover the costs of medically necessary health care services. If we agree that health care is a basic good, and if individuals have entrusted a portion of their resources to the pool in order to assure themselves reasonable access to that basic good, the holder of the pool (whether a for-profit or a nonprofit managed care organization) has ethical obligations to be a good fiscal steward and a good steward of both individual and population health.

As this dual steward, a managed care organization's priority must be to provide medically necessary care for individuals in the context of limited resources and population-based rationing decisions. Hence, the ethical framework that informs rationing decisions must balance concerns for patient autonomy and justice, providing for the judicious and equitable use and distribution of resources. In such an arrangement, the requirements of the principles of autonomy and beneficence are legitimately constrained by the requirements of justice. Thus, coverage restrictions arrived at through rationing choices at the policy level constrain the exercise of individual autonomy on the part of patients, as well as the exercise of autonomy and beneficence on the part of providers. Doing so in an ethical way requires a procedurally fair and principled balancing of individual and population health care interests.

Three ethical concerns loom large when an individual's coverage and thus access to health care services are determined on the basis of coverage rules developed from a populationwide resource management perspective. These concerns track commonly voiced worries of the public about managed care—worries focused on changes in the provider-patient relationship and fear of abandonment through the denial of coverage. When fleshing out an ethically acceptable balancing of individual and population interests it is important to ask: (1) Is patient advocacy and the fiduciary nature of the physician-patient relationship preserved? (2) Are members of vulnerable populations treated fairly and respectfully? and (3) Are there reasonable provisions for making coverage exceptions?

PRESERVATION OF THE PHYSICIAN'S FIDUCIARY RESPONSIBILITIES

The rise of managed care has meant the shifting of power, money, and influence from the delivery sector to the financing sector of our health care system. While physicians have constituted the wealthiest and least regulated profession in our history, and great wealth has been consolidated on the delivery side, the delivery sector has also lived under the ethos of fiduciary obligations. The primary health care relationship between physician and patient has been understood as a trust or fiduciary relationship, the qualities of which are often likened to the qualities associated with a covenantal relationship. Managed care organizations have introduced mechanisms of influence and oversight into the health care provider and patient relationship that threaten to change the professionalism of the health care provider and these fiduciary obligations.

A major strategy for achieving cost-containment goals involves managing the behavior of physicians. Physicians used to manage patient care on the basis of their individual knowledge of medicine and assessment of their patient's need. Now they are often required to play gatekeeping roles, defend their treatment choices and referrals on the grounds of medical necessity, order treatments consistent with practice guidelines and drug formularies, and conform their treatment decisions and practices to the determinations of nonphysician case managers and utilization reviewers. Many uncertainties continue concerning the scope of a health care professional's responsibilities for patient advocacy within the matrix of decision making and decision makers in managed care organizations. While the need for patient advocacy increases under managed care, physicians may be less motivated as well as less able to be advocates, because of performance and financial pressures managed care organizations may place on them.

The responsibilities toward the sick implied by the fiduciary model should not be unduly restricted by the contractually based and contractually bounded responsibilities of the managed care organization toward the sick enrollee. The challenge is to preserve the vitality of the fiduciary responsibilities of the caregiver to the patient, and thus the patient's trust.

FAIRNESS TO VULNERABLE POPULATIONS

Managed care's approach to the financing and delivery of health care was inspired by the earlier successes of HMOs with predominantly healthy populations. Yet increasingly, managed care organizations are being approached to manage the care of vulnerable populations because of the promise of cost containment. The question arises, can managed care develop the techniques as well as the sensitivity to address the needs of populations with more diverse, extreme, and costly health care requirements?

Managed care has yet to give significant attention to its capacity to support the health care needs of the chronically ill and disabled among us. The adequate provision of health care to those of us with complex health needs often requires interrelated medical and nonmedical services. There is no evidence that premium costs are currently developed with extremely expensive enrollees in mind, or that the cyclical losses posted by insurers take into account, in appropriate ways, the costs of extremely expensive populations. Since managed care has undermined the ability of providers to shift costs to offset the expenses associated with care of the chronically and seriously ill, and lean definitions of medical necessity often define many of the needs of these persons to be outside managed care's realm of responsibility, there is serious concern about whether market-based managed care has the potential to meet the health care needs of everyone in our society. How should the concept of medical necessity be interpreted by physicians, case managers, and medical directors so that the cracks some of us presently fall through when we need and seek health care do not become chasms too wide to bridge by any resources?

COVERAGE EXCEPTIONS

Managed care organizations typically exclude coverage for investigational interventions, due to the absence of adequate safety, efficacy, and cost-effectiveness data.

This is a reasonable constraint to place on the allocation of pooled and limited resources, since they should neither be knowingly wasted nor unknowingly spent. While the human inclination is to try to rescue individuals in dire circumstances, it is clear that doing so as a general rule would be both a poor expenditure of shared resources and unaffordable.

But blanket contractual exclusions for coverage of investigational interventions, based on the claim that there is insufficient evidence of safety and efficacy, can ring callous when a person's life is on the line and research has progressed in a positive direction. Is it not ethically required to consider when, if ever, rescue efforts, and thus exceptions to the general rule, ought to be undertaken by managed care organizations? Is it not a reasonable demonstration of a commitment to improving the quality of health care that promising research, particularly for those in dire need, be supported by managed care plans? Most plans rule out coverage for investigational interventions by requiring that the intervention satisfy a high standard of evidence to support coverage. A remaining challenge for managed care organizations is to set the evidentiary bar so that it fulfills an appropriate requirement of fidelity to the sick and the dying and an appropriate commitment to stewardship of the plan members' limited health care resources.

Exceptions to coverage policies require complex value-laden judgments. Trust may well depend upon the extent to which a managed care organization shares the substance of these ethical choices around coverage for investigational interventions with those on behalf of whom it stewards health care resources, elicits the values of those affected, and prices its insurance to conform to the enrolled population's values concerning such coverage policies and exceptions.

ACCOUNTABILITY AND ETHICS RESOURCES

At a minimum, the complex web of parties responsible for the quality of health care delivered to a patient and to a population includes the purchasers (employers and government), managed care plans, provider organizations, professionals, and enrollees. It is critical to clarify who bears responsibility for what decisions and to develop accountability measures for each of these key players.

Further, managed care arrangements challenge us to develop and integrate new ethics resources and skills. Many clinical situations are now encumbered by organizational and business interests that must be identified and incorporated into the ethical analysis of a problematic situation. Multiple organizations may be involved in a single situation, or different functions of one and the same organization may generate conflicts with ethical dimensions. This requires (1) a suitable moral compass—a set of fundamental value commitments—to direct the structuring of the integrated organization and the key relationships within it, (2) frameworks of ethical principles suitable to the issues that arise within integrative health care organizations, (3) guidelines that provide concrete advice for ethical decision making for all components of the organization and between components, (4) procedures for resolving ethical challenges that are not well handled by simple application of ethical principles, rules, or guidelines, and (5) the individuals, materials, and other resources necessary to support ethical reflection throughout the organization.

COMMUNITY RESPONSIBILITIES

Our current debate about health care financing is largely a middle-class debate around health care for the already insured. In its market-based form, managed care fails to speak directly to important societal health care goals—coverage for the uninsured and underinsured and the maintenance of strong health care education, research, and public health initiatives. Managed care organizations have little incentive to promote these broader societal goals since there is arguably little direct profit, but rather increased financial outlay, associated with them. Further, managed care's cost-containment strategies increasingly dismantle the financial arrangements that used to support these endeavors.

Managed care organizations now largely command and distribute the contents of our societal health care purse. They also reap the benefits of tax and other governmental subsidies for health care coverage that accrue to both their privately and publicly insured enrollees. To what extent, then, should they embrace responsibilities to the community to promote the fundamental needs of a progressive health care system and a healthy society, and what specific responsibilities should this entail? These are important questions, since they determine the range of ethical responsibilities of a managed care organization beyond the confines of its contracts with enrollees and its obligations to its shareholders.

Any business organization has obligations to its community simply by virtue of its dependency on its surrounding environment to be able to have and maintain a business. But such prudential considerations are not the sole basis of managed care organizations' responsibilities to the broader community. Due to reasons deriving from the kind of "business" they are in, managed care organizations can be argued to be stewards of a resource crucial to the flourishing of their enrollees. Beyond this, it can be argued that managed care organizations have the ability and the responsibility to support community goals that cannot be fully captured in or reduced to the content of a health insurance contract. By virtue of the "product" they deliver, a product that meets universal human needs, as well as their control of the resources presently being expended to address those needs in our society, managed care organizations may have some responsibility to shape our societal health care "product" and to contribute to the building and maintaining of the best possible system of responses to the varied needs of the sick within the constraints of finite resources. Thus, they can be argued to have responsibilities to the uninsured, the underinsured, the chronically ill, health care education and research, and the overall health of the population at large. If it is not possible for managed care organizations in a market-based system to garner and manage resources to effectively promote societal health care goals, they at least have a duty to contribute to broader societal discussion of strategies to meet these societal needs, as well as to participate in or support the strategies selected.

While it is by putting cost containment and improved quality into vital tension with one another and endeavoring to make that tension a constructive and affordable one that managed care does right by individuals and its enrolled populations, it is by taking the initiative to examine the grounds and extent of their ethical responsibility to promote crucial societal health care goals that managed care organizations will earn a favored place in our health care history.

PART ONE

Rationing Shared Resources

1

Balancing a Plan's Obligations to Individual Patients and Its Enrolled Population

CASE STUDY _____

The Benefit Committee at DesertHealth, a for-profit HMO, must decide whether or not labs should be reimbursed for a new test called PUREPAP. Currently, reimbursement is not included in the fee the plan pays to the lab or the provider. Some physicians, as well as some members, have appealed DesertHealth's current position.

PUREPAP is an advanced computerized tool used to rescreen Pap smears. It was recently approved by the Food and Drug Administration (FDA) as a quality assessment tool. This means that the test is approved only for rescreening for the purposes of quality-assessment, not for use as a diagnostic tool for initial screening.

The scientific literature recognizes errors in the detection and interpretation of cervical smear abnormalities as a leading cause of false-negative findings. This is seen as an unavoidable consequence of manual screening: one slide has 50,000 to 300,000 cells, and one technician might review a hundred slides in one day. PUREPAP pinpoints, magnifies, and rank orders abnormal cells that may have been missed by initial microscopic screening, especially cells that are hard for the human eye to detect. It uses computers to identify and magnify images of the 128 highest-ranking abnormal cells on any one slide.

Presently, plans submit 10 percent of their negative slides to a legally required manual rescreening, which detects approximately 8 percent false-negatives. PUREPAP provides a computerized rescreening process that is about 7 percent more effective in detecting false-negatives than manual rescreening of negative Pap smears. In other words, if 10 percent false-negatives are detected under the current manual rescreening system, 10.7 percent would be detected using PUREPAP. For example, if manual rescreening detected 8 false-negatives out of a 100-slide pool, PUREPAP would detect 8.56.

DesertHealth pays for about ninety-five thousand Pap smears per year. The usual charge for a PUREPAP rescreening is $80. If 85 percent were negative and all were rescreened using PUREPAP, the cost to the plan would be $4.8 million, even assuming the 25 percent discount typically applied in contracts between the plan and service providers. The plan's underwriters estimate that PUREPAP would cost approximately $30,000 to detect one false-negative.

The medical director of DesertHealth Laboratories, a division of DesertHealth, believes that PUREPAP should not be covered because its efficacy has not been scientifically proven and it is not considered the recognized standard of care in the practice of medicine for rescreening in cervical and vaginal cytology. A high number of the detected abnormal cells will resolve without treatment, meaning the abnormality is either harmless or temporary, and no further treatment is necessary. Therefore, the reported 7 percent increase in detection does not reflect a commensurate increase in the detection of cervical cancer. Numbers demonstrating the efficacy of PUREPAP with respect to the detection of cancer are not yet available. DesertHealth's medical director points out that the American Society of Cytopathology recommends additional studies to determine the efficacy and cost of the test.

DesertHealth's Medical Policy Committee also recommends against reimbursing PUREPAP because it is not a recognized standard of care and because additional study is recommended. The committee stresses that most cervical cancer grows slowly over the course of ten to fifteen years, and that the implications of a false-negative are greatly overstated. In other words, the detriment to the patient of not catching an abnormal cell in the early stages of development is not as medically significant as may be supposed by the public. In addition, the committee points out that new and more promising technology, although not yet approved by the FDA, will probably make PUREPAP obsolete.

One other committee at DesertHealth, the Consumer Affairs Committee, has weighed in on the issue. This committee includes consumer representatives and representatives from the medical board. This committee also argues against covering PUREPAP; instead, the plan should spend the resources that would be spent on PUREPAP to promote regular Pap tests, because this would ultimately save more lives and be more cost-effective.

Due to extensive marketing through medical literature, the Internet, and women's magazines, public awareness of and demand for PUREPAP rescreening has grown. However, the public broadly believes that it can and should be used to actually detect cancer rather than for its currently more limited and approved use in rescreening. Women have brought articles to their physicians, requested the rescreening, and appealed DesertHealth's denials. They have argued that PURE-PAP should no longer be considered experimental and that the marginal increase in efficacy is worth it, not only to those additional women with false-negatives identified by PUREPAP but to all women.

A few physicians have likewise advocated for members, arguing that this test should be considered medically necessary and is worth covering. In particular, physicians have complained about DesertHealth's current policy to "cover" PUREPAP but not adequately reimburse for it. Technically, rescreening is covered and a provider can use the appropriate billing code for any rescreening test. The provider, however, will be reimbursed at the rate of the cheaper existing test regardless of which test is actually used. In effect then, PUREPAP is covered but not adequately reimbursed. Because it is technically "covered," a provider cannot "balance bill" the member. That is, under state law, a provider in an HMO cannot bill a member for the unpaid balance of covered services after the HMO has paid the provider the agreed-upon rate. As a result, the provider cannot agree to allow the member to pay for it out-of-pocket. In short, any provider ordering a PUREPAP rescreening will absorb the cost and is in this way discouraged from doing so.

Finally, DesertHealth recently received a letter from the state Department of Insurance, the agency responsible for regulating HMOs, questioning why the test should not be considered a "preventive service" and therefore within the related state mandate for all such services. There is a state HMO law requiring "coverage of all preventive services, including screening for cancer."

The Benefit Committee must consider these competing interests and must decide whether the benefit of this new technology is outweighed by its cost to the plan.

Questions for Consideration

➤ How should DesertHealth balance its obligation to its enrolled population to distribute resources fairly against its obligation to provide medically necessary care to an individual member?

➤ How might the plan defend the position that the benefit of the test is outweighed by the costs?

➤ When, if ever, might the plan have an ethical obligation to provide coverage for PUREPAP, or offer PUREPAP on a fee-for-service basis? Why?

➤ Under what conditions, if any, might a plan give preferential treatment to a particular group of enrollees?

➤ Does a physician have any duty to the plan's enrolled population that would mitigate the duty to advocate for an individual patient?

➤ How, if at all, should the state mandate be qualified or changed to take into account a cost-benefit analysis of a test such as PUREPAP? What are the ethical implications of the plan's policy to cover but not to fully reimburse?

COMMENTARY

Leonard M. Fleck, Ph.D.

The two immediate ethical questions raised by this case are: Is a just and caring managed care plan morally obligated to cover PUREPAP rescreening? Are physicians who care for women who receive Pap smears morally obligated to advocate for such coverage? Below these immediate questions are two deeper questions. First, what does it mean to be a "just and caring" managed care plan when you have only limited resources to meet the virtually unlimited health needs of members of the plan? Second, what does it mean to be a "just and caring" physician when you have only limited resources to meet the health needs of the patient before you now?

Several presuppositions built into these two questions need to be made explicit. (1) It really is the case that plans have only *limited resources*. In the final analysis those limits are determined by plan members, all of whom have other needs and wants on which they would prefer to spend their money. Employers who provide health benefits to their employees are the proximate determiners of those limits; but if employees are willing to sacrifice take-home pay, then those limits can always in theory be moved upward. Alternatively, if employees are not willing to make those sacrifices, then those limits establish de facto budgets for managed care plans.

(2) The domain of *health needs* is constantly expanding with emerging medical technologies, PUREPAP being a perfect example of such expansion (Callahan 1990). That is, we know that if Pap smears are done on a population at low risk for cervical cancer, the result will be some number of false-negative results. What "false-negative" means is that the smear contained abnormal cells, possibly indicative of cancer, that were missed in the lab analysis. In a small number of such cases, failure to detect may mean progression to an advanced cancer and a fatal outcome that might otherwise have been averted. Hence, we *need* to do some rescreening to pick up those false-negatives, possibly saving some lives. Further, if we can devise an improved rescreening procedure, even if only very modestly improved (as in PUREPAP), then we *need* to adopt that improvement. This is the logic of technological dissemination in health care. My intent at this point is not to endorse that logic, just to describe it as accurately as possible.

(3) If plans (and patients) have only limited resources to meet an expanding array of presumptive health needs, then health care rationing and need prioritization are inescapable. What "health care rationing" means is that "we" judge some possible health interventions as yielding, or likely yielding, too little benefit at too great a cost. That is, these interventions are not cost-effective enough. We judge that there are other interventions that are likely to yield more in the way of health benefit at a lower cost than this one, and hence we assign this latter intervention a lower priority. Here is the core of the moral problem.

If we cannot meet all health needs of all plan members because of limited resources, then how should we fairly or justly determine which needs *will* be met? And who has the moral right to make such decisions? Is this a pure medical judgment (and a matter of medical ethics) for physicians to decide? Is it a pure business judgment (and a matter of business ethics) for CEOs to decide? Or is it a collective judgment that plan members need to make regarding what they judge to be the cost-effective and just claims that they may make on common plan resources through a process of rational democratic deliberation (Fleck 1994)? Or is this the sort of judgment that individual plan members ought to be allowed to make in consultation with their physicians? If we were to endorse this last option, then how would we mitigate the understandable tendency of ill and fearful patients to make decisions about their own health needs that were neither fair nor cost-effective from the collective perspective? Should we insist instead that if patients are going to make individualized rationing and prioritization choices they would need to make these from an impartial and broadly rational point of view when they first joined the plan in a healthy state? That is, they would have to be largely ignorant of their own future health needs.

The heterogeneity of health needs further complicates this discussion of rationing and prioritization. Some individuals are nearly perfectly healthy all their lives and then drop dead suddenly at age ninety. Others have multiple chronic health needs for most of their lives. Men have no need for Pap smears; women have no need for prostate tests. The costs of addressing these different health needs also vary enormously, as will the likelihood of a good outcome from various health care interventions, such as autologous bone marrow transplants for various cancers. How then can we make fair rationing and prioritization judgments in accessing limited health resources when we have such heterogeneity and uncertainty? More specifically, how can we make a just and caring decision about coverage of the PUREPAP rescreening test?

The PUREPAP test should not be a covered benefit. This judgment is supported by a number of moral considerations. First, the fact is that the Consumer Affairs Committee of this managed care plan is recommending against funding. If this committee is in fact fairly representative of the plan membership as a whole, if they have had access to all the information they need to make an informed decision, and if their judgment has not been distorted by biased or misleading information, then their judgment has substantial moral weight. More precisely, the most salient moral fact is that they are making this rationing decision for themselves and for those they care about who are members of the plan. They are not some outside group of experts or executives who are making a rationing decision whose consequences they will not have to bear for individuals to whom they have no emotional ties. In other words, this is properly viewed as an exercise in moral autonomy (Menzel 1990).

Second, they are supported in their judgment by the Medical Policy Committee and the relevant medical literature. That is, PUREPAP rescreening increases by only 7 percent the number of false-negatives that would otherwise be identified by current rescreening methods. Further, the cost of detecting this extra false-negative by this method may be as high as $30,000. If detecting such a false-negative meant, each and every time, that a woman's life would be saved who otherwise would die of cervical cancer, then it could be argued (and many on that Consumer Affairs Committee might argue as well) that this was a reasonable expenditure, especially if what we were saving involved twenty to thirty high-quality life years per woman saved.

But this is a false assumption. All we would be detecting would be abnormal cells. Some of these abnormal cells would not be indicative of any serious disease process. Their abnormal state resolves without any medical intervention. Others might represent early stages of cancer. For most people this is a scary thought. However, the best medical knowledge now suggests that cervical cancer develops very slowly, over roughly a ten- to fifteen-year period. This has the practical moral implication that if these cells are missed on the current screening, they may well be picked up a year later on a future Pap smear, or a year after that.

We should not conclude from this analysis that there is no risk of premature death if we fail to approve PUREPAP rescreening. On the contrary, what we probably ought to assume is that some lives will be lost to cervical cancer that could have been saved if we had used PUREPAP to rescreen all the negative Pap results. Official statistics in this matter have not been found, but we can at least make some hypothetical moral judgments. What is most likely is that the number of saved lives will be small, and the cost of saving each of those lives might be more than $1 million. As the case itself points out, in order to maximize the likelihood of saving such lives all the negative Pap smears would have to be rescreened at an increased annual cost to the plan of $4.8 million. It looks as if we would be purchasing a very marginal benefit at a very high cost.

At this point two objections might be raised: (1) Human life is priceless. If we have the capacity to save a life, then we are morally obligated to do so. It is both unjust and uncaring simply to accept passively these deaths that could be averted. (2) It is the lives of *women* that are being devalued by failure to do PUREPAP rescreening. There are all sorts of studies indicating that women's health needs are systematically ignored in our health care system (Steingart et al. 1991). This is another example of this sort of injustice; and therefore, it is strongly morally objectionable that our managed care plan would refuse to fund PUREPAP.

To the first objection a reasonable response is to point out that human life is not priceless. That is, each of us places a limit on what we are willing to spend to save our life from some increased risk of death. If we were really committed to the belief that human life is priceless, we would insist that cars be built that could withstand a head-on collision at fifty miles per hour. But only a small fraction of the population would be able to afford such cars. So we make a trade-off: affordable cars for an increased risk of death. We likewise limit the capacity of government to tax us to fund an unlimited number of possible public programs that could reduce risks in a variety of settings and increase the number of lives saved. And we do this so that we can spend that money on frivolous personal preferences, some of which may be detrimental to our health, such as the $4 billion we spent last year on potato chips in America. Yet very few people see these decisions as either unreasonable or morally objectionable.

Despite appearances, the pricelessness of human life is not a worthy moral ideal. If taken seriously, it would distort our spending on health care in ways that were neither just nor caring. For example, given all sorts of advances in contemporary medicine that permit us to prolong life, we could spend virtually limitless sums prolonging the lives of the terminally ill by extra days or weeks or months. Such individuals would have a first and an unlimited claim on all health resources. Practically, little or no medical relief would be available to sufferers from arthritis or to individuals with disabilities who could achieve substantial functional restoration with a variety of medical assistance devices, since in neither case is life itself at risk. Such an outcome would seem flawed both as a matter of justice and as a matter of compassion (Fleck 1990). A more reasonable approach to these issues would counsel that if there are only limited resources to save lives and meet health needs, then we ought to save those lives or those life years that are less expensive rather than more expensive. There are likely to be numerous less expensive ways of saving lives or life years in our managed care plan than what PUREPAP offers.

As to the second objection: *women's* lives are being sacrificed. Is there not something presumptively discriminatory in this outcome? However, the basis for the moral objection can be obviated if the Consumer Affairs Committee of our managed care plan is sensitive to this issue. Specifically, the dollars saved by not purchasing PUREPAP can be allocated to meet what women in the plan regard as their own higher-priority, more cost-effective health needs. For example, many women in the plan may not be getting their Pap smears in a regular enough or timely enough manner, if at all. If so, that might represent a more just and a more prudent use of those resources.

Still, some women will die "unnecessarily" as a result of this decision. These deaths are correctly described, morally speaking, as unfortunate, not unjust. No one is morally blameworthy for those deaths. Women themselves in the plan, or their morally appropriate representatives, assumed this risk for themselves. These women did not select out some subgroup of women in the plan and judge that their lives and health were not worth the added expense. Rather, we can imagine a Women's Health Benefit subcommittee making the PUREPAP decision. They would be making a trade-off decision, knowing that they all would be more or less equally vulnerable to dying prematurely from cervical cancer. But they would collectively judge that there were other health benefits that they would rather purchase for themselves that were more costworthy (Eddy 1996). Hence, their choice to exclude PUREPAP is both just and rationally autonomous.

A broad conclusion might need some important qualifications. For example, some women may be at substantially greater risk for cervical cancer or for a variant of it that might progress much more rapidly than normally expected (perhaps because of genetics, perhaps because of personal health history), and they might be relatively easily medically identified. They might have a claim to rescreening of their negative Pap results that was both just and cost-effective. This is not something that can be settled in the abstract. The empirical details will likely be decisive in these cases. This is morally analogous to the decision of what dye to use for CT scans. We can use either a high osmolar contrast agent (HOCA) at $10 per procedure or a low osmolar contrast agent (LOCA) at $120 per procedure. That more expensive dye reduces by a factor of ten the risk of anaphylactic shock, roughly a chance in a thousand with HOCA. A test can identify *some* individuals ahead of time at risk of shock; they will be given the more expensive agent, which is both just and cost-effective. The rest of us will need to assume the risk, or else at an aggregated national level accept increased costs for CT scanning of about $2 billion per year.

There is another critical moral qualification that must be noted. We need a managed care plan that is "leakproof." More specifically, the savings generated by any particular rationing protocol must be captured and redirected to meet what plan members regard as other, higher-priority health needs. If those savings leak out of the care budget and into the advertizing budget, or into enhanced salary and benefits for upper-level management, or into higher dividends for shareholders, that is morally objectionable. It is *marginal* benefits that are being given up, but they are *benefits*. Physicians fail as fiduciary agents of their patients if they implement rationing protocols that permit savings to leak out of the care budget (Daniels 1986).

There is yet another perspective we ought to consider. Most of these matters involve collective policy decisions, as opposed to letting individuals decide as individuals. Does true respect for patient autonomy entail allowing individuals to decide for themselves what is or is not costworthy care, so long as it is their own resources they are using? In the final analysis, of course, individuals are free to spend their personal funds as they wish, no matter how foolish the expense. However, the matter is not quite that simple so far as the moral responsibility of physicians is concerned; and the matter may not be that simple so far as social justice is concerned, either.

Suppose a patient requests a PUREPAP retest of a negative Pap smear. A just and caring physician would probably inquire what rational basis the patient had for the request and then point out why this would most likely be a waste of money. In terms of social justice, the problem is that individuals may take a tax deduction for medical expenses beyond what their health insurance covers. This is fair and reasonable for individuals who must purchase health insurance out-of-pocket, as opposed to having it provided as a tax-free benefit by their employer. But for individuals who are already insured, this tax deduction amounts to a federal subsidy of health care judged by experts, as well as their fellow plan members, to be noncostworthy. Given massive unmet health needs in our society that could easily be met in a costworthy fashion, such subsidies are both unjust and inefficient. If individuals wish to purchase PUREPAP to allay their own anxieties, then such expenses should be entirely unsubsidized.

This brings us back to another feature of this case that is morally problematic. It seems that the managed care plan "covers" rescreening as part of the benefits package but reimburses providers only for the less expensive method of rescreening. In effect, this shifts the burden of making a rationing decision down to the level of individual providers. This is a serious moral problem itself. In competitive markets managed care plans will want to avoid creating the public impression that they engage in rationing. Not funding PUREPAP may be too explicit and visible a case of rationing from the perspective of organizational self-interest. Shifting the decision to the doctor-patient relationship may effectively hide this from public view. In some circumstances such a shift is morally and medically warranted; for example, when a highly individualized medical judgment is required, when hard-and-fast practice guidelines are likely to prove too crude. At present, however, there is no evidence that such individualized judgment is required for PUREPAP.

What happens then, when such decisions are shifted to individual physicians, is that patients have the impression that physicians ought to be making individualized decisions. Moreover, if physician income is linked to such decisions through a capitation mechanism, for example, and if patients are aware of this link, then patients will suspect that denial of access to this test is driven by physician self-interest rather than the best interests of the patient. This is a surefire prescription for eroding trust in the doctor-patient relationship. There is no obvious justification for managed care policies that would create such a climate of distrust.

In this case the evidence is very strong that PUREPAP yields only a very marginal benefit at best; and consequently, there ought to be a policy in the plan that simply denies access to the test for all.

What is described here is an idealization. No managed care plan has committed itself to making this idealization real; if consumers were suitably informed and empowered, however, this ideal could be realized. There are powerful considerations of justice to warrant this, especially in our existing fragmented and competitive health care system. Our health care system is inundated with marginally beneficial, noncostworthy care. PUREPAP is a good example. But the task of deleting such care from the system is not merely an economic challenge; it is a moral challenge as well, since the care being deleted is potentially beneficial to some. This is not a personal but rather a collective moral challenge. It requires creating organizational structures and social practices that will make possible deep moral conversation among plan members so that their rationing and prioritization decisions reflect their shared sense of what a just and caring managed care plan ought to be.

References

Callahan, D. 1990. *What Kind of Life: The Limits of Medical Progress.* New York: Simon and Schuster, especially chapter 2, "On the Ragged Edge: Needs, Endless Needs."

Daniels, N. 1986. "Why Saying No to Patients in the United States Is So Hard." *New England Journal of Medicine* 314, no. 21:1380–83.

Eddy, D. 1996. *Clinical Decision Making: From Theory to Practice.* Boston: Jones and Bartlett Publishers, especially chapters 11–15.

Fleck, L. M. 1990. "Pricing Human Life: The Moral Costs of Medical Progress." *The Centennial Review* 34 (Spring):227–54.

———. 1994. "Just Caring: Oregon, Health Care Rationing, and Informed Democratic Deliberation." *The Journal of Medicine and Philosophy* 19 (August):367–88.

Menzel, P. 1990. *Strong Medicine: The Ethical Rationing of Health Care.* New York: Oxford University Press, especially chapters 1–3.

Steingart, R. M.; Packer, M.; Hamm, P.; Coglianese, M. E.; Gersh, B.; Geltman, E. M.; Sollano, J.; Katz, S.; Moyé, L.; Basta, L. L.; Lewis, S. J.; Gottlieb, S. S.; Bernstein, V.; McEwan, P.; Jacobson, K.; Brown, E. J.; Kukin, M. L.; Kantrowitz, N. E.; and Pfeffer, M. A. 1991. "Sex Differences in the Management of Coronary Artery Disease." *New England Journal of Medicine* 325, no. 4:226–30.

COMMENTARY

Mitchell Sugarman, M.B.A.

One can approach the question of automated Pap smear rescreening from many perspectives: the individual patient, the patient population paying health care costs, the physician, the laboratory, the health care plan, and the manufacturer of the technology. For the sake of this discussion, let us assume that DesertHealth is leaning toward *not* covering or paying for PUREPAP, as seems apparent from the case. If DesertHealth decides to pay for PUREPAP, there will be little controversy. The controversial issues would still exist, but DesertHealth, its members, its providers, and the technology manufacturer would not be wrestling with it. Rarely do such parties object to an excess of coverage even if such an excess contributes indirectly to a lack of resources for some other service. In essence, DesertHealth could conceivably *purchase* the avoidance of the conflict by paying for PUREPAP. It ought to be obvious to most, however, that such a management style would soon make any health plan unprofitable.

The introduction of the modern-day Pap smear in the 1940s has reduced the incidence of death from cervical cancer among women who regularly receive Pap smears in the United States by 70 percent. Yet remarkably, perhaps only 15 percent of American women regularly receive Pap smears (Garnick 1997). It would be reasonable to conclude that those deaths that do occur from cervical cancer occur much more frequently among those women who are not regularly screened with a Pap smear, and that if the number of women being screened could be significantly increased, the incidence of death from cervical cancer could be further reduced. Although what is immediately at issue in the case of DesertHealth is whether the HMO should pay for automated Pap smear rescreening, these observations immediately raise the intuitive question of whether it would be more cost-effective to apply resources toward the PUREPAP technology or toward efforts to increase the number of women currently being screened in the first place. DesertHealth's Consumer Affairs Committee raises just this issue. On the surface, cost-effectiveness would seem to be an issue only for the health care plan, DesertHealth; but since all costs are eventually passed on, the rest of the stakeholders are affected by this issue as well. The one exception would be PUREPAP's manufacturer.

Based on this discussion, let us return to the DesertHealth case and note that the "plan's underwriters estimate PUREPAP would cost approximately $30,000 to detect one false-negative." A natural question would be whether this false-negative would significantly alter the health outcome of the individual patient concerned. Pap smears are classified using the Bethesda System (National Cancer Institute Workshop 1989), established in 1988 at the National Institutes of Health in Bethesda: ASCUS (atypical squamous cell of undetermined significance), LSIL (low-grade squamous intraepithelial lesions), and HSIL (high-grade squamous intraepithelial lesions). A fourth diagnostic category would be the adenocarcinoma-in-situ and cancer of the cervix, often abbreviated HSIL+. Pathologists are far more concerned with HSIL and HSIL+ lesions than they are with ASCUS and LSIL. This is because these are the lesions most likely to advance to a dangerous state, while an estimated 85 percent of

LSIL lesions regress on their own. ASCUS are usually identified as LSIL after further evaluation or else remain as cells of undetermined significance. Furthermore, there is no clear evidence that missed false-negatives would not be picked up later in a subsequent Pap smear while intervention could still be effective. The actual cost of catching a false-negative that might have a *significant* effect on health outcome might be far more than $30,000. This argument is essentially the one made by the medical director of DesertHealth Laboratories.

DesertHealth's Medical Policy Committee makes a similar argument and goes a step further by stating that, "new and more promising technology, although not yet approved by the FDA, will probably make PUREPAP obsolete." In fact, consideraton of the current state of the technological environment is a key element in the determination of whether or not to cover a new technology. While PUREPAP is intended for rescreening, the anticipation of new technologies that would perform initial or primary screening is a valid reason to wait before investing in PUREPAP. Even though DesertHealth is not considering purchasing the PUREPAP technology for use in its own laboratories, once the HMO begins covering PUREPAP by paying for it through its providers, it would find it very difficult to stop, even in light of the availability of a new, improved technology; rather, the likelihood is that the newer technology would simply come at an added cost. Another new technology that changes the way Pap smears are prepared, and thus makes them easier to read, might also influence DesertHealth's decision. In fact, both such situations exist in the cytological technology market.

DesertHealth cannot ignore the arguments made by the "public" that believes the test should be provided. Regardless of what the scientific evidence might show or not show, it is the public that will ultimately choose DesertHealth or not, based on the perception of whether or not the HMO provides quality health care. Therefore, if DesertHealth decides not to pay for PUREPAP, it must communicate clearly why this decision is sound and why it does not compromise the quality of the health care DesertHealth's members receive.

Providers who complain that they cannot bill patients for the additional costs of PUREPAP under state law, for their part, bear the responsibility for showing why PUREPAP *should* be covered. To do so they would need to provide clinically sound documentation (usually in the form of peer-reviewed, published clinical trials) demonstrating a worthwhile benefit from the use of PUREPAP.

All this leads back to the evidence: What do we know about what happens when PUREPAP is used, and how does that change things in a meaningful way for patients? Technology assessment is designed to measure the benefits and harms of a technology and then compare them to see if the benefits outweigh the harms. If there is a net benefit from the intervention, the next step is to evaluate the *relative value* of that benefit. This generally involves more abstract reasoning and is therefore more difficult to do. As a measure of benefit, years of life saved (YLS) is one possible way of looking at the benefit of a health intervention, at least in terms of its ability to increase life expectancy. YLS looks at a particular intervention, let's say a hypertension guideline, and calculates the number of individuals likely to be affected by the guideline within a given population. If implementation of the guideline resulted in three individuals in a thousand living an extra ten years, one could say that the intervention adds thirty YLS (ten years multiplied by three individuals) for that population of one thousand individuals. In a cost-effectiveness model, then, one could look at the incremental cost per YLS. So in the previous example, if the hypertension guideline cost $100 per individual to implement, the overall cost would be $100,000 ($100 multiplied by one thousand individuals), and the incremental cost would be about $3,333 per YLS ($100,000 divided by thirty YLS).

Another consideration is that you may conclude that allocating resources for intervention A (automated Pap smear screening) would not provide as much benefit as taking those same resources and applying them towards intervention B (education programs for increased awareness of the value of initial Pap smear screening). The question then arises: Will the resources, if not used for intervention A, actually get used for intervention B? Lacking a better model, this "alternative-use" model is often cited.

The problem DesertHealth faces is that arguments about why it should or should not pay for PUREPAP are being made in the absence of data. As previously stated, significant gains in the detection and prevention of death from cervical cancer have already been made by the Pap smear as it is currently performed. Nonetheless, it is also reasonable to conclude that a reduction in false-negatives will add some benefit since a small number of these false-negatives could represent the rare case of high-grade squamous cell carcinoma. But scientific data about PURE-PAP's effect on the lives and the health of DesertHealth's patient population do not exist. Moreover, this data will probably not exist for some time to come, if ever, even if the appropriate clinical trials are designed, enrolled, and completed. In order to measure the only meaningful outcome—YLS from using PUREPAP compared to YLS from *not* using PUREPAP—clinical trials would have to compare outcomes for a minimum of fifteen to twenty years, the length of time it takes for rates of cervical cancer and death from cervical cancer to be measured.

Complicating matters is the fact that the outcome from increasing the frequency of Pap smear screening, perhaps from every three years to every two years or annually, would also be a valid alternative to compare to PUREPAP. So would an increase in manual rescreening from the current legally mandated 10 percent to a rate of 50 or 100 percent. For that matter, the overall quality of a cervical cancer screening program might well be improved by *twice* rescreening 100 percent (that is, 200 percent rescreening) of the negative slides. No one knows quite where to locate the point of diminishing returns. Using PUREPAP may very well take plan, providers, and patients beyond that point.

An alternative argument for the use of PUREPAP and other automated Pap smear rescreening technologies is that there is a genuine shortage of qualified laboratory cytology technologists. The number of schools in the United States currently training individuals to become cytology technologists has dwindled drastically, and experts are predicting a near-crisis in the future with respect to replacing retiring technologists. Furthermore, a machine does not get tired or retire: it screens the one-hundreth slide as effectively as it screened the first. Given the routine nature of Pap smear reading, the same cannot be said for the human examining Pap smear slides.

So how should DesertHealth balance its obligation to its enrolled population to distribute resources fairly against its obligation to provide medically necessary care to the individual member? The key to this question lies in answering the question, What is meant by *medically necessary*? Lacking sufficient evidence that PUREPAP will significantly improve the health outcomes of a given member or significant percentage of a population of members, it would be difficult to argue that the use of PUREPAP is medically necessary.

State laws make it difficult for DesertHealth to institute a copayment that members would pay when they insist on PUREPAP's use, but DesertHealth could explore this possibility further as a means of managing this issue while it awaits some of the new technologies expected to obviate the need for PUREPAP. "Additional rescreening" might be looked at as a separate service from initial screening and legally mandated rescreening for quality purposes. In so doing, DesertHealth could state that this new service is *not covered* and thus allow providers to balance their billing with out-of-pocket payments from members. The state's laws may not be meeting the needs of citizens if they set up a catch-22 here.

Educating its members through brochures or seminars to the facts about PUREPAP's relatively weak benefits when compared to initial Pap smear screening would also be in DesertHealth's best interest. This has become especially important in order to balance the trend of aggressive marketing tactics used by proponents of a new technology—most often the manufacturers—to sway the public. DesertHealth's best defense is to expose the facts as they exist, which would include a frank discussion of cost versus benefit. Members who insist on receiving the potential additional benefit from the automated Pap smear rescreening should be provided with a mechanism for paying for PUREPAP on their own.

DesertHealth also needs to work closely with its providers so that, like their members, they will understand that DesertHealth's decision is based principally on a thorough examination of the scientific evidence about both care *and* benefit. If

DesertHealth ultimately decides not to cover PUREPAP, the decision should not undermine its relationships with its providers, who might otherwise perceive the decision as significant interference in the patient-provider relationship. Again, developing a mechanism whereby members can choose to use PUREPAP and pay for all or a part of it themselves would go a long way toward preserving the relationship DesertHealth has with its providers. While the inherent inequities of a self-pay model, where some individuals can afford to purchase "better" or at least what is *perceived* as better health care than others are obvious, such inequities have been and probably always will be a fact of health care in the United States. The advantage, however, is the ability to manage the realities of needing to get along with the public, members, potential enrollees, and providers.

Another option DesertHealth might wish to consider is an algorithm that ranks women by risk, perhaps based on family history, previous histological abnormality, or other evaluative method, and only offer coverage for PUREPAP to these women. An argument for this type of selective use of an expensive technology has been made with other technologies such as low osmolar contrast media (LOCM), used in imaging studies. While the incidence of serious adverse effects from conventional contrast media is low, and death as a result is even lower (Jacobson and Rosenquist 1988), large-scale clinical studies did show that the use of LOCM could reduce the incidence of serious effect and death even further. However, LOCM may cost seven or eight times as much as conventional imaging media, and switching to it universally would be terribly expensive. Given this scenario, it is now widely accepted practice to use LOCM only on those patients who would be most likely to suffer the greatest harm from an adverse event while undergoing contrast imaging studies: the very old and frail, the very young, and those individuals who have a history of experiencing moderate to severe adverse effects from contrast media. In this way, the relative value of using an expensive new technology is increased. Selective use of PUREPAP might similarly increase its relative value.

Finally, there is the issue of the state law that mandates the "coverage of all preventive services, including screening for cancer." First, DesertHealth would make a valid argument that it is already meeting the state mandate by performing what is generally accepted to be the appropriate screening for cervical cancer, that is, routine Pap smears at regular intervals with a legally mandated 10 percent manual rescreening. Second, a public policy that provides for unlimited coverage for all preventive services without consideration of the limits of resources and what makes sense would always be at odds with the practical management and solvency of health care carriers.

Situations like the one described in this case will arise as long as new medical technologies are available and aggressively marketed before good clinical data have been gathered that demonstrate their safety, effectiveness, and overall value. The test of time in the form of long-term outcomes should eventually determine which technologies add value and which ones do not. However, the interim use of technologies that eventually prove to be of little or no value (and in some cases even harmful) will continue to add to the rapidly increasing cost of health care in the United States.

References

Garnick, M. B. 1997. "Gynecologic Cancer." In *Scientific American Medicine*, pp. 1–20. Edited by D. C. Dale and D. D. Federman. New York: Scientific American.

Jacobson, P. D., and Rosenquist, J. 1988. "The Introduction of Low-Osmolar Contrast Agents in Radiology." *Journal of the American Medical Association* 260, no. 11:1586–92.

National Cancer Institute Workshop. 1989. "The 1988 Bethesda System for Reporting Cervical/Vaginal Cytologic Diagnoses." *Journal of the American Medical Association* 262, no. 7:931–34.

2

Coverage of Emergency Services

CASE STUDY _____

Most managed care plans treat emergency services differently from other care. Some plans require preauthorization for coverage of emergency services. Others require authorization within twenty-four or forty-eight hours. Still others require that the injury be "life or limb threatening" in order to be covered. And some require a "reasonable belief" that the emergency was real, with "reasonable" defined either by the plan or by the member.

Public pressure and some state legislatures have forced managed care organizations to reexamine their policies relating to coverage for emergency services. In response to increasing denials of coverage, some state statutes now prohibit use of a preauthorization requirement, prohibit nonpayment based on a failure to notify the plan within a certain time period, or set a "prudent layperson" standard for determining what constitutes an emergency.

Lawrence Care is a licensed HMO in a state that has not yet enacted such legislation. Nonetheless, Lawrence Care's policy committee has been asked to consider when and if authorization should be required for emergency services, what the definition of "emergency" should be, and who should determine when an emergency exists.

The committee has identified three categories of problem cases the new emergency care policy must address. First, there are cases when use of the emergency department is objectively not necessary and is an inappropriate use of resources, for example, when members go to the emergency department for a common sore throat rather than to an urgent care center or their primary care physician. Second, there are cases of what might be termed a "questionable emergency," for example, when a member slips on the ice, hurts a wrist, and, unsure whether it is sprained or broken, goes to the emergency department. Third, there are cases that qualify as emergencies, but the member fails to obtain timely authorization from the plan, for example, when a member is in a car accident and suffers severe head injuries, and the spouse fails to obtain authorization within the requisite twenty-four-hour time period for what turns out to be a two-week admission.

Lawrence Care's current definition of "covered emergency" includes "medically necessary health services for unforeseen illnesses or injuries that are threatening to life or limb and require immediate medical attention as determined by Lawrence Care." Preauthorization is generally required under the plan unless the situation meets this definition. Even if the definition of "emergency" is met, authorization must still be obtained within twenty-four-hours of treatment.

One recent incident, in particular, has caused Lawrence Care to reexamine its coverage for emergency services. Mr. and Mrs. Lane, in their early sixties, are both retired and live in a small house in Winston, just forty miles south of the large town of Fort Lawrence. In the five years they have been members of Lawrence Care, they have had two serious health incidents, both of which led to disagreements with Lawrence Care.

In the first incident, Mr. Lane slipped in the driveway while shoveling snow early one Sunday morning. His wrist seemed to be broken, and he also hit his head on the driveway. Mr. Lane's wrist caused him considerable pain, and he was disoriented and felt nauseous. Mrs. Lane immediately called 911 for an ambulance, which took Mr. Lane to Winston General Hospital, five miles from their home. Mr. Lane's wrist was X-rayed and found to be severely sprained. Mrs. Lane was given instructions to monitor him for signs of a concussion. She forgot to call the plan before she dialed 911, but she did call to report the event and services within twenty-four hours.

The next month the Lanes received a letter from Lawrence Care explaining that the ambulance charge and emergency department services would not be covered because they were not "threatening to life or limb" and should have been treated by urgent care only after obtaining preauthorization from the plan. The Lanes appealed, and eventually Lawrence Care agreed to pay the emergency department fees but not the ambulance charge. The Lanes learned a costly lesson: if a medical problem arises, first call Lawrence Care, and then dial 911, if authorized.

A few months later, Mrs. Lane contracted what turned out to be meningitis. The Lanes had spent the day together doing yard work and then went out for dinner. Mrs. Lane felt fine when she went to bed. The next morning, she awoke with a severe headache, a stiff neck, and a fever. Mr. Lane called the Lawrence Care twenty-four-hour nurse hotline. He spoke with a nurse who asked him a number of questions and ruled out anything more serious than the flu, which was making the rounds in the community. She suggested fluids and rest for Mrs. Lane and told Mr. Lane to call if her condition worsened.

By noon, Mrs. Lane was vomiting and breathing irregularly. Again, instead of calling 911 or proceeding to the hospital or urgent care center, Mr. Lane called the nurse hotline. This time the nurse felt she should consult with a physician and call the Lanes back to instruct them. After about thirty minutes, she called the Lanes and advised them to go to Baptist Hospital in Fort Lawrence about fifty miles from their home. The nurse explained that this was the only hospital where they would be fully reimbursed for services.

The Lanes set out immediately. Mr. Lane considered driving to Winston General Hospital but recalled the trouble they had been through with the previous hospitalization and reasoned that it was probably just the flu. Baptist Hospital is on the far north side of Fort Lawrence. By the time the Lanes neared the outskirts of Fort Lawrence it was apparent that Mrs. Lane's condition was worsening rapidly. Still, Mr. Lane was determined to follow the instructions of the plan and twenty minutes later pulled into Baptist Hospital. Mrs. Lane was admitted and diagnosed. She died that evening of irreversible effects of meningitis. The emergency department physician explained to Mr. Lane that with this type of condition a few hours can make the difference between life and death.

When Mr. Lane explained the events of the day, the physician became irate that the plan did not send Mr. Lane and his wife to Winston General, only five miles from their home. Mr. Lane regrets that he did not just stop at Winston General and claims that the plan was negligent in its referral policies and actions. Mr. Lane has hired an attorney to litigate these claims.

Lawrence Care's policy committee must draft a provision for coverage of emergency services that addresses not only the Lanes' situation but the other types of recurrent emergency department scenarios outlined previously.

Questions for Consideration

➤ How are emergency department services different from other health care services?

➤ In light of these differences, what requirements, if any, should managed care organizations attach to accessing, authorizing, and covering emergency department services?

➤ What definition of "emergency" best balances the interests of the member against those of the plan population?

➤ Should the determination that an "emergency" exists be at the discretion of the plan or left to the judgment of the member? Why?

➤ Is coverage policy for emergency care best addressed by government regulation? Why?

COMMENTARY

E. Haavi Morreim, Ph.D.

The United States' health care economy is in the midst of an extraordinary transition. After decades of costs rising out of control, the businesses and governments that directly pay for most health care have mandated major cost control. From the lavish practices of the past, medicine is being rewritten from the ground up, virtually overnight. Among a variety of economizing moves, health plans have especially targeted the most obvious areas in which money appears to have been wasted. Emergency care is one of them. Charges for emergency care usually run high, and many patients use emergency departments as their major source of primary care, rather than reserving them only for emergent or urgent conditions. Some visits are plainly not for emergency problems, as when a family simply leaves a frail elderly parent at the emergency department, hoping that someone else will now take responsibility for care.

Accordingly, many health plans, including the Lanes' plan, have instituted preauthorization requirements as a kind of preemergency triage to reduce unnecessary emergency department use. Such emergency department restrictions can also encourage members to seek ongoing care from their primary care physicians. Continuity in this relationship has a significant positive value for patients' overall health and health care (Blumenthal 1996; Safran, Tarlov, and Rogers 1994; Grumbach and Bodenheimer 1995). Not incidentally, a reduction in nonurgent emergency department use can also help staff to focus its attention on those who need it most (Steinbrook 1996).

Problems

Unfortunately, these preauthorization requirements, along with retrospective refusals to pay for emergency services, have placed many emergency departments in a significant financial pinch. Federal law (Emergency Medical Treatment and Active Labor Act, P.L. 99-272, 42 U.S.C. § 1395dd) requires emergency departments to screen and stabilize all patients who present themselves. Yet when health plans deny payment, and when patients also are unwilling or unable to pay, emergency departments usually must absorb the cost—cumulatively a substantial problem for many emergency departments.

More important, patients can suffer serious adverse consequences. Some patients have been denied preauthorization for conditions that later turned out to be major illnesses, including ectopic pregnancy, pulmonary embolus, acute myocardial infarction (heart attack), and sepsis (massive infection). In other cases, bureaucratic delays cause the problems. One study showed that the time required to complete authorizations can range from twenty minutes to over two-and-a-half hours (Derlet and Hamilton 1996). Still other deleterious delays can arise as patients avoid needed care because of payment fears, as exemplified by the Lanes' situation.

There are further problems with emergency department preauthorization requirements and unpredictable retrospective payment denials. First, the savings may not be substantial. Emergency care only constitutes about 2 to 5 percent of U.S. health care dollars (Burke, Yeh, and Karcz 1997; Hyman 1998). Hence, "unnecessary" emergency care may only represent a relatively small portion of the total spectrum of "inappropriate" and costly medical care that may rightly warrant trimming. Further, although emergency department charges are often high, actual incremental *costs* of providing nonemergency care in the emergency department are often relatively low, leading some researchers to conclude that diverting nonurgent care to other settings will not necessarily achieve significant savings (Williams 1996). To some extent those charges are high because emergency departments are only able to collect about half of their charges, requiring them to make up for lost income by charging paying patients more.

Another problem with tight emergency department utilization management is the dearth of high-quality guidelines by which to make decisions. Throughout medicine, health plans have responded to wide variations in physicians' practices by creating guidelines that purport to summarize appropriate care for specified indications. However, many of these guidelines are based on relatively little sound empirical evidence. More commonly they are the product of data and methodology that are fraught with flaws, or they are the consensus products of clinicians chosen because their clinical views already reflect the health plan's cost-conserving goals (Soumerai et al. 1993; Epstein 1995). And often they are created by entities that have a significant conflict of interest in the results of their outcomes, studies, and guidelines creation: insurers and managed care organizations, employers, manufacturers of drugs and devices, and corporations that develop and sell guidelines for profit.

This is not to say that such guidelines are invariably defective. Some can be quite helpful, as for instance the guidelines that have substantially reduced adverse anesthesia events during surgery (Eichorn 1989). Still, inadequate guidelines clearly pose a problem. In the Lanes' case, one must question the validity of any guideline that fails to identify high fever, severe headache, and stiff neck as a potential meningitis—and later fails to pick up the same patient's irregular breathing and changes in mental status as a sign of acute deterioration.

Beyond this, restrictive policies like Lawrence Care's fail to address the reasons people seek nonurgent care from emergency departments in the first place. Aside from situations posing obvious peril to life and limb, fear and uncertainty pervade many decisions to visit an emergency department. When Mr. Lane injured his wrist and struck his head on the driveway, he and his wife had no way to know whether his wrist was broken or how severe his apparent concussion might be. He also was in significant pain that deserved prompt relief. And when they sought ambulance transportation, they may well have deemed this safer than expecting Mrs. Lane, in her late sixties and perhaps unaccustomed to driving on snowy roads, to drive him to the hospital herself.

Emergency department visits are also prompted by a lack of alternatives. For people in inner-city neighborhoods, for instance, the hospital emergency department is often far more accessible than a primary care physician's office, which may be distant (requiring costly cab fare or a lengthy bus ride) or whose schedule may require the patient to take precious time away from work or to pay for child care. The emergency department is always open. Although on-site waiting times may be lengthy, appointments need not be made weeks in advance. And many emergency departments are less likely than primary care physicians to insist on payment, while some even provide free medications upon discharge.

Personal values can also prompt emergency department use. Many people do not immediately seek medical treatment at the first sign of ailment, preferring instead to "tough it out" and hope the problem will disappear on its own. When the patient finally decides this approach has failed, it may be late at night. Although health care providers may be annoyed to see such problems at these hours, when ostensibly the patient could have sought help earlier, it is not clear that this pattern is actually so costly in the final analysis. Because these patients only come to medical attention when their preference for holding off has failed, it is not known how often the strategy has in fact worked well in the past for self-limited problems, saving considerable expense for providers. Many primary care physicians in managed care rely often on the watch-and-wait approach. Indeed, patients are given mixed signals. On the one hand, they are criticized for attempting to self-diagnose or self-medicate instead of seeking care. At the same time, other patients are equally criticized for being frivolous, demanding treatment for every little sniffle. People with limited medical knowledge can be forgiven if they find this confusing.

Resolutions

In the final analysis, it may be best for Lawrence Care to downplay preauthorization requirements and post hoc payment denial as its principal approaches to reducing emergency department costs. These tactics can imperil patients, expose the health plan to greater legal risks, and ultimately may save little money relative to their administrative costs. At the very least, if Lawrence Care retains the option to deny payment, its decisions should be based not on a patient's final diagnosis but on presenting symptoms and on whether a prudent layperson would reasonably judge those symptoms to constitute an emergency (Steinbrook 1996). Several states have enacted legislation to this effect, and several more are considering the same (Burke, Yeh, and Karcz 1997). Such standards may be difficult to interpret and may actually help emergency departments more than patients, since the departments rather than patients are usually left holding the financial bag (Hyman 1998). But they do represent a conceptual shift that could ameliorate the problem and leave people like the Lanes in less fear of misjudging their own medical problems.

At the same time, it seems essential to search for safer, more effective ways to encourage prudent judgment. Some practical problem solving is in order. First, better outcomes studies and guidelines are needed throughout medicine if health care is to be more evidence-based and rely less on anecdote, intuition, happenstance, and local medical fashions. Next, health plans like Lawrence Care need to address the underlying needs that give rise to ostensibly unwarranted emergency department use. Lawrence Care should ensure that the offices of primary care physicians are conveniently available, with hours that permit working people to receive care without forfeiting income. They might, for instance, pay physicians an extra fee, such as $15 for each office visit after 5 P.M., to encourage them to offer longer hours (Lowes 1996). Twenty-four-hour urgent care must likewise be available for nonemergency problems. If clear access to such facilities had been available for Mr. Lane's sprained wrist, the couple might have avoided the earlier battles that rendered them so reluctant to visit the emergency department for Mrs. Lane's illness.

If high emergency department charges are a problem, then Lawrence Care should try to negotiate better rates. For example, if most of its patients use a particular emergency department, the plan might negotiate a capitated arrangement to encourage that department to be more judicious about the high levels of testing and hospital admission that are often the most significant source of emergency costs. Alternatively, fee discounts might be arranged.

If high use is a problem, Lawrence Care could place its own internists or case managers into emergency departments at the times its members are most likely to appear. Some health plans have instituted twenty-four-hour telephone assistance to help (not require) members to discern what sort of help they may need. Others have initiated home-based interventions that can keep problems from developing in the first place, such as visits to the home of an elderly person to remedy the most likely causes of in-home falls and accidents (Jahn 1996).

Patients could still be held accountable but in better ways than retrospective surprise denials of coverage. Lawrence Care might, for instance, tune its financial penalties to each patient's own history of unwarranted emergency department use.

The bare fact that someone like Mr. or Mrs. Lane occasionally misjudges the need for emergency care does not mean that the patient is a problem.

Indeed, health plans have already made an important discovery about physicians, which may be relevant to patients who use emergency departments: most of the unnecessary care is provided by a relatively small number of physicians, not by the great majority who generally practice very reasonably. Hence, many health plans now focus their cost-containment efforts on this minority of physicians who systematically overuse resources. By analogy, Lawrence Care might focus on those patients who tend to abuse the emergency department, perhaps tuning financial incentives like higher cost-sharing to each patient's individual history of emergency department use. Instead of penalizing a first-time "offender" the same as a chronic abuser, each demonstrably inappropriate visit might warrant a demerit of some sort, such that a patient who collects a certain number of demerits over a period of time might receive further education from the primary care physician or perhaps an increasing level of cost-sharing.

Even better, Lawrence Care might try to listen to those who chronically (over)use emergency departments. Any such situation may well reflect an underlying unmet need that, if properly addressed, could not only reduce visits but also improve the patient's health and reduce the need for health care overall. Health plans that have developed disease management programs for illnesses such as asthma and congestive heart failure, for instance, have markedly reduced emergency department visits and improved patients' health by helping them to function as active partners in the management of their own diseases (Epstein 1996; Harris 1996). Such positive approaches are preferable to the punitive, unpredictable, and sometimes harmful constraints that Lawrence Care now uses.

References

Blumenthal, D. 1996. "Effects of Market Reforms on Doctors and Their Patients." *Health Affairs* 15, no. 2:170–84.

Burke, M. C.; Yeh, C.; and Karcz, A. 1997. "The Myths of Emergency Medical Care Access in the Managed Care Era." *American Journal of Managed Care* 3, no. 9:1316–20.

Derlet, R. W., and Hamilton, B. 1996. "The Impact of Health Maintenance Organization Care Authorization Policy on an Emergency Department Before California's New Managed Care Law." *Academic Emergency Medicine* 3, no. 4:338–44.

Eichorn, J. H. 1989. "Prevention of Intraoperative Anesthesia Accidents and Related Severe Injury through Safety Monitoring." *Anesthesiology* 70, no. 4:572–77.

Epstein, A. 1995. "Performance Reports on Quality—Prototypes, Problems, and Prospects." *New England Journal of Medicine* 333, no. 1:57–61.

Epstein, R. S. 1996. "From Outcomes Research to Disease Management: A Guide for the Perplexed." *Annals of Internal Medicine* 124, no. 9:832–37.

Grumbach, K., and Bodenheimer, T. 1995. "The Organization of Health Care." *Journal of the American Medical Associaton* 273, no. 2:160–67.

Harris, J. M., Jr. 1996. "Disease Management: New Wine in New Bottles?" *Annals of Internal Medicine* 124, no. 9:838–42.

Hyman, D. A. 1998. "Consumer Protection in a Managed Care World: Should Consumers call 911?" *Villanova Law Review* 43, no. 2:409.

Jahn, M. 1996. "Keeping Outpatients from Becoming Inpatients." *Medical Economics* 73, no. 14: 81–93.

Lowes, R. L. 1996. "Here Comes Managed-Care Medicaid: Should You Hop Aboard? " *Medical Economics* 73. no. 9:60–73.

Safran, D. G.; Tarlov, A. R.; and Rogers, W. H. 1994. "Primary Care Performance in Fee-For-Service and Prepaid Health Care Systems." *Journal of the American Medical Association* 271, no. 20:1579–86.

Soumerai, S. B.; Ross-Degnan, D.; Fortess, E. E.; and Abelson, J. 1993. "A Critical Analysis of Studies of State Drug Reimbursement Policies: Research in Need of Discipline." *Milbank Quarterly* 71, no. 2:217–52.

Steinbrook, R. 1996. "The Role of the Emergency Department." *New England Journal of Medicine* 334, no. 10:657–58.

Williams, R. M. 1996. "The Costs of Visits to Emergency Departments." *New England Journal of Medicine* 334, no. 10:642–46.

COMMENTARY

Karen A. Jordan, J.D.

This case presents the unique dilemmas posed by the use of managed care strategies to constrain health care costs incurred in the provision of emergency care. Administrators of managed care plans perceive the emergency department setting as creating even stronger justifications for the infusion of strategies to control provider and enrollee behavior. Because expensive, specialized equipment and highly trained staff must be maintained, emergency department visits generate higher charges than comparable visits to physicians' offices (Young et al. 1996). Moreover, some patients use emergency departments for their primary care needs (Hurley, Freund, and Taylor 1989). Lastly, a patient arriving at an emergency department may be assigned to a physician who is not participating in the managed care plan, thereby lessening the plan's control over the cost of care for the enrollee (Hoffman 1997). However, whether the use of managed care strategies is justified depends on whether and to what extent the provision of emergency care fits into the managed care model.

The key premise underlying managed care is that costs can be constrained by eliminating the provision of unnecessary health care services and, further, that given the unique nature of health care, both patients and providers of health care need help in making the determination as to what care is medically necessary. Managed care plans therefore use strategies designed to restrain the use of unnecessary diagnostic tests and to encourage the most efficient treatment protocols. These strategies, including preauthorization and utilization review, have the potential to be effective in reducing costs. Utilization review broadens the circle of decision makers, thereby tempering uninformed decisions of patients and medically questionable decisions of providers. Preauthorization ensures that the need for especially costly medical procedures is reviewed before the care is provided, thereby lessening the likelihood that the patient or the provider will be left bearing the cost after the plan denies coverage.

However, managed care involves trade-offs. If utilization review and preauthorization procedures are performed by competent reviewers, the potential to identify unnecessary care is arguably enhanced. But the autonomy of both patient and provider is adversely affected. Further, even competent reviewers may be influenced by conflicts of interest inherent in the managed care setting, thereby creating the potential for denials of some necessary care (Peeno 1998). Nonetheless, although perhaps disfavored by providers and enrollees for these reasons, managed care arguably presents an acceptable balancing of interests in nonemergency situations, where its impact is less critical.

When the patient's medical condition falls into the category of "emergency," however, the trade-off may become unacceptable. The potential presence of a condition seriously threatening to life or bodily function inevitably changes the dynamics. For example, as Mrs. Lane's situation illustrates, time is often of the essence. Further, the practice of emergency medicine has a unique focus. The purpose of emergency medicine is to evaluate, stabilize, and treat illnesses and injuries that require immediate attention (Brenner and Simon 1984). Emergency department physicians must be able to differentiate patients experiencing an emergency condition from those who have similar symptoms but who are not suffering from an emergency condition. Perhaps more important, physicians must be able to identify patients who are candidates for sudden deterioration. Thus, the emergency setting requires that the uncertainties inherent in medicine be confronted with a dramatically different approach. Practitioners in other fields, such as internal medicine, seek to identify conditions in the order of probability, with the most likely diagnosis listed first. In contrast, emergency department physicians must identify conditions in the order of the worst possible diagnosis, thereby often requiring diagnostic tests not as readily performed in another setting to rule out life-threatening possibilities.

Managed care's underlying premise is therefore severely compromised in the emergency setting. Rather than ensuring an efficient provision of appropriate medical care, preauthorization and utilization review may pose obstacles to the appropriate practice of emergency medicine. Preauthorization may unreasonably delay access to care. Utilization review performed in hindsight—and from an internal medicine rather than an emergency medicine perspective—may label as "unnecessary" diagnostic and treatment services needed to rule out life-threatening conditions.

Moreover, managed care strategies may not effectively constrain health care costs. If patients do not receive appropriate care quickly in the emergency department, the patient's condition may deteriorate and become more costly to manage in the long run. Further, state and federal laws, such as the Emergency Medical Treatment and Active Labor Act (P.L. 99–272, 42 U.S.C. § 1395dd), which imposes various duties on providers of care in the emergency setting, require that patients who arrive at the emergency department receive an appropriate screening examination; and if an emergency condition is identified, the patient must receive treatment necessary to stabilize the condition. Thus, preauthorization and utilization review strategies often will not prevent the patient from receiving care deemed appropriate by the emergency department physician. As a result, although the managed care plan may avoid the direct cost of these services, the cost is indirectly passed on to other payers as the hospital raises charges to offset the lack of reimbursement.

In sum, the provision of emergency services does not readily fall within the managed care model, and the use of traditional preauthorization and utilization review strategies in the emergency setting can be challenged as inappropriate. Indeed, in the emergency setting, managed care is often less about managing health care costs than about shifting the burden of the cost to the provider, the patient, or society at large. However, this does not mean that the provision of emergency services is completely unmanageable. Rather, emergency care should be managed using strategies tailored to the unique characteristics of the emergency setting.

The issue then is whether government regulation is necessary or whether managed care plans will voluntarily modify their practices, as Lawrence Care appears ready to consider. This depends on two factors: (1) the market power of consumers of managed care plans and (2) whether managed care plans can be held legally responsible for harm resulting from unreasonable policies and procedures. As to the first factor, it seems unlikely that a proper balancing of interests will emerge in the absence of governmental intervention. Although some private purchasers of health care coverage, such as large employer groups, are seeking to increase their bargaining power, the majority do not have sufficient market power to compel managed care plans to modify their current practices. Further, purchasers of health plans are often more interested in price than in details such as obstacles to emergency care (Matthew, 1996). The second factor is more influential. Indeed, the fact that some managed care plans, such as Lawrence Care, may be rethinking their policies probably reflects the increasing likelihood that managed care policies that cause poor medical outcomes, such as in the Lanes' case, may result in tort liability for the managed care organization.

The increasing likelihood stems from recent case law developments. First, tort theories that impose a direct duty of reasonable care on managed care entities are emerging. For example, in *Harrell v. Total Health Care, Inc.* (1989 Westlaw 13066 [Mo. Ct. App. 1989], *affirmed*, 781 S.W. 2d 58 [Mo. 1989]), the court extended the doctrine of institutional negligence to the defendant HMO because it had assumed the traditional role of a hospital. That is, the court viewed the HMO as a comprehensive health center with responsibilities for arranging and coordinating the total health care of patients. The concept of institutional negligence encompasses various duties, including the duty to select competent physicians, to monitor physician performance, and to formulate, adopt, and enforce policies that help ensure the provision of quality care to patients.

Second, developments in the law of the Employee Retirement Income Security Act of 1974 (ERISA) (P.L. 93–406, 29 U.S.C. § 1001 ct. seq.), render it less likely that managed care organizations will be shielded from such liability. ERISA contains a clause that provides that state laws are superseded if they "relate to" the benefit plans provided by most private employers (29 U.S.C. § 1144[a]). Historically, courts broadly viewed ERISA as preempting, and thus precluding, all tort and contract claims brought against insurers or managed care entities. For example, in *Kuhl v. Lincoln National Health Plan of Kansas City* (999 F. 2d 298 [8th Cir. 1993]), the court barred a suit based on an HMO's preauthorization procedures that caused a significant delay in the member's care and ultimately in his death. In *Corcoran v. United Healthcare, Inc.* (965 F. 2d 1321 [5th Cir. 1992], *cert. denied*, 506 U.S. 1033 [1992], the court held that ERISA preempted a claim based on an allegedly negligent utilization review determination denying hospitalization for an at-risk pregnancy that resulted in the death of the fetus.

In more recent decisions, however, courts are more carefully scrutinizing tort claims against insurers and managed care organizations. Although a claim such as the Corcorans' is likely still to be preempted because the plaintiff is essentially challenging a benefit determination (and thus the quantity of care received), some claims challenging negligent policies and procedures may be allowed to proceed. For example, in *Ouellette v. The Christ Hospital* (924 F. Supp. 1160 [S.D. Ohio 1996]), the plaintiff alleged that she was prematurely and negligently discharged from the hospital because the policies and incentives used by her managed care plan undermined the quality of care provided by the hospital. The court found that the claim did not arise from the process of benefit determination, and thus was not automatically preempted, because the plaintiff was not challenging the quantity of care but rather the quality of care that she received. In *Pappas v. Asbel* (675 A. 2d

711 [Super. Ct. Pa. 1996]), the court more definitively held that ERISA did not preempt a claim against an HMO based on the delay in care resulting from allegedly negligent preauthorization procedures.

To the extent ERISA's protective shield erodes, courts would be free to adopt tort theories that could be used to impose a duty of reasonable care on managed care plans. This increased potential for tort liability may exert a significant influence on the policies and procedures adopted by managed care plans. Importantly, however, although the potential for tort liability is increasing, judicial regulation through tort law is a case-by-case and state-by-state proposition. Thus, managed care plans could postpone modifications to their policies until such time as the states in which they operate have expressly recognized the tort theories discussed here.

Legislation may therefore provide a more timely resolution to the problem. Further, a legislative solution arguably positions the debate in a more appropriate forum. As discussed shortly, difficult questions must be addressed in determining the extent to which the provision of emergency services should be managed. Notably, the debate is ultimately about who pays for emergency care. Limiting the use of managed care strategies collectively spreads the risk of emergency services more broadly across the community. That is, to the extent laws require managed care plans to cover emergency services, the risk is spread among all policyholders. All of those who pay premiums for health coverage are asked to absorb the costs. The legislative process is a more effective forum to discuss and resolve these types of policy-laden issues.

Moreover, federal legislation arguably provides a better solution than state legislation for two reasons. First, state legislation, similar to judicial regulation, permits managed care plans to continue operating as usual until the state in which they operate enacts legislation. While many states are moving forward with consumer protection laws for persons in managed care plans, others may be unable to act on this volatile issue given the powerful interest groups affected. Second, state legislation is vulnerable to ERISA preemption. ERISA's savings clause exempts from preemption state laws that, although "relating to" employee benefit plans, regulate "the business of insurance" (29 U.S.C. § 1144[b]). Many courts, however, take a narrow approach to the analysis and refuse to save state laws that regulate HMOs, Blue Cross and Blue Shield plans, or plans offered by the variety of emerging managed care organizations. Thus, state laws regulating the use of managed care in the emergency setting may offer limited protection.

Whether addressed voluntarily by managed care plans or through legislation, the central issue becomes how managed care strategies should be tailored for the emergency care setting. Several interests must be balanced. Managed care plans cannot be mandated to cover, without limitation, all services provided in the emergency department. On the other hand, enrollees are entitled to coverage of services necessary to treat perceived emergencies. Similarly, hospital emergency departments, which are required under federal law to provide certain screening examinations and stabilizing care, cannot be left without reimbursement given the increasing difficulty of shifting the cost of uncompensated care onto other payers. A reasonable balancing would hold managed care plans responsible for coverage of services necessary to treat potential emergencies, providers responsible for costs beyond what is necessary to treat such emergencies, and enrollees responsible for the costs associated with emergency department visits that are obvious nonemergencies (Hoffman 1997).

The key questions are those Lawrence Care has elected to consider. What definition of emergency should be used? Who should determine when an emergency exists? When should the determination be made? Should members be required to obtain preauthorization before accessing care in emergency situations? In considering these questions, it is useful to look to existing legislative provisions designed to address the problem of managed care and emergency services.

Legislators have generally adopted a "prudent" or "reasonable" person standard. For example, proposed federal legislation requires plans to cover and make reasonable payments for "items and services that are necessary for the diagnosis, treatment, and stabilization of an emergency medical condition" (Patient Access to Responsible Care Act, 1997 Cong. H.R. 1415, § 2771[(b)(1)(C) and (2)(B)]). Emergency medical condition is defined as a condition "manifesting itself by acute symptoms of sufficient severity (including severe pain) such that a prudent layperson, who possesses an average knowledge of health and medicine, could reasonably expect the absence of immediate medical attention . . . to result in (i) placing the patient's health in serious jeopardy, (ii) serious impairment to bodily functions, or (iii) serious dysfunction of any bodily organ or part." (§ 2771[(b)(2)(A)]). The prudent person standard protects the enrollee's entitlement to services necessary to treat perceived emergencies by recognizing that managed care plan members should not be put in the position of making quasi-clinical evaluations of their conditions.

In addition, by requiring coverage of all health care services "necessary for the diagnosis, treatment, and stabilization" of the emergency condition, the definition protects the interests of both the hospital and the managed care plan. The hospital will receive reimbursement for providing services required by federal law and by the unique characteristics of emergency medicine. Yet the managed care plan may withhold payment for services beyond those that are necessary, even in the emergency setting.

The proposed federal provision also appears to prevent a denial of coverage based on "hindsight." Some states have more expressly precluded hindsight denials by mandating that managed care plans base their determination on the member's presenting symptoms and conditions, not on the diagnosis established after the medical evaluation. These principles are also reflected in the federal guidelines used in the Medicare program. Guidelines issued by the Health Care Financing Agency, addressing emergency care for Medicare managed care beneficiaries, provide that plans may "not retroactively deny a claim because a condition, which appeared to be an emergency, turns out to be non-emergency in nature" (Commerce Clearinghouse, Inc. [CCH] 1997). Further, the guidelines provide that all procedures performed during evaluation and treatment of an emergency condition related to the care of that condition must be covered.

Provisions such as these would allow utilization review in the emergency setting in a manner that reflects a responsible balancing of interests. The provisions protect the interests of the enrollees and the providers, and they do not impose an undue burden on the interest of managed care plans. Plans could, of course, more expressly protect their interest by providing that if it is clearly a case of routine illness where the patient's medical condition never was, or never appeared to be, an emergency, the plan is not responsible for payment of claims for the services.

Although utilization review can be tailored to fit the emergency setting, the use of preauthorization may be categorically unjustified, given the serious consequences associated with an inappropriate delay in the provision of emergency services. It seems entirely unreasonable to require enrollees to obtain authorization before proceeding to an emergency department when their symptoms suggest the presence of an emergency condition. Most states that have addressed the issue and the proposed federal legislation prohibit the use of preauthorization requirements for emergency care. The federal proposal states that plans shall "require no pre-authorization for items and services furnished in a hospital emergency department to an enrollee with symptoms that would reasonably suggest to a prudent layperson an emergency medical condition" (1997 Cong. H.R. 1415, § 2771[(b)(1)(B)]).

Some states, however, have permitted a limited use of preauthorization. For example, an Arizona provision states that a health plan "may require as a condition of coverage prior authorization for health care services arising after the initial medical screening examination and immediately necessary stabilizing treatment" (West Supp. 1997, Ariz. Re. Stat. Ann. § 20–2803[C]). Because this use of preauthorization would not cause a delay in getting to the emergency department, nor in the provision of immediate care, it may reflect an acceptable balancing of interests.

To temper the harmful consequences associated with even this more limited use of preauthorization, the plan's response time could be restricted. Arizona, for example, provides that prior authorization is granted unless denied or unless the direction of the enrollee's care is initiated by the plan within a "reasonable period of time after the plan receives the prior authorization request" (West Supp. 1997,

Ariz. Re. Stat. Ann. § 20–2803[C]). Still other states require that, if the plan uses any type of preauthorization for emergency services, for example, for poststabilization treatment, the plan must provide twenty-four-hour telephone access in order to respond to requests in a timely manner. Whether requiring a response within a "reasonable" time or in a "timely" manner affords sufficient protection to enrollees, given the ambiguity of the terms, should be further examined.

These legislative solutions represent a careful tailoring of managed care strategies in light of the unique characteristics of the emergency setting. Although designed to temper the adverse impact on enrollees such as the Lanes, they permit managed care plans to "manage" coverage of emergency services to the extent reasonable. Given the heightened potential for tort liability for unreasonable managed care policies, Lawrence Care should seriously consider these legislative solutions in formulating its policy provisions for coverage of emergency services.

References

American College of Emergency Physicians. 1994. "Policy Statement: Definition of Emergency Service." *Annals of Emergency Medicine* 23, no. 6:1397.

Brenner, B. E., and Simon, R. R. 1984. "The Specialty of Emergency Medicine." *Journal of Emergency Medicine* 1, no. 4:349–352.

Christakis, A. 1997. "Emergency Room Gatekeeping: A New Twist on Patient Dumping." *Wisconsin Law Review* 1997:295–320.

Commerce Clearinghouse, Inc. (CCH). 1997. *Medicare and Medicaid Guide*, P 13,960.22. 3:5841–43.

Hoffman, D. B. 1997. "Emergency Care and Managed Care—A Dangerous Combination." *Washington Law Review* 72:315–407.

Hurley, R. E.; Freund, D. A.; and Taylor, D. E. 1989. "Emergency Room Use and Primary Care Case Management: Evidence from Four Medicaid Demonstration Programs." *American Journal of Public Health* 79, no. 7:843–46.

Jordan, K. 1997. "Tort Liability for Managed Care: The Weakening of ERISA's Protective Shield." *The Journal of Law, Medicine and Ethics* 25, nos. 2–3:160–79.

Matthew, D. B. 1996. "Controlling the Reverse Agency Costs of Employment-Based Health Insurance: Of Markets, Courts, and a Regulatory Quagmire." *Wake Forest Law Review* 31:1037–73.

Peeno, L. 1998. "What Is the Value of a Voice?" *U.S. News & World Report* March 9, 1998: 40–46.

Steinbrook, R. 1996. "The Role of the Emergency Department." *New England Journal of Medicine* 334, no. 10:657–58.

Young, G. P.; Wagner, M. B.; Kellerman, A. L.; Ellis, J.; and Bouley, D. 1996. "Ambulatory Visits to Hospital Emergency Departments: Patterns and Reasons for Use: 24 Hours in the ED Study Group." *Journal of the American Medical Association* 276, no. 6:460–65.

3

Coverage of Investigational Interventions for Life-Threatening Conditions

CASE STUDY

Coverage for Simultaneous Kidney-Pancreas Transplants

In 1975, John Ryan, then a thirty-three-year-old supervisor in his state's Department of Revenue, was diagnosed with diabetes. For many years he successfully managed his disease with insulin injections. However, in November 1993, he initiated dialysis for kidney failure and, at the same time, agreed to be placed on a waiting list for a kidney transplant.

Based on discussions with his physician and his transplant surgeon, Mr. Ryan asked to become a candidate for a simultaneous kidney-pancreas transplant. His physicians believed that transplanting only a kidney would likely lead to recurrent failure of the new organ, since his original disease (insulin dependent diabetes mellitus, IDDM) would remain unchanged.

Mr. Ryan submitted a written request for a simultaneous kidney-pancreas transplant to his insurer in January 1994. The insurer denied the request, stating that it does not cover pancreas transplants because it considers them to be "investigational, and not a proven form of treatment." In the state's contract with Mr. Ryan's health plan, "investigational medical procedures" are defined as "those techniques or services that have been confined largely to laboratory and/or animal research or have progressed to limited human application and trials, but lack wide recognition as proven and effective measures in clinical medicine."

At the time of the denial, coverage for pancreas transplants in the state was inconsistent. A majority of insurance carriers and health plans provided coverage in some circumstances (most often for simultaneous kidney-pancreas transplants for patients with IDDM). On the other hand, Medicare and the state's Medicaid program did not cover pancreas transplants under any circumstances. When he resubmitted his request for coverage, Mr. Ryan cited this variation in coverage to support his contention that by not paying for the transplant, the health plan would be outside of mainstream medical opinion, out-of-date, and arbitrary. Furthermore, he claimed, such a decision would deny him generally accepted medical care that he could receive if he belonged to any number of other health plans.

The health plan again denied the request, this time citing a technology assessment of pancreas transplants completed the previous year by the plan's own Center for Technology Evaluation. The center was created in 1990 to develop practice guidelines and to conduct assessments of the safety and effectiveness of selected technologies. The center's assessments are conducted by small work groups whose members are selected for their expertise in the technology under study and who are typically drawn from the various primary and specialty medical departments in the health plan. The center itself does not make coverage decisions; however, the health plan noted that its Benefits Committee's decisions not to cover pancreas transplants were based largely on the center's assessment.

As additional support for denying Mr. Ryan's request again, the plan stated that it has an obligation to the employer (in this situation, the state) to uphold the contract for its entire term. In response, Mr. Ryan argued that the contract language itself should not impose a restriction on an enrollee to obtain medically necessary care if, as Mr. Ryan maintained happened here, the status of an intervention (such as simultaneous kidney-pancreas transplants) changes from investigational to therapeutic midway through the contract period.

For at least the past two decades, the state has offered its employees a choice of five health plans. Mr. Ryan has not changed his health care coverage during the past ten years. Each year, a few weeks before open enrollment, the state provides all employees a booklet with information and comparisons of the health plan (and other employee benefits) options available. This information does not indicate which health plan, if any, covers pancreas transplants. The employee learns whether he or she has coverage only after joining a plan and receiving its certificate of coverage.

Coverage for ABMT for Scleroderma

Lois Washington, a woman in her late forties, was diagnosed four years ago with scleroderma. There is no cure for scleroderma, an autoimmune disease affecting the skin and internal organs that eventually leads to death through organ failure (usually kidney or lung failure). Treatment with chemotherapeutic agents slows disease progression, but there is a 50 percent mortality rate within five years of diagnosis.

Ms. Washington was covered through an HMO that had a contractual arrangement with her clinic and physician. The HMO paid the clinic on a discounted fee-for-service basis. Thus, the HMO, not her physician, bore the full risk for the cost of Ms. Washington's care.

Since her diagnosis, Ms. Washington benefitted from all standard therapies available. However, standard treatments were no longer proving efficacious. Were there a promising therapy on the horizon, Ms. Washington's physician assured her, he would advocate on her behalf for her HMO to cover the experimental intervention. Since he knew of no promising intervention, however, the physician urged her to work with him on a care plan directed at her maximal function and comfort as the disease progressed.

Ms. Washington chose to travel to a distant cancer research center at her own expense to be evaluated for inclusion in an experimental trial. When she returned, she requested that her HMO cover her participation in the center's current research on scleroderma, which involves an autologous bone marrow transplant (ABMT). The cancer research center would not initiate the intervention unless the patient provided $75,000 up front.

The research center provided no data but sent a letter stating that some patients treated with allogeneic bone marrow transplants (that is, transplants of *donor* bone marrow rather than the patient's own bone marrow) for other conditions, who also happened to have scleroderma, experienced an improvement in their scleroderma. The center also sent three case reports on patients in Europe who had undergone ABMT for scleroderma within the previous six months, from which there was little data as yet. The research protocol was a pilot study to determine whether the intervention was safe enough to qualify for a phase I experimental study.

Because ABMT for scleroderma had not even entered the experimental phase, the HMO concluded that there was insufficient reason to believe it would offer Ms. Washington any therapeutic benefit and, therefore, that an exception to her coverage contract was unwarranted. The HMO's coverage denial was upheld by a second medical director review and the appeals committee of the HMO.

Ms. Washington's lawyer then served the HMO with a one-week notice to appear at a temporary injunction hearing, at which a judge would hear both sides of the coverage dispute and determine whether the HMO would be required to pay for the intervention desired by the patient. At the hearing, Ms. Washington's lawyer argued that ABMT for scleroderma was an "off-label" use of an accepted intervention and that the cost of treatment would equal only a few cents per HMO member per month. He implied that the HMO was making a self-serving, financially motivated decision and that the HMO had a duty to attempt to rescue patients in such dire need.

The HMO argued that the intervention fit its stated definition of experimental treatment (and therefore should not be covered under the terms of the plan), pointed out that the cancer research center admitted that the procedure had never been done in the United States on a human being, explained that the research center was pursuing only a pilot study to explore whether there was a sufficient rationale for a phase I study, and indicated that the cancer center's consent form clearly stated that the procedure was experimental and of unpredictable outcome. The HMO also noted that there appeared to be no balanced presentation of Ms. Washington's expected quality of life with or without the intervention.

The HMO argued further that covering experimental interventions like the one in question would eventually lead to unaffordable insurance costs, since it would require the pricing of health insurance products at levels most payers would be unwilling, if not unable, to bear. Further, the HMO reminded the court, it would be unfair to HMOs to require coverage for such interventions, whether by state court order or legislation, when the Employee Retirement Income Security Act (ERISA) protects self-insured payers from these additional burdens.

The patient's attorney exhorted the judge, "The patient's life is in your hands." The attorney emphasized the patient's 50 percent chance of death within five years if treatment was not pursued. The judge ruled that if an "off-label" use of an approved procedure was at issue, and a reputable cancer research center has said the patient needs that procedure, then the patient should have it. The judge ordered the HMO to pay the cost of the procedure.

Questions for Consideration

➤ Should Mr. Ryan's health plan add simultaneous kidney-pancreas transplants to its covered services? Should Ms. Washington's health plan cover ABMT for scleroderma? Why?

➤ When, if ever, should HMOs make compassionate exceptions to clearly stated and clearly applicable benefit exclusions? When is an exception to a benefit exclusion fair or unfair to the other members of an HMO?

➤ What obligations, if any, does Mr. Ryan have to choose the plan most appropriate to his long-term condition?

➤ What concerns, if any, are raised by the variation in coverage for pancreas transplants across health plans?

➤ Who should make coverage decisions for emerging technologies and procedures? What criteria should be used? What process should be followed?

➤ What information regarding coverage should health plans provide to enrollees and potential enrollees?

COMMENTARY _____

William T. McGivney, Ph.D.

Denials by health plans of requests for the coverage of investigational technologies for patients have generated contentious debate, public criticism, and adverse legal judgments for such plans. They also have created consternation, anger, and, in some cases, significant hardship for patients and their families. All of this has been sparked by the implementation of a stipulation, the investigational exclusion, that has been present in health plan language for decades.

In the past, indemnity health insurance plans did not invoke the investigational exclusion to nearly the degree that managed care plans have recently. Indemnity plans were not charged with nor did they assert that they would be specifically "managing" the care of members. Rather, the administrative role of indemnity plans was mainly to serve as a financing mechanism (for example, claims payer) and as a network builder for the employers that used them as a vendor.

Indemnity plans were indeed charged with carrying out the terms of the payer-employer contractual agreement. However, when they did interpret and apply the term "investigational," they focused generally on whether the technology was "widely accepted" by practicing physicians or whether or not it was a "standard of practice." Plans usually made this determination by relying on the existence or absence of a CPT code (a code assigned by a committee of the American Medical Association for reimbursement purposes). This left the matter squarely in the hands of the practicing medical community, which determined when a technology should receive a CPT code.

With the advent of the managed care movement in the mid- to late 1980s, health care companies began to move aggressively to control the costs of health care for large employers which were very concerned about the steep rise in such costs. Since the use of medical technology was the factor at once most responsible for, and most controllable with respect to the rate of rise of health care expenditures, managed care companies focused especially on controlling the use of health care technologies. "Utilization management" became a major department of all managed care companies. Those programs implemented requirements that long lists of existing technologies with significant variations in use and new expensive technologies be preapproved as covered before the particular technology or service was rendered to the patient. With these requirements, hospitals, physicians, and other providers were subject to the coverage criteria and processes for decision making put in place by the plans.

Most significantly, the contractual definition of "investigational" shifted from one based on physician opinion or acceptance to one based on the availability of clinical outcomes data. Most often physician opinions of the safety and effectiveness of established technologies were not based on data from formal studies, as such data did not exist. Managed care plans increasingly assumed responsibility for making such determinations and set up formal technology-assessment programs that evaluated the available scientific evidence about the safety and effectiveness of a particular technology for a specified clinical indication. Based on these evaluations, the plan then defined the technology either as investigational (not covered) or established (covered).

Tenets of Decision Making in Beneficent, Well-Managed Plans

The technology-assessment processes of managed care companies are founded on the need to orient medical decision making more to outcome-based determinations. Indeed, a major contribution of the managed care industry to the health care system has been to promote and sometimes force outcome-based decision making; that is, decisions based on scientific results and not just opinion, no matter how expert. In a beneficent, well-managed health plan, the technology-assessment process and the coverage policy-setting process should proceed from seven basic tenets:

1. The managed care plan supports the technological imperative of medicine but seeks to avoid technological Armageddon.
2. Whether one is patient, physician, or payer, one wants proof that the intervention one is about to undergo, prescribe, or pay for is proven safe and effective.
3. The coverage decision-making process must be consistent with the binding contractual language, and the language used in the communication of a decision must be consistent with both the contractual language and the decision-making process.
4. Clinical decision making and coverage decision making constitute risk-benefit analyses; that is, the more severe and life-threatening the disease or condition, the less the degree of certitude about effectiveness and the greater the risk of harm that patient, physician, and payer should be willing to accept.
5. The proponent of the technology has the primary responsibility for the development of clinical data to support the use of that technology. As the entity that requires data to support an affirmative coverage decision, the payer should support the patient care costs of well-designed clinical trials that aim to develop such data.

6. Those in responsible decision-making positions should use processes and make decisions that they feel would be appropriate for themselves or their loved ones.

7. In close calls, always favor the position of the patient.

Simultaneous Kidney-Pancreas Transplant

The case of John Ryan illustrates violation of tenet number 3. The failure of health plans to ensure basic consistency and communication across people and processes to those who develop the contractual language, to those who evaluate technologies and set coverage policy, and to those who communicate decisions to beneficiaries is the most common deficiency in decision making in health plans.

In the present case, the plan denies Mr. Ryan's request initially on the basis that pancreas transplants are "investigational, and not a proven form of treatment." The contractual definition of the term "investigational" does not support the language the denial relies on. The definition stipulates "investigational" as "those techniques or services that have been confined largely to laboratory and/or animal research or have progressed to limited human application and trials, but lack wide recognition as proven and effective measures in clinical medicine." According to this definition, a denial might be appropriate in three areas:

1. if the procedure has basically been or is primarily being studied in animal models;

2. if the procedure has limited human application or is confined to limited, early human trials; or

3. if there is no group or body that recognizes it as proven and effective.

Number 3 is the major point of contention in that this segment of contractual language has ceded authority for recognizing a particular technology as investigational to bodies outside the health plan. The general nature of the contractual statement permits a wide range of groups to be considered, including the practicing medical community, the transplant community, or just those who perform simultaneous kidney-pancreas transplants. Another potential source of recognition could come from payers themselves. That a majority of plans and carriers in the state provide coverage for pancreas transplants constitutes recognition by a very conservative group that simultaneous kidney-pancreas transplants are indeed recognized as "proven and effective." Two other minor points are worth noting: (1) if the denial specified only pancreas transplant, it would have referred to the wrong procedure; and (2) the second area for denial is somewhat unclear in using a positive term, "progressed," in a negative context.

The fact that upon appeal the health plan consults its own technology-assessment process is also irrelevant. The contract contains no stipulations according to which the plan would make its own determination of what the scientific data says. Such an outcome- and data-based evaluative process is not explicitly supported by the contractual language.

The contractual language of this plan dictates that the plan's policies reflect current thinking on simultaneous kidney-pancreas transplant and other technologies. Unless there were a specific exclusion for simultaneous kidney-pancreas transplants, the plan's obligation to the employer to uphold the contract for its duration entails keeping up with changes in the "recognition" of this type of transplant as "proven and effective." Thus, Mr. Ryan is correct in arguing that the consideration of the status and the setting of coverage policy for a medical technology must be ongoing.

Finally, plan information for members, detailing coverage contractual language and explaining the processes used to determine coverage and coverage policies for specific technologies, is notoriously deficient. The fact that such material has been presented to members and that members have reviewed it clearly does not constitute an informed decision by a member to forgo coverage of certain types—including transplants.

ABMT for Scleroderma

The case of Lois Washington exemplifies the true extreme of decision making in a managed care plan. The recommendation is an expensive, investigational therapy for a life-threatening disease for which there is no effective treatment. Furthermore, the treatment—ABMT—has never been provided in the United States and has only been provided to three patients in Europe, with little data available. The treatment is being offered to Ms. Washington within the context of a "pilot study" to determine if the procedure is safe enough to justify a phase I study. Unpublished case reports apparently are available that indicate some improvement in patients' scleroderma when they were treated with allogeneic bone marrow transplant for some unnamed primary condition.

The health plan appears to have been faithful to the basic tenets of plan decision making mentioned previously, which are process-oriented, outcome- and data-based, flexible, and humanistic. The judge, for his or her part, has decided that a "liberal" interpretation of the plan's coverage contractual language is appropriate in this case of a woman in her forties afflicted with a life-threatening illness. The liberal interpretation, resulting in an order to pay, reflects the judge's application of the prevailing societal sentiment that dying patients should receive any treatment that has any theoretical potential to be beneficial. In rendering this decision, the judge has invoked another insurance contract definition, "medical necessity," by calling on the health plan to pay for a technology that the patient "needs."

While the case does not provide the specific contractual definition of "medical necessity," the application of this concept by the judge illustrates an important distinction in plan language and decision making that goes to the heart of decisions about payment for the use of investigational technologies in life-threatening illness. The investigational exclusion relates to the establishment of global policies about whether technologies will be paid for when requested for certain diseases or conditions. The definition and application of medical necessity gets down to the individual patient level. In the present situation, the decision maker (for example, the judge) focuses not on the general coverage policy (for example, investigational versus established) that applies to all plan members. Rather, the judge focuses on how the individual patient with specific clinical needs can be best treated at the particular point in time. At this level of decision making for a dying patient, contractual language regarding the definition of investigational becomes just so much vaporous verbiage to most judges. These judges are holding the plan accountable to indicate how it has assessed the situation and needs of the member as a patient and whether it has carried out that assessment in an unbiased way.

For health plans, the solution is simple and straightforward when one pursues a decision making process that is moral and that is true to the sixth and seventh tenets as stated previously. William McGivney and Grace Powers Monaco established a process for a major national health plan in September of 1991, at the height of the high-dose chemotherapy/bone marrow transplant controversy (McGivney 1994). The process they outlined—known as the McGivney and Monaco process—was the model for California legislation (Friedman-Knowles Experimental Treatment Act of 1996) mandating an external review process when patients appeal the denial of the use of investigational technologies in "fatal" illnesses. The California bill then formed the basis for legislation passed in Texas and Ohio; it is being considered in other states as well.

The McGivney and Monaco process was more progressive and liberal than that mandated by the legislation that followed it. In this process, no request to the health plan for coverage for bone marrow transplantation could be denied without having gone through an external review process at the outset. Briefly, the health plan asked a nationally known patient advocate, Grace Powers Monaco, to gather a panel of leading oncologists to review difficult cases. In each case, the patient advocate picked three reviewers to look at the documentation submitted by the attending physician. The health plan had nothing to do or say about either who was on the panel or which experts were chosen to review individual cases.

The review panel asked two questions. First, were the proposed treatments "promising"? This was to make the process consistent with the concept of "promising" that the plan had introduced into its contractual language to bridge the large gap between "investigational" and "established" and to allow payment for promising, yet investigational, technologies. The second pivotal question was "is the present treatment likely to be effective for the patient whose records you have sitting in front of you?" The reviewer had to define what he or she thought was the appropriate definition of "effective." If one of the three reviewers indicated that, "Yes, the treatment was likely to be effective," the health plan paid for it.

This model process responded to the needs of all parties. The decisions were clinically and legally defensible because the process used unbiased experts whose sole interest was the direction of appropriate treatment. The process was purposely biased toward decisions favoring the position of the patient, as a minority view of one oncologist would result in payment.

The process was not "rocket science." The decision-making process was simple, straightforward, and made sense to all parties. It was fair, and all involved were comfortable with the process being applied in their individual cases. Most importantly, it was a moral process in that it sought to do what was right. This model process is one that could and should have been applied in the Washington case.

References

Friedman-Knowles Experimental Treatment Act of 1996, chapter 979, section 1370.4 California Public Health and Safety Code and division 2, part 2, chapter 1, article 2.5, section 10145.3 California Insurance Code.

McGivney, W. T. 1994. "Autologous Bone Marrow Transplantation: A Microcosm of the U.S. Health Care System." In *Adopting New Medical Technology*, pp. 109–16. Edited by A. C. Gelijns and H. V. Dawkins. Washington, D.C.: National Academy Press.

COMMENTARY _____

Gwen Wagstrom Halaas, M.D., M.B.A.

The cases of John Ryan and Lois Washington raise especially challenging issues in health care because they involve an individual's request for rescue from a devastating disease, very complex scientific information, and little clarity on costs and benefits. These are the cases that end up on the front page of the newspaper or in a court of law.

Simultaneous kidney-pancreas transplants and ABMT for scleroderma are interventions that are done in research centers with ongoing clinical investigation. Among the solid organ transplants, pancreas transplants are newer. Bone marrow transplantation has been done primarily for cancer and disease of the bone marrow. As transplantation techniques improve, physicians may recommend transplantation of other organs and for a wider range of conditions. While both solid organ transplantation and bone marrow transplantation have been done for decades, health plans cover them only for certain conditions.

There are two types of coverage decisions. Most coverage decisions are guided by coverage policies that apply to all health plan enrollees and define what interventions the health plan will or will not pay for. These policies are developed by medical staff at the health plan and are based on scientific evidence; they often include specific criteria for coverage. The policies guide clinics and physicians in providing referrals and in directing some requests to the health plan for a coverage decision on behalf of an individual patient—the second type of coverage decision. Certain case-specific requests require prior authorization from the health plan because they are experimental, complex, or require referral to a center of excellence for treatment and case management. The authorization for coverage is given by the plan's medical director, based on scientific evidence of the intervention's safety and effectiveness, and guided by the plan's benefits contract language.

Many insurers have contract language that specifically excludes experimental interventions from coverage. The contract usually includes the plan's definition of experimental, a definition that differs among insurers. As in these two cases, the issue is whether the intervention in question meets the contractual definition of experimental and, even if it does, whether a reasonable case can be made for granting coverage as an exception.

Contracts are legally binding documents between health plans and purchasers that direct the business of paying for health care. Purchasers of health care coverage and regulators expect health plans to base their coverage decisions on that contract language. Making coverage decisions that reflect contract language depends on fair and consistent application of the language. The term "experimental" needs detailed clarification. The U.S. Food and Drug Administration (FDA) distinguishes between different phases of trials of drugs and medical devices; cancer researchers base distinctions between phases on evidence of safety and efficacy. There is no consistent staging, however, to help determine when a new intervention should no longer be considered experimental but deemed safe and reasonably effective for coverage. If health plans continue to deny coverage for experimental interventions, there needs to be a universally accepted definition of experimental, with criteria that determine when coverage is appropriate. An alternative would be for health plans to clearly specify the level of experimental care covered in each of their contracts and the price of that coverage. Employers or individuals can then choose to pay for a specific level of coverage.

Coverage Exceptions in These Two Cases

In Mr. Ryan's case, the plan denied his request for a simultaneous kidney-pancreas transplant as investigational, defined in the contract as "those techniques or services that have been confined largely to laboratory and/or animal research or have progressed to limited human application and trials, but lack wide recognition as proven and effective measures in clinical medicine." Who should define "limited application," "wide recognition," and "proven and effective?" In this case, the decision was based on the findings of the health plan's own Center for Technology Evaluation. This is reasonable if the group evaluating the intervention is representative of experts in the field and if the findings are based on current peer-reviewed medical literature. Variations in coverage by other local health plans, however, support Mr. Ryan's argument that the transplant is no longer experimental. This is a situation where the most current evidence available on the outcomes of simultaneous kidney-pancreas transplant is critical to making a fair decision.

Is an exception appropriate in Mr. Ryan's case? To answer this question, the medical director must be certain that all pertinent clinical information about Mr. Ryan is known and considered and that the current evidence available on the safety and effectiveness of the transplant is thoroughly reviewed. There is no specific clinical or other situation indicated that sets Mr. Ryan apart from others who have requested this type of transplant. The one source of controversy appears to be the variability in coverage within the community. To support its denial of coverage, the health plan cites the technology-assessment report but does not specify the findings that lead to that decision. If the technology-assessment report used by Mr. Ryan's health plan was not current, and a review of the current literature suggests the intervention is more promising, then it is likely that an exception should be made and the policy revised. The argument about honoring the employer's contract does not preclude making an exception (unless this is a self-insured product, in which case the employer, not the plan's medical director, is the only one allowed to grant exceptions).

Exceptions to benefits should be made by a medical director or other designated staff of a health plan under the supervision of the medical director. Medical directors are physicians with practice experience as well as experience and/or education in the business of providing health care services to a population. These medical directors are supported by nurses, lawyers, and others who can provide the necessary information to support these complex decisions. Decisions are made based on the scientific evidence available, within the limits of the contract language, and within an appropriate time frame.

Reasons for making exceptions include a unique individual clinical situation that is compelling, new evidence about the procedure in question, or a perceived better use of resources than the standard covered procedure. For example, an individual at significantly increased risk from surgery might be granted coverage as an exception for a new intervention that has proven safe and has some evidence of effectiveness rather than the standard covered surgical treatment. These decisions are made as exceptions only for that specific situation or clinical condition until the contract language is changed.

Exceptions are intended to give the medical director some flexibility in the face of the unique aspects of an individual case. However, once the exception to cover is made, that decision sets a precedent; any request for coverage of that benefit for another individual with the same circumstances should be covered in the future. For example, making an exception for Mr. Ryan would require revision of the policy to cover any similar request for a simultaneous kidney-pancreas transplant in diabetics with renal failure. Arbitrary or inconsistent exceptions raise legal and ethical concerns. To make exceptions based purely on the persistence of the patient or the intervention of others on behalf of the patient is not fair to the others insured by the plan. From a population perspective, paying for exceptions to benefits that results in a lack of funds to pay for covered benefits is also unfair. If, for example, the decision were to pay for simultaneous kidney-pancreas transplants, and this resulted in insufficient funds to pay for routine care for diabetes or for dialysis for kidney failure, then a few would benefit at the expense of many. Some health plans have written guidelines for making exceptions, which include reasons such as those described, that help medical directors be consistent and equitable and help document the reasons for making the exception.

In selecting a health plan to offer to employees, the premium cost is of great importance to the employer, but offering health care coverage that is comparable within the community is also important for attracting and retaining employees. New devices, new procedures, or new medications often cannot be anticipated or clarified in detail in a contract or in materials that inform employers and employees. However, the health plan and employer have an obligation to inform employees and members of the details of coverage in an understandable and inclusive manner. How much information should be provided to potential health plan members before their employer has selected a health plan as an option is still uncertain. Once an employer selects the health plan options, it must provide convenient ways for employees to be familiar with the basic information of what is covered and how health care services should be accessed. In turn, individual employees such as Mr. Ryan are obligated to review the options for coverage with their employer and to select the health plan that best meets their individual or family's current and anticipated needs. It is difficult to review completely all details of a health plan contract, however, and there are always unknown factors that affect health status in the future.

What about the case of Ms. Washington? Clearly, ABMT for scleroderma is much more experimental than simultaneous kidney-pancreas transplants, having been done on only three human beings, and none in the United States. ABMT for scleroderma was described as a pilot study to determine whether the treatment was safe enough to even qualify for a phase I trial. This is about as experimental as it gets, and the mortality risk of five to ten percent is not insignificant. Although scleroderma is a miserable disease, a 50 percent risk of dying in five years must be weighed against the risks of the proposed intervention, which are unknown. Understanding the real effectiveness of this intervention is going to take years; studies will need to include enough treated patients over a long enough period of time to determine whether ABMT offers any benefit over currently available treatments.

Although we do not have the contract language for this HMO, it is quite clear that this procedure was being done in a research setting under a specific protocol intended to determine the safety of the procedure. Thus, the health plan's denial was clearly based on the experimental nature of this intervention. The remaining question is whether an exception is appropriate. The typical reasons for making an exception to benefits are not met in this case. There is no available evidence to support the effectiveness or cost-effectiveness of ABMT for scleroderma. There is no unique clinical situation with Ms. Washington, although scleroderma is a compelling disease with no known successful treatment.

The Rule of Rescue and Justice

The problem with saying no to Ms. Washington is that American patients, families, and physicians do not accept defeat easily, and disease is seen as an enemy that demands full-scale warfare—without regard to cost or risk. Are the chronically ill or dying a vulnerable population for whom denial of coverage of any treatment would be morally unfair? Today in America, the rule of rescue appears to be the trump card that overcomes any contract language or process intended to guide decisions by evidence of safety or effectiveness. If society supports the rule of rescue as foremost in coverage decisions, then health insurance contracts must change to reflect that belief, and the price of providing rescue must be included in the premiums. If not, then guidelines need to be created to help make decisions that are fair to all the insured members, while maximizing the opportunity to receive the treatment resulting in the best outcome that is affordable for all.

Should a health plan cover all rescue treatments? Or should a health plan establish a threshold level of safety and efficacy before new procedures are covered? In Ms. Washington's case, the temptation is to invoke the ethical principle of nonmaleficence: First, do no harm. From the individual perspective, there is clear harm that can be the direct result of this intervention—and unknown benefit. From the population perspective, coverage of this clearly experimental intervention may cause harm to other enrollees in the health plan because without carefully crafted criteria, covering this particular intervention would set a precedent for coverage of other equally experimental interventions that may involve significant risk and unknown benefit.

Covering the high cost of this particular intervention and others in the future may limit resources available for other needs. Although resource allocation is currently not explicit, the cost of high-technology rescue interventions is a significant factor in the decision not to invest in maximizing preventive services or not to cover things such as the nicotine patch to aid in stopping smoking. Also, if the cost of these experimental interventions results in increased premiums, access to health care coverage might be reduced as small employers choose to drop unaffordable options.

What about justice? Is Ms. Washington being treated fairly? She has received all the interventions recommended by her physician. Eventually, those interventions were no longer helpful, and her physician knew of no other promising options. Perhaps her physician was aware of the ABMT research but had significant concerns about safety and real doubts about any benefit. Note that the health plan did not deny Ms. Washington access to the research, it only refused to pay for it. Its denial of payment was based on the experimental nature of the intervention, which is quite clear in this case.

Funding Research

Who should pay for research? Much of the ongoing clinical investigation of drugs and new procedures is covered by health plans. It often takes years to clearly understand the appropriate dose or combination of drugs or the appropriate candidates for new surgical procedures. Who should pay for research at an earlier stage—on the first individuals, before safety and effectiveness are even established? In most instances, these studies are funded by grants from organizations supporting research or by the companies involved in the development of drugs or devices. Some are funded by the institutions that employ the physicians doing the research. All of those funding sources are facing tighter budgets, as are health plans. Is it appropriate for researchers to demand $75,000 from the first individual with scleroderma who will receive this procedure in the United States, when the safety and efficacy of this procedure for this condition are still unknown?

What is fair for all the other members of the health plan, whose premiums contribute to the pool the plan uses to pay members' health care services? For instance, would it be fair for a health plan to provide access at no cost to a member to a procedure with no known benefit but with a known mortality risk or with other unknown risks? Since there are no explicit societal norms, health plans have developed processes to make decisions based on specific contract language. When the contract language is not clear and there is no known scientific evidence, but the situation is compelling, as for Ms. Washington, the health plan may ultimately respond to public pressure or the threat of going to court or being mandated by state legislatures.

Is it fair to the members of a health plan to pay for research because it is the only option that holds some small possibility of rescue, or because it is required by a judge or mandated by the legislature? Fairness in this situation can be determined only on the basis of an understanding of the potential benefit, the potential cost, and the total resources available to meet the costs of essential health care for all members in the health plan, including appropriate preventive services. A clearer social mandate about investing resources at the end of life, or for futile care, would be helpful. Also, health plans would benefit from a clear and consistent set of ethical principles to guide coverage decisions that are then considered by the courts and legislatures.

Conclusion

Discussions about nonmaleficence, justice, cost-effectiveness, and the role of scientific evidence in coverage decisions must occur among all stakeholders apart from individual cases. These discussions must include the population perspective typically left out by researchers, providers, and the public. Insurers have considered the population perspective for actuarial purposes in insuring against the costs of illness but not for investing in wellness and determining the value of certain health care services in maximizing health. The high investment in medical care and poor showing in health statistics in the United States make it imperative for health plans to consider cost-effectiveness and the population perspective. Although aspects of this problem are unique to the United States, it is also a global problem, resulting from rapidly improving technology in the diagnosis and treatment of disease and broader access to health care services within populations.

There will never be a right answer for all of these decisions. Clearly, however, the decision making process must be improved. Decisions must be based on scientific evidence that is readily available, with data on effectiveness and outcomes. There must be useful cost-benefit or cost-effectiveness analysis to allow reasoned comparison of available treatment options. Research scientists and prescribing physicians must be actively involved in the decision making process. Members and patients must be better informed about the process and about what the evidence shows. Purchasers and members must understand what is and what is not covered in their insurance plan. There must be an understanding of value for the purchase price and of available options for members and families in different circumstances.

Difficult decisions for individuals struggling with devastating illness will always remain. Those decisions can be made easier with clear information that is understood by all. When informed discussions occur on a regular basis, when contract language is clarified and read by those who are affected by it, and when researchers, physicians, payers, and the public can collaborate on important issues in health, then the debate will turn from the individual's desperate plight to successful outcomes and improved health.

| 4

Coverage of Complementary Health Care

CASE STUDY _____

Ultra Health System, a nonprofit health care delivery system located on the West Coast, has recently opened a for-profit complementary health care clinic. Ultra Health System's new clinic, AltCare, offers services and products ranging from acupuncture, massage, yoga, chiropractic care, and pedicures to nutritional supplements, herbalist consultations, aromatherapy, and upscale personal care products. AltCare advertises to the public and publishes a fee schedule for the services it offers.

A growing number of health plans have begun to offer insurance products that include coverage for complementary health care, and Ultra Health has sold several such service contracts to health plans. AltCare receives a large proportion of its clients on referral from both primary care physicians and specialists from contracted health plans, in addition to its sizable private pay contingent. Clients who lack a referral to AltCare pay the full fee for service out-of-pocket.

Ultra Health is a delivery system engaged in direct contracting, a unique form of managed care based on the principle of careful care management directed by the physician rather than by a health insurance carrier or plan. Ultra Health's approach to managing care and containing costs is based on the use of care delivery teams schooled in clinical care pathways. In direct contracting, a self-insured employer or the government contracts directly with a delivery system to provide a defined health care benefits package for an enrollee for an agreed-upon price. Ultra Health receives payment on a fee-for-service basis for each health care service it provides. Its direct contracting agreement includes a risk-adjusted target budget for the covered population. If costs exceed the budget target for a given quarter, Ultra Health is penalized by receiving lower fees for service in the following quarter. Thus, it is in the interest of Ultra Health to control costs and "hit the target."

Although AltCare is directed by a physician who is skilled in both Western and complementary approaches to healing, the addition of AltCare has been a source of deep discontent among the majority of physicians employed by Ultra Health. Their view is that Ultra Health should not attach its name to AltCare, thereby endorsing the services offered, since the empirical support for the use of these services does not meet Western standards. They object that AltCare seems to have no ethic for determining what therapies should and should not be offered through AltCare. What sells, rather than what evidence says works, seems to them to be AltCare's principle of selection. A smaller group of physicians associated with Ultra Health remains open to some of the complementary modalities.

Ultra Health is located in an area with a large east Asian population. Mr. Chow, a patient suffering from chronic and now severe lower back pain, is experiencing serious disability. He is employed by one of the businesses in the direct contracting consortium and chose the direct contracting option from among his coverage choices because it allowed him to self-refer within Ultra Health. Mr. Chow, an immigrant, appreciates his open access to caregivers because it has enabled him to find physicians who treat him with respect, support his use of Chinese medicine, and—given his difficulties with English and the cultural challenges of Western health care—go the extra mile to help him understand his condition and his options.

For a number of years, Mr. Chow has been a patient of Dr. Young, an orthopedic specialist in the Ultra Health network. Dr. Young belongs to several health plan networks in the area and is involved in a number of reimbursement arrangements. Several years ago, Dr. Young convinced Mr. Chow to undergo a CAT scan and a myelogram, which enabled Dr. Young to diagnose degenerative disc disease. Although Mr. Chow felt these diagnostic techniques, particularly the myelogram, to be very painful with no observable return, he has followed Dr. Young's advice and worked diligently with physical therapists and the exercise regimens they have recommended. Until recently, this effectively managed Mr. Chow's pain. Dr. Young then decided that Mr. Chow needed a more aggressive approach to healing that would involve, first, spinal injections of cortisone and, if necessary, a surgical spinal fusion.

Mr. Chow opposed Dr. Young's recommendations. He recalled the painful, unproductive injections he endured during his myelogram and he feared any cutting of his body. He told Dr. Young that a relative had received lots of help from acupuncture for a back problem and that he preferred to try this method.

Dr. Young agreed to refer Mr. Chow to AltCare's acupuncturist and, as he had with a previous patient, consulted with the medical director of AltCare to ensure good communication between them as Mr. Chow's treatment proceeded. He discovered that although AltCare was Ultra Health-owned, Ultra Health's direct contract with Mr. Chow's employer covered no services at AltCare. Ultra Health's own physicians and clinics had pressured Ultra Health to not enter into direct contracting agreements that provide AltCare coverage for patients receiving primary care through Ultra Health's clinics. This was the only way those Ultra Health physicians who opposed the system's creation of AltCare felt they could discourage their patients who can self-refer from using AltCare. Dr. Young realized, then, that while other patients he referred to AltCare had coverage for these services, Mr. Chow could only access AltCare on a private pay basis. For Mr. Chow, whose income was just sufficient to meet the needs of his large family, paying AltCare out-of-pocket was an insurmountable hurdle to accessing acupuncture treatment.

Questions for Consideration

➤ What criteria should be used when deciding whether to offer coverage for complementary health care?

➤ How, if at all, should coverage policy regarding complementary health care differ from coverage policy for other interventions?

➤ Under what conditions should professional and/or ethical objections affect whether a delivery system offers complementary health care and whether such services are covered?

➤ Should Dr. Young appeal Ultra Health's refusal to cover acupuncture for Mr. Chow? If so, what arguments should he bring to the appeal process?

➤ What obligations does Ultra Health have to networked physicians and patients, such as Mr. Chow, who can self-refer?

➤ What ethical issues are raised when a nonprofit health care system develops a for-profit complementary health care clinic?

COMMENTARY

Daniel O. Dugan, Ph.D.

Mr. Chow's low back pain is getting worse, and for good reason. He has degenerative disc disease. Dr. Young believes that Mr. Chow's decision to try acupuncture treatments as an alternative to spinal injections and surgery is both medically appropriate and consonant with Mr. Chow's self-defining spiritual values. Dr. Young also believes that Mr. Chow's acupuncture treatments should be covered by his health insurance plan. Dr. Young's professional ethical standards encourage him to honor his patient's rights—including information about reasonable alternatives to high-risk, questionable outcome procedures—and to advocate for the best interests of his patient (American Medical Association 1995). Dr. Young should be particularly energetic in his advocacy in this managed care environment, in which political and economic agendas have created a conflict between his patient's interests and those of the Ultra Health System physician group and delivery system.

Beyond the ethical issues in the individual patient-physician relationship are larger organizational ethical concerns, including (1) the responsibilities of corporate executives in arranging health care insurance for their employees, (2) the rationale and fairness (consistency) of the Ultra Health physician group's insistence that access to AltCare services not be included in the direct contract arrangement with Mr. Chow's employer, and (3) Ultra Health's responsibilities to its members, patients, primary care physicians, customers, and community.

Corporate Responsibilities

Most Americans obtain health care services through insurance plans provided by their employers. Most employers offering insurance offer only one plan, chosen on the basis of cost savings. More than 75 percent of employees who have employer-arranged health insurance—along with rapidly increasing numbers of Medicare and Medicaid enrollees—receive health care services through one of one thousand HMOs and other kinds of managed care organizations. By providing more than one reputable health care insurance option to its employees, Mr. Young's employer demonstrates a laudable ethical commitment to employee choice and well-being.

A corporate framework for negotiating managed care contracts that identifies employers' ethical commitments to employee and community well-being should also include provisions requiring managed care organizations to develop consistent standards for measuring the quality of their services, "report cards" showing performance data compared to other area health plans in detailed and under-standable terms, and formal ethics standards protective of patients' rights and welfare (Biblo et al. 1995).

Still, most employees need more assistance than they receive from companies and insurance plans to understand the plan provisions and rules used to decide covered benefits. They also need copies of the entire contract, counseling assistance in selecting a plan, and interpreters' assistance when necessary. Further, when they become patients, they need the help of independent advocates to assist them in using the insurance plan's mechanisms for resolving complaints and appeals regarding denials of reimbursement for services (Annas 1998).

Mr. Chow's company draws its labor force from a community with a large Asian population, many of whom have limited understanding of English. Mr. Chow's unpleasant discovery, as a distressed and therefore vulnerable patient at a time of need, that his choice (to eschew powerful drugs and major surgery and seek palliation and rehabilitation through a trial of acupuncture) is not a covered option in the plan he selected is a common experience. This corporation should demonstrate respect for the cultural values of the large Asian population by advocating specifically, in its contracting for health care services, for access to acupuncture and other non-Western therapies that are well known within Asian communities to be effective. This form of corporate advocacy might be particularly effective with Ultra Health. AltCare already owns and provides acupuncture by a qualified and state-licensed practitioner.

Such advocacy also makes sense economically. Mr. Chow is strongly motivated to try to manage his pain so as to maintain a normal level of functioning. Short-term, noninvasive, effective approaches to chronic problems like Mr. Chow's promise to benefit his employers by minimizing lost productivity time.

Health Delivery Systems' Responsibilities in Direct Contracting Arrangements

Administrators and physicians in horizontally integrated provider-hospital systems like Ultra Health have now had more than twenty-five years' experience with HMOs and have learned about cost-saving strategies such as gatekeeping, prospective and retrospective payment denials, concurrent utilization review, case management, capitation arrangements, risk-sharing, and outcome-based care pathways. Increasingly, they are eliminating HMO plans and contracting directly with employers (Beckham 1997).

Direct contracting arrangements arguably benefit providers and self-insured employers alike. They promise to encourage competition, allowing smaller employers and smaller provider groups to compete. They may also increase the range of consumer choices by providing more information about available options in the health care marketplace to employees, thereby pressuring providers to be more accountable for cost and quality.

Of particular ethical concern in Ultra Health's direct contracting arrangement is that, while physicians had more influence at the policy level on defining covered benefits for *plan members* than usual in HMOs, *patients* and their physician-advocates at the clinical level are less audible and influential. In HMO plans, patients and physicians together contend with plan administrators. In direct contract plans, patients contend with plan administrators—now possibly including their own physicians. Conscientious primary care physicians like Dr. Young may therefore face the same barriers in direct contracting arrangements in seeking effective and beneficial treatments for their patients as they do in conventional HMOs.

Dr. Young's effectiveness in advocating for Mr. Chow in this case will depend, in large part, on the ethical infrastructure of the Ultra Health plan. Apparently Mr. Chow's employer has ratified the contract with Ultra Health that excluded acupuncture as a covered option.

The contract between the Ultra Health plan and Mr. Chow is an arms-length business relationship. The plan is obliged to abide only with the terms of the contract. When plan members become patients, however, the fiduciary duties of health care providers to their patients move to the forefront.

At this point Dr. Young should present the case to the hospital's ethics committee and seek its support of Mr. Chow's rights, a health plan member who is now a patient in need. Mr. Chow deserves timely access to an external appeals mechanism, independent of the health plan, to address this denial of a medically recommended alternative to a more expensive conventional treatment approach that does not work for many patients, and that offers greater risks and burdens than benefits to the patient.

Mr. Chow should have received counseling and education in his own language regarding the provisions of the plan for covered benefits and the procedures for timely resolution of complaints and denials in an impartial forum. If he did not, Dr. Young's appeal has strong ethical merit. It is even stronger if Mr. Chow was not informed upon enrollment of provisions encouraging his physician to limit or restrict treatments and/or recommendations of medical specialists' services.

Short of national health care reform, federal legislation is probably necessary to define and protect the rights of patients in the patient-physician relationship, as well as the rights of health plan members to information, counseling, and fair processes of dispute resolution. Such protections are needed to provide the context in which physicians like Dr. Young can advocate more effectively for their patients (Annas 1998).

Criteria for Coverage of Complementary Health Care Therapies: Process and Selection Principles

PROCESS

Dr. Young's advocacy in this case goes beyond the argument that the plan has been unfair to his patient by virtue of its failure to provide education, counseling, and assistance with appeals. He also challenges the stated rationale of the plan's denial of acupuncture as a covered benefit. Ultra Health sells its complementary therapy services in the marketplace, on a fee-for-service basis. Moreover, Ultra Health includes AltCare services in some of its other managed care contracts. This inconsistency is unfair. Its tolerance by the Ultra Health medical group suggests that lack of empirical evidence of benefit of AltCAre services is not the real reason for this inconsistency. If the reason is that the Ultra Health physician group wants more control of the flow of patient referrals, the real agenda is power, that is, politics, not patient-centered care.

How should plans like Ultra Health's make decisions regarding covered benefits? One principle is that the process ought to be open, not hidden from the scrutiny of the public. Physicians who take care of patients should actively participate in developing policy decisions, practice guidelines, and clinical pathways. Policies should be explicit, clearly stated, and understandable (Perkel 1996). Patients and the community, as recipients and beneficiaries of health care services, ought to be involved. The preferences and values of those persons whom the rationing decisions will most directly affect should be identified and articulated through town meetings (American Medical Association 1995).

A process reflective of a moral concern for community needs and values will "consider cultural and spiritual population differences" in determining the meaning of quality health care services. "These differences include health-related beliefs and values, disease incidence and prevalence, as well as treatment efficacy" (Bruton 1996). Clinicians know the importance of respecting patients' and families' culturally based requests regarding treatment decisions and information sharing in the acute care context. These values, particularly in communities with large ethnic and/or immigrant populations, are equally important to take into account in determining what services are provided to groups. For the models persons hold of health, illness, medicine, and healing determine the care that they choose (Rossman 1997).

SELECTION PRINCIPLES: A WORKING FRAMEWORK

Managed care organizations in increasing numbers are adding complementary therapies to their arrays of health care services. Until societal and professional consensus on criteria for including such therapies emerges, it seems reasonable that they be evaluated individually—like conventional medical therapies—through a process open to considering the interests of all stakeholders in the health plan, in terms of their safety, practitioners' qualifications, evidence of their efficacy and benefit, their fair distribution, and their cost effectiveness.

QUALIFICATIONS AND SAFETY

There are currently at least ten thousand individuals actively providing acupuncture in the United States, about half of whom are licensed physicians. Nonphysician practitioners are credentialed through either the National Commission for the

Certification of Acupuncturists (NCCA) or programs provided by individual states. At present, there are at least seventy schools of acupuncture with curriculums developed for the education of nonphysician providers, thirty-four of which are accredited by the National Accreditation Commission of Schools and Colleges of Acupuncture and Oriental Medicine (Lytle 1997).

Of the nine to twelve million acupuncture treatments yearly in the United States, about 70 percent are for pain control. Although piercing with acupuncture needles always has potential risk, adverse outcomes from acupuncture are infrequent (Lytle 1997).

EFFECTIVENESS

The claim that acupuncture's unproven efficacy renders it "experimental" seems naive. Acupuncture has been practiced by Chinese physicians for more than twenty-five hundred years. Its positive effects have been experienced, observed, and reported by physicians and patients alike for that long (Wolpe 1990). Still, it makes sense to consider acupuncture's mounting claims of efficacy according to accepted standards of empirical research. Managed care organizations should make their determinations regarding covered benefits by evaluating such claims. This is preferable to the stance of orthodox U.S. medicine generally for two decades, labeling acupuncture a heresy, and arbitrarily attributing claims of effectiveness and benefit to "placebo effect," "suggestion," and "self-limiting problems" (Wolpe 1985).

The task of identifying health technologies that work, in conventional as well as unconventional medicine, is in its initial stages in this country; "twenty percent of the medical treatment we use is supported by good scientific evidence of benefit, let alone more benefit than burden or risk" (Ross 1994). Efficacy, of course, is particularly problematic in conventional medicine in the treatment of chronic pain, including chronic low back pain. "It is interesting, that the two areas for which most acceptance [of acupuncture] has come from the orthodox [medical] establishment—chronic pain and substance abuse—are two of the most intractable problems in medicine. Acupuncture has had its greatest success in those areas where American medicine is most frustrated with its lack of effectiveness" (Wolpe 1990).

A study conducted on back pain found that patients receiving acupuncture showed significant reductions in visual analog scale (VAS)–assessed pain, activity pain scores, and clinical signs compared with those treated at the same acupoints with a disconnected transcutaneous electrical nerve stimulation unit. Using this study design, acupuncture given as adjunctive treatment to standard rehabilitation to patients with low back pain "was found to significantly improve the treatment outcome when compared to effects of the rehabilitation program administered alone. Many more of those who received acupuncture as supplemental care were able to return to their previous type of employment" (Birch and Hammerschlag 1996; Gunn et al. 1980).

BENEFIT

High customer satisfaction ratings and data demonstrating growing numbers of Americans seeking access to alternative therapies (including acupuncture) for chronic pain problems are well known and documented. Because pain and satisfaction are both subjective experiences, measurable in adults only by report and by inference (for example, increased functional ability and increased use of services), patients' and communities' assessments of benefits, based on personal, economic, cultural, and religious values, should have considerable weight in health plans' determinations of covered benefits.

MEDICAL NECESSITY

Chronic pain is a fundamental harm both to individual sufferers (patients) and to society at large. If acupuncture offers a reasonable likelihood of effectiveness and benefit in terms of some measure of pain relief and of increased functional ability, a strong case may be made to classify acupuncture as a covered benefit when medically recommended and supervised.

FAIR DISTRIBUTION

As is the case with other treatments, primary care physicians are capable of and responsible for recommending suitable alternative therapies, based on careful needs assessments. In this case, trusting Dr. Young to recommend acupuncture when medically indicated for his patient would promote fairness, for all patients would have similar access to acupuncture through their physicians.

COST-EFFECTIVENESS

Most complementary therapies, again including acupuncture, are relatively inexpensive, particularly in comparison to the costs of potent medications and of surgical procedures. The cost-effectiveness of alternative therapies, acupuncture included, in fact, is commonly cited by consumer groups, legislators, and managed care organizations that provide them.

Conclusion

Ultra Health should develop and publicize (1) the principles that guide its decisions in entering into contracts with employers, health plans, and its own medical staff; (2) the criteria and data upon which it bases its decisions regarding coverage of benefits; (3) its efforts to educate its staff, employers, employees, and the community regarding the specific provisions of those contracts; (4) the methods and mechanisms in place to assess the quality of its services and their outcomes for patients; and (5) the processes and mechanisms available to patients, families, and physicians for obtaining clarification of coverage allowances and for appealing denials of service in particular cases in open and fair forums.

A large group of Ultra Health physicians have not endorsed Ultra Health's decision to provide complementary services through AltCare. AltCare's for-profit status has raised understandable ethical concerns by these physicians that the move is purely economic in its motivations. Both nonprofit and for-profit health care organizations, of course, must generate revenues exceeding their expenditures. From an ethical perspective, the key issue is how profits are distributed. If AltCare's profits are invested in improving patient care services or in providing community health benefits, rather than in disproportionate administrative salaries or investment returns to shareholders, AltCare's priorities are ethically defensible.

At the very least, Ultra Health's communications with its own medical staff have been inadequate. Dr. Young can acknowledge and support the ethical bases of the medical staff's concerns. At the same time, he might challenge their current position on at least two grounds. First, he might question the scientific basis of the treatment decisions by Ultra Health's physicians in their current management of patients in the intensive care unit. The widely acknowledged prevalence of overuse of highly invasive and extremely expensive treatments in end-of-life care in acute care hospitals is well known.

Second, Dr. Young might remind his peers that the American Medical Association, in concert with scores of prominent physician-ethicists, has recommended strong physician representation on authoritative committees in managed care organizations—to support physicians advocating for their patients on grounds of respect for patient autonomy and duties of nonmaleficence and beneficence. How, he might ask them, has such strong physician participation in shaping policies in Ultra Health's direct contracting arrangement with employers in the community not only failed to support his efforts to advocate for his patient but frustrated them?

As Mr. Chow's physician, Dr. Young has witnessed his patient's conscientious compliance with his recommendations for pain management over the course of many years. Knowing Mr. Chow well, Dr. Young respects the ethical rationale underlying his patient's decision to seek palliation and rehabilitation before (or instead of) submitting himself to a course of conventional treatment whose efficacy is questionable, whose side effects are considerable, and whose expense is high. Why should Dr. Young have to fight the system to support a decision by his patient that is medically appropriate, economically responsible, and reflective of the deep cultural values that shape his patient's definition of quality of life?

Ultra Health's current stance sends a confusing message to the community as well. On the one hand, by opening AltCare and its services to private-paying patients and to members of HMOs, Ultra Health conveys an endorsement of the safety, effectiveness, and benefits of those services for patients and the community. By restricting covered access to AltCare services in its direct contracting arrangement, however, Ultra Health seems to devalue its stated commitments to preventive health and to promoting safe and cost-effective treatments, and capitulating to physicians' demands on political rather than either ethical or economic grounds.

Dr. Young should advocate vigorously on behalf of Mr. Chow's choice of acupuncture in this case.

References

American Medical Association, Council on Ethical and Judicial Affairs. 1995. "Ethical Issues in Managed Care." *Journal of the American Medical Association* 273, no. 4:330–35.

Annas, G. J. "A National Bill of Patients' Rights." 1998. *New England Journal of Medicine* 338, no. 10:695–99.

Beckham, J. D. 1997. "The Beginning of the End for HMOs: The Awakening Market." *Healthcare Forum Journal* Nov.-Dec.:44–47.

Biblo, J.; Christopher, M.; Johnson, L.; and Potter, R. L. 1995. *Ethical Issues in Managed Care: Guidelines for Clinicians and Recommendations to Accrediting Organizations.* Kansas City, Mo.: Bioethics Development Group.

Birch, S., and Hammerschlag, R. 1996. "Acupuncture Efficacy: A Summary of Controlled Clinical Trials." Tarrytown, N.Y.: National Academy of Acupuncture and Oriental Medicine, p. 15.

Bruton, H. D., M.D. 1996. *Report of the Executive Council: Ethics in Managed Care.* Raleigh, N.C.: North Carolina Medical Society.

Gunn, C. C.; Milbrandt, W. E.; Little, A. S.; and Mason, K. E. 1980. "Dry Needling of Muscle Motor Points for Chronic Low-Back Pain." *Spine* 5:279–91.

Lytle, C.D. 1997. "Safety and Regulation of Acupuncture Needles and Other Devices." In *NIH Consensus Development Conference on Acupuncture.* Edited by D. Ramsey, M.D. Bethesda, Md.: National Institutes of Health, Office of Alternative Medicine.

Perkel, R., M.D. 1996. "Ethics and Managed Care." *Medical Clinics of North America* 80, no. 2: 263–78.

Ross, J. W. 1994. "Ethical Decision Making in Managed Care Environments." *Bioethics Forum* (Fall):22–26.

Rossman, M., M.D. 1997. "Alternative Therapies: Who Will Manage What, and How?" *Alternative Therapies* 3, no. 3:63–66.

Wolpe, P. R. 1985. "The Maintenance of Professional Authority: Acupuncture and the American Physician." *Social Problems* 32, no. 5:409–24.

Wolpe, P. R. 1990. "Acupuncture in American Medicine in the 1990s." *The Academy of Medical Acupuncture Review* 2, no. 2:23–29.

COMMENTARY

Martin Gunderson, Ph.D., J.D.

It is easy to sympathize with Mr. Chow. He needs care for severe and chronic lower back pain, but the treatments recommended by Dr. Young, his physician at Ultra Health, are not acceptable to him and may be contrary to his deeply held cultural values, which include a preference for Chinese medicine. Mr. Chow believes that acupuncture might help, and Dr. Young is willing to refer him. Unfortunately, although Ultra Health's new clinic, AltCare, provides this treatment, Mr. Chow's Ultra Health contract does not cover such services. The case is especially poignant since Mr. Chow chose Ultra Health because it allowed him to self-refer and thereby find physicians sympathetic to his cultural needs. His plight raises significant issues concerning appropriate health care, respect for persons, and the integrity of health care delivery systems.

Appropriate Health Care

Health care is not an end in itself but a means to health, which includes physical, psychological, and spiritual dimensions. What constitutes psychological, spiritual, and sometimes even physical health depends, in part, on a person's values. Mr. Chow's case makes clear how differently we can view the health needs of individuals. It also shows that a Western view of a patient's physical health needs may conflict with the patient's psychological or spiritual health concerns. Insofar as Mr. Chow's fear of being cut and his desire for Chinese medicine reflect deeply held cultural values, complementary health care that reflects those values may be important for Mr. Chow's psychological and spiritual health even if there is little evidence that the complementary care sought will change the underlying physical condition that causes his pain.

Nonprofit managed care organizations such as Ultra Health ought to serve the health care needs of the community. When the community has a large population with cultural values that are best served by complementary health care such as Chinese medicine, there is reason for making such complementary care available. Of course, managed care organizations must also provide the sorts of medical treatment that have been shown to be effective on the basis of Western science. Respect for individual patients requires making available a range of health care services that fit with individual values. Coordinating these services also requires sensitivity to the integrity of health care delivery systems. Both of these need to be looked at in more depth.

Respect for Persons

For the past thirty years respect for persons has been one of the central themes in biomedical ethics. Typically respect for persons is interpreted in terms of respect for individual autonomy—the capacity for self-governance, which includes being free from the controlling influences of others and being able to make decisions that are informed and reflect one's own values. The general principle of respect for persons has been used to support the principle of informed consent, which provides that patients have a right to refuse treatment. Dr. Young is right to respect Mr. Chow's refusal of spinal injections of cortisone and surgical spinal fusion.

If patients are to be self-governing regarding their health care, they need to be able to work with their physicians to choose from an array of relevant options. This gives health care providers reason to offer a variety of services. In the case of communities with a large Asian population, it may provide reason to offer alternative care that includes such practices as acupuncture. Moreover, the strength of this reason will grow to the extent that Ultra Health comes to dominate the market, since it may then be difficult to obtain complementary care elsewhere.

In light of the principle of respect for persons, the pressure brought by physicians at Ultra Health to prevent their organization from entering into direct contracting agreements that allow coverage for AltCare is troubling. They are acting to restrict the autonomy of patients, employers, and physicians who might want to contract for that coverage. Such an interference with liberty requires a strong justification, but it is doubtful that the physicians at Ultra Health can provide an adequate justification. The physicians claim that the treatments offered by AltCare are not justified in terms of the empirical standards of Western science. In the case of acupuncture it is clear that many people find great comfort in the practice even if it does not cure underlying physical conditions. In the case of Mr. Chow it may also have a cultural significance that is important for his spiritual health. In the case of pedicures and upscale personal care products, there may be less cultural significance, but there seems little harm in allowing people to contract for coverage of such things.

Of course, Ultra Health should not offer treatments that can be shown to be unsafe or make claims about treatments that are misleading. In particular, patients must not pass up necessary care offered by Western medicine because they mistakenly believe that complementary care will be equally effective when that is not the case. Patients need to be well informed of the limits of complementary care both when they choose to sign health care contracts and when they decide on specific treatments. In this respect, Ultra Health is wise to have selected a director for AltCare who is a physician skilled in both Western and complementary approaches to healing.

Patients in the Ultra Health system may, however, be misled into thinking that the practices at AltCare are supported by the evidentiary standards of Western medicine. In particular, they might be misled because the majority of physicians at Ultra Health are committed to Western medicine and Ultra Health lends its name, and hence its reputation, to AltCare. Ultra Health's physicians have reason to worry about whether they are portrayed as endorsing practices they do not accept.

Many physicians at Ultra Health also claim that AltCare has no ethic for determining what treatments should be offered. As will be argued in the next section, AltCare does need to develop a principled way of determining what services it will offer. This is not, however, an insuperable problem.

Aside from providing adequate information about the nature and limits of various treatments such as complementary care, Ultra Health must not mislead potential enrollees about what services are available. Unfortunately, Ultra Health's ownership of AltCare is likely to create the false expectation that referrals can be made to AltCare. The very name "Ultra Health" seems to indicate that a full range of health care services will be available. In addition, the self-referral provision of contracts like the one Mr. Chow accepted might lead to a reasonable expectation that patients may refer themselves to health care providers at AltCare. Unless Ultra Health makes it perfectly clear that neither referrals nor self-referrals to AltCare can be made for patients involved in direct contracting with Ultra Health, respect for the autonomy of those who sign contracts with Ultra Health will be undermined.

People who enter into contracts with health care providers may agree to limits on coverage, and such agreements can justify withholding coverage at a later time. Limiting coverage in such circumstances is compatible with respecting the patient's autonomy. If those who sign contracts with Ultra Health are misled, however, the physicians at Ultra Health cannot argue that the organization respects the autonomy of those who sign health care contracts that limit coverage. In addition, to the extent that Ultra Health physicians unjustifiably pressure Ultra Health not to enter into contracts that provide coverage of AltCare, they cannot argue that the contracts limiting coverage respect the autonomy of their patients.

Of course, physicians, as well as patients, are persons and ought to be respected. It would interfere with their autonomy to require them to provide treatments that they believe are unsound or unethical. In addition, physicians need to be represented in the decision making at Ultra Health. The case makes it clear that the physicians who oppose complementary care are not forced to support it and are even in a position to have their will enforced throughout the organization.

On the other hand, it is not clear that physicians who support complementary care and other health care providers at AltCare have sufficient representation.

From the point of view of the managers at Ultra Health, what is needed is an organizational structure in which the physicians who are committed to Western medicine can provide the services they advocate without being required to support complementary care, while at the same time those who practice complementary health care are allowed to practice their craft. Designing health care systems that respect both health care professionals and patients requires addressing issues of professional and institutional integrity.

Integrity of Health Care Delivery Systems

"Integrity" may mean simply honesty. It may also be used to signal wholeness or integration. Ultra Health has concerns about integrity in both these senses. It is clear from the previous section that Ultra Health's ownership of AltCare is likely to mislead people. This presents Ultra Health with a dilemma. If the organization fails to make it clear that the physicians at Ultra Health do not support many of the practices at AltCare and that referrals will not be made to AltCare, it is being less than honest. On the other hand, if the organization makes it clear that the majority of its physicians do not support AltCare and that there will be no referrals to AltCare, it undermines the wholeness and integration of the Ultra Health system.

Furthermore, if the physicians at Ultra Health are right that AltCare has no ethic for determining what treatments are offered and is motivated purely by the pursuit of profit, then there is another threat to the integrity of Ultra Health. Part of Ultra Health is presumably guided by strong principles of professional ethics such as the codes and guidelines propounded by the American Medical Association and standards of scientific medicine such as reliance on empirical evidence and efficiency, while another part of the organization, AltCare, lacks ethical principles of medical practice. AltCare needs to develop coherent underlying principles that do not undermine the rest of the Ultra Health organization.

The integration and wholeness of Ultra Health is also threatened because it is a nonprofit organization and AltCare is a for-profit organization. Nonprofit organizations typically have as part of their mission serving the good of the community, while for-profit organizations are typically public corporations that need to serve the interests of shareholders. This can create a conflict of interest in the managers of Ultra Health, who have an ethical obligation to serve the community good while also having a fiduciary obligation to the shareholders of AltCare. This problem is exacerbated if the managers are paid in part from the profits of AltCare. The managers will then have an incentive to emphasize contracts favorable to AltCare even when it is contrary to the physicians who practice medicine in other parts of the Ultra Health system.

Ultra Health has, however, managed to minimize one sort of conflict of interest that threatens the professional integrity of physicians. It is sometimes claimed that fee-for-service arrangements create conflicts of interest for physicians because they create incentives to overtreat but that the alternative of financing by capitation, in which physicians receive a set payment for a range of future services, also leads to a conflict of interest by creating incentives to undertreat. Since the purchasers pay a fee-for-service to Ultra Health, there is some incentive to provide treatments. Ultra Health, however, has adopted as part of its contract a target budget that limits the extent to which its fee-for-service arrangement provides an incentive to overtreat. In general the practitioners at AltCare and the physicians at Ultra Health need to be brought into sufficient coordination that Ultra Health can remain an integrated whole.

Resolving the Ethical Issues

Above all, Ultra Health needs to make certain that the people who sign contracts are not misled. People will likely assume that referrals, including self-referrals, can be made to AltCare. Ultra Health needs to make it clear whether such referrals will be covered. The easiest way to avoid misleading people would be to provide coverage. The pressure for integrity in the sense of the system's integration provides an additional reason for providing coverage and for working with the physicians in Ultra Health to make AltCare more acceptable or at least tolerable to them. The principles undergirding the practice of Western scientific medicine can, for instance, be used to set limits on what is offered by AltCare. Practices that are shown to be either harmful or wholly ineffective can be eliminated. It is too much to demand, however, that all the practices offered be proven to be effective. After all, many of the procedures that make up the standard practice of medicine have not been shown to be effective. This is why there is such a need for outcome studies. Ultra Health should use outcome studies for both treatments offered by the physicians at Ultra Health and the treatments offered by AltCare, and the results should be made available to patients and physicians.

Outcome studies need to consider more outcomes than physiological changes, however. Given the cultural values that support Chinese medicine, such practices as acupuncture can have beneficial effects on spiritual and psychological health even if they do not resolve the underlying physical disease or injury. Such positive effects should not be ignored by Ultra Health physicians who practice Western medicine, though they would be right to argue that practices of complementary medicine that can be shown to harm a patient's health should not be tolerated. In general, practices that create a positive effect without producing overriding harm should be covered. In this way, Ultra Health can achieve a fair bit of integration and wholeness by using standards of Western medicine to set limits on complementary medicine, while not allowing the standards of Western medicine to completely supplant the theory and practice of the complementary medicine offered by AltCare.

5

Coverage Exceptions for Contractually Excluded Benefits

CASE STUDY

Request for Coverage for Benign Gynecomastia

Fifteen-year-old Jim has lived for over ten years in the same midwestern suburban community with his parents and two brothers. At age twelve, Jim's breast tissue became enlarged. His pediatrician acknowledged Jim's concern about his appearance and assured Jim and his family that the condition would probably resolve itself as he completed puberty. Two years later, however, Jim's breasts appeared even more enlarged and his pediatrician referred him to a pediatric endocrinologist, who confirmed the pediatrician's diagnosis of benign adolescent gynecomastia. He also noted that Jim's pubertal development has been normal otherwise and his medical history unremarkable.

Gynecomastia is typically self-correcting within two to three years; treatment options include waiting for resolution of the condition with the aid of the drug Tamoxifen and surgical excision (mastectomy). Both Jim's pediatrician and his endocrinologist recommended Tamoxifen and argued against surgery, believing his condition would correct itself. When, at the family's insistence, Jim's pediatrician referred him to a surgeon (within the family's health plan's network), she agreed with the other physicians' recommendations.

Jim's parents have noted that his appearance has had an effect on his activities and behavior. For example, Jim, along with his brothers (one two years older than Jim, the other two years younger), had always been active in sports. Beginning with the last school year, however, he became embarrassed to take off his shirt and refused to go to gym or to participate in school sports. His parents have also reported a marked decline in his self-confidence and self-esteem. Jim started to gain weight and now, at 190 pounds, is overweight for his five-foot, nine-inch frame.

From the start Jim has clearly expressed his desire for surgery for his condition, saying he felt and looked "like a freak." At his urging, his parents had him examined three months ago by a surgeon outside their health plan's network. The surgeon concluded that since Jim's condition had progressed for over two years and had not improved despite treatment with Tamoxifen, bilateral mastectomy should be done, in his words, "as early as reasonably possible to prevent any permanent damage to Jim's development."

Jim was covered under his father's group plan, provided through his father's employer, a twenty-person graphics design firm. The employer offered its employees only one option—an HMO with no out-of-network coverage. The plan paid for Jim's Tamoxifen; however, the plan's certificate of coverage specifies "surgical correction of male breast enlargement" on its itemized list of services not covered. Nonetheless, armed with the out-of-network surgeon's recommendation, Jim and his parents requested coverage for the procedure. The health plan denied the request. In accordance with the plan's appeal process, Jim requested a written reconsideration of the denial. To support his request for coverage, Jim obtained a recommendation from a second out-of-network surgeon, who agreed that bilateral mastectomy was indicated. The health plan again denied the request for coverage.

Relevant state statutes and rules provide that:

- Managed care plans may limit or exclude coverage for cosmetic surgery.
- Managed care plans must provide reconstructive benefits when such service is performed because of a congenital disease or anomaly that has resulted in a functional defect as determined by the attending physician.
- Managed care plans must provide "medically necessary care," defined as health care services that are appropriate in terms of type, frequency, level, setting, and duration of the enrollee's diagnosis or condition, and diagnostic testing and preventive services. Medically necessary care must be consistent with generally accepted practice parameters as determined by health care providers in the same or similar general specialty as typically manage the condition, procedure, or treatment at issue; it must also help restore or maintain the enrollee's health, prevent deterioration of the enrollee's condition, or prevent the reasonably likely onset of a health problem or detect an incipient problem.

Request for Coverage for Electric Wheelchair

Ruth Meyer is a forty-one-year-old employee of the public library in a small southwestern city. She is a widow with no children and has no close relatives living nearby. In 1987 she developed multiple sclerosis. The disease progressed rapidly, so that within three years Ms. Meyer needed a wheelchair for mobility. A manual wheelchair met her needs at the time. She continued to live alone and was able to continue to work full-time. In early 1993, however, Ms. Meyer was losing strength in her upper body and could no longer push herself easily in her manual wheelchair; she experienced significant pain in her shoulders as a result. Her doctor then prescribed an electric wheelchair. Ms. Meyer's request that her health plan pay for the electric wheelchair was denied. She appealed this decision with documentation from her physician and an occupational therapist about the medical need for the chair but was again denied.

Several months later, Ms. Meyer's pain immobilized her and she was taken to a hospital by ambulance. She underwent rotator cuff surgery to repair two torn tendons in her shoulder. After the surgery she was transferred to a transitional care center for rehabilitation. Her health plan paid for the surgery and for the first four weeks of her stay at the transitional care center. When she reached her coverage limit, however, Ms. Meyer did not feel she was ready to go home, since she lived alone and was not yet strong enough to move about easily. She remained in the center for additional rehabilitation for two more months and spent nearly $15,000 of her own money.

After Ms. Meyer returned home, she needed assistance with transfers in and out of the wheelchair, cooking, other home health care services, and transportation to and from her job at the library, which now had been reduced to half-time. The plan would not pay for any of these services. Instead, funding for them and for a part-time personal care attendant initially came through a special state program. Once funding for this program ran out, Ms. Meyer picked up these expenses as well.

Getting around in the manual wheelchair became increasingly difficult for Ms. Meyer. At work, she relied on her coworkers to push her wherever she needed to go. Her employer, however, became more and more concerned with this arrangement, and Ms. Meyer believed that her job was in jeopardy. Weekends were the worst, according to Ms. Meyer, because on those days she could find no one to assist her.

Her doctors again prescribed an electric wheelchair, arguing that without such a chair, Ms. Meyer would probably reinjure her shoulder. The request was again denied. The health plan maintains that its decisions comply with the contract it has with Ms. Meyer's employer. Under the terms of the contract, coverage for "durable medical equipment" is limited to $2,000 per item, skilled nursing facility care is limited to four weeks, and home health care, including a personal care attendant, is not covered.

In August 1995, Ms. Meyer's story was publicized by a columnist in her city's daily paper. Shortly thereafter, the health plan approved the request for the electric wheelchair, but only up to $2,000, the limit under its contract. Public reaction to the column, however, generated more than enough contributions to pay the balance of the wheelchair's $10,000 cost.

The cost of Ms. Meyer's surgery and related services and the health plan's share of her rehabilitation stay had easily exceeded the cost of an electric wheelchair.

Questions for Consideration

➤ Does Jim have a health problem? Is a bilateral mastectomy "medically necessary"? Why?

➤ Is the plan justified in excluding coverage of Jim's condition? Why?

➤ Should Ms. Meyer's health plan have paid for the electric wheelchair when it was first prescribed? Should it pay for the chair now? Why? How should transportation and other ancillary support services that Ms. Meyer needs be paid for? Is a $2,000 limit for durable medical equipment reasonable and acceptable?

➤ How should coverage exceptions be decided?

➤ Is the state's definition of medically necessary care useful? Why?

➤ Why might a plan cover treatment with Tamoxifen but not cover surgical treatment for the same condition? Why might a plan cap services such as durable medical equipment, skilled nursing facilities, and home health care?

➤ What is the media's role and responsibility in publicizing Ms. Meyer's case (or other cases of denied or uncovered services)? Does the media have any responsibility to individuals whose cases it does not publicize?

COMMENTARY _____

David Mechanic, Ph.D.

Health care has always been rationed in one way or another. Rationing refers to various processes of allocating limited resources among competing demands. In traditional insurance the primary form of rationing occurs by means of benefit design and the types of coverage and exclusions that define the health insurance policy.

Benefit design influences the price of an insurance policy. In principle, health insurance can cover any conceivable service, but few purchasers would be willing to pay the necessary premium. Some services, in particular, involve what economists call "moral hazard," an inclination to use more of the service than is optimal when it is insured. This would certainly apply to health spas, for example, and more conventional services such as psychotherapy. When insurers provide for such services, they seek mechanisms to restrict wider use: for example, they may require that the enrollee have a defined diagnosis of particular severity, set expenditure limits, require high coinsurance, or use some combination of these measures. To survive financially, insurers have to make reasonably good actuarial predictions of what services they can cover at what premiums.

HMOs also have to design their benefits, but they generally offer a much wider scope of coverage under the concept of "medical necessity." They then control expenditures through a variety of arrangements. These include sharing risk with physicians, other financial incentives and penalties, such as bonuses and withholds, and maintaining administrative oversight of physician practices. Typically, they also require that primary care physicians authorize any expensive tests or referrals to specialty care as a way of reducing the use of expensive services. When individuals join HMOs, they generally are led to believe that they will receive whatever services are necessary for their health and welfare; they are unlikely to have a clear conception of what these services or their needs might be in the future. There is, of course, much uncertainty in medicine and concepts of medical necessity can differ widely. Even if contracts specify beforehand that certain medical interventions are excluded from coverage, most consumers at the point of plan enrollment are unlikely to understand any but the obvious exclusions (such as cosmetic surgery, dental care, optometry services, drugs). Managed care organizations have a responsibility to inform enrollees clearly about their coverage.

Realistically, the contract between an enrollee and an HMO involves the enrollee's agreement to accept rationing by health care providers, although the contract is almost never presented in these terms. In return for enhanced coverage or lower price, the enrollee agrees to give plan providers discretion to withhold services if they are of little or no benefit to the enrollee's health or to substitute less costly services for more expensive ones when there is no evidence that the more expensive intervention would yield a better health outcome. Thus, the HMO might substitute nurse practitioner care for physician care in managing chronic disease, might use home care or outpatient services instead of inpatient care, or might substitute generic for brand-name drugs. The understanding that all necessary care will be provided does not permit substitution of an inferior intervention for a more effective one, although there might be disagreement about the effectiveness of available alternatives. Moreover, effectiveness may be viewed from a narrower medical perspective or from broader psychosocial ones. Although medical care traditionally has been narrowly focused, psychosocial factors and mental health are central to distress and disability, the course of illness and dysfunction, and successful treatment and rehabilitation.

Jim's family, enrolled in an HMO, is justified in assuming that family members would receive all services needed to maintain function and prevent deterioration since this is the way HMOs characterize their services. Initially, three physicians in the plan seem to agree that gynecomastia is self-correcting with Tamoxifen, and this appears consistent with existing medical knowledge.

Jim's condition has not improved over two years with Tamoxifen and, in the judgment of at least one surgeon, it has progressed. Moreover, there is increasing evidence of deterioration in personality, behavior, and self-esteem attributable to the progression of the condition. These serious consequences can affect Jim's future social development and function. Two outside surgeons now recommend bilateral mastectomy. Given these facts, and the understanding that behavioral outcomes are as important as physical ones, one can reasonably argue that in this case bilateral mastectomy falls within a reasonable definition of "medical necessity." At the very least, the request for the surgery should be heard by an impartial panel whose members have expertise in both medical and developmental aspects of the condition. It is appropriate to have an outside review body of disinterested physicians to whom Jim's family could appeal the decision, a process now required in the state of New Jersey and some other states. Such mechanisms give consumers greater assurance that they are not being denied care because of cost-containment interests or financial incentives and provide for a more neutral judgment in contested cases. New Jersey regulations do not require the insurer to conform with the appeal body's judgment, but the threat of negative publicity in failing to do so should serve as a deterrent to not doing so.

The certificate of coverage explicitly excludes "surgical correction of male breast enlargement"—a justifiable exclusion if the surgery is viewed simply as cosmetic. Even if Jim's parents had had a choice of insurance policy—which they did not in this case because the employer selected the plan—it would be unreasonable to expect them to have anticipated that what appears as a cosmetic surgical exclusion could have implications for providing their son a medically necessary treatment.

We are told that three physicians in the plan opposed the surgical treatment initially. Given the facts over the subsequent two years, it is reasonable to believe their judgments might have changed. For this, among other reasons, implicit rationing can be strongly supported, which leaves such clinical judgments in the hands of the providers involved in the ongoing care of the patient (Mechanic 1997a). It is extraordinarily difficult to write explicit rules that cover all contingencies and needed exceptions as the individual circumstances of a medical condition evolve.

The case of Ruth Meyer is somewhat different. Although the case description is consistent with both managed care and indemnity coverage, let us assume that she had indemnity coverage that contains costs through benefit design. Unlike a capitated organization, which can balance different types of costs against one another, traditional indemnity plans pay only for the services covered, no matter how irrational the overall pattern of care. To the extent that the indemnity insurers used a utilization review organization and assigned a high-cost case manager to Ms.

Meyers, it might have been possible for the case manager to provide some noncovered services as a way of preventing use of expensive covered services, but such arrangements apparently were not operative in this case.

Function is what good medical care is all about, although physicians still have much to do to incorporate this idea into everyday practice. For Ms. Meyer the prescription of an electric wheelchair would be medically necessary because it allowed her to retain function and to slow deterioration in her function over time. Nonetheless, no indemnity insurance program is required to provide all care that is medically necessary—however medical necessity is defined. Such plans provide what the benefit design of the plan calls for and no more. Many states have mandated that all insurance programs cover particular benefits. Such mandates have two difficulties: under the federal Employee Retirement Income Security Act (ERISA), self-insured employers need not conform to such mandates (an incentive for employers to self-insure); mandates also drive up the cost of health care premiums, leading some employers either to drop health insurance completely or to hire less-than-full-time workers who would not be eligible to receive health benefits.

In indemnity insurance, the key issue for management is whether the patient's illness justifies a particular intervention. Initially, Ms. Meyer's request for an electric wheelchair was seen as unjustified, despite support from her physician and an occupational therapist. Most wheelchair-dependent persons would likely prefer an electric wheelchair to a manual one, and plans must monitor their expenditures to keep costs and premiums under control. At this stage it would have been desirable for Ms. Meyer to have access to a review procedure with decision makers who have no financial interest in either denying or granting her request for the more expensive intervention.

After the fact we are led to infer that it would have been economically advantageous in this case for the insurer to pay for the electric wheelchair; however, the insurer had no way of knowing this ahead of time. Moreover, preventive measures taken to avoid future costs do not necessarily result in lower costs for the insurer, even in the aggregate (Russell 1986). If the insurer provided an electric wheelchair to everyone who made a good case for one, they might incur greater costs than they would in providing whatever future care was needed.

It seems clear that the insurer should have authorized $2,000 toward the purchase of an electric wheelchair. The insurer is not liable for the other $8,000, however, since the contract specifically limits its responsibility. Such limitations allow lower premiums for the employer and/or employee and may make it possible for the employer to purchase health insurance for employees in the first place.

Why argue that it was unrealistic to expect that Jim's parents could assess his future need for a medically necessary bilateral mastectomy and not make a similar argument for Ruth Meyer? In Ms. Meyer's case the exclusion was a conventional one that most people can readily understand: Once an insurer sets a payment ceiling, that is all they plan to pay. Perhaps Ms. Meyer could not foresee her need for an electric wheelchair or, if she did, did not realize how expensive it would be. Such judgments, however, are within the context of everyday decision making and not very different from decisions to take collision insurance on one's car or fire insurance on the contents of one's apartment.

The case tells us little about Ms. Meyer's economic circumstances except that she is employed and has no dependents. We are told that after being denied an electric wheelchair, she suffered consequences that immobilized her and required her to spend $15,000 of her own funds for extended rehabilitation. This implies that Ms. Meyer had the financial means to purchase the wheelchair and chose not to. Thus, Ms. Meyer must share responsibility for her subsequent problems, since she could have taken measures to prevent them. Knowing of the inadequacies of her health insurance program, Ms. Meyer might also have purchased secondary insurance to fill its gaps.

Media coverage of Ms. Meyer's plight led to contributions to enable her to purchase an electric wheelchair. Such appeals have a triple function. They provide help in particular instances; they allow members of the public to reaffirm community-helping values; and they also put insurers on notice that certain practices will not be tolerated and will harm public trust in their enterprise. Recent publicity given to "gag rules," "drive-through deliveries," and "assembly line mastectomies" suggests that media dramatization arouses public concern and often results in legislative or regulatory initiatives. However, media attention often treats anecdotes as a representative picture of reality and is a poor way of formulating health policy (Mechanic 1997b). It is not even a particularly good way of giving assistance to those most in need. While the insurer may relent to a particular instance of negative publicity, one episode is unlikely to lead to any serious improvement of basic operations. Whether a person receives assistance is simply an accident of media interest, and such cases rarely receive the media's attention.

The case of Ruth Meyer reflects the character of the U.S. health care system with its employment-based coverage, broad range of exclusions, lack of choice among health care plans, and large number of uninsured and underinsured persons. Further, it illustrates U.S. medicine's strong acute care, technical orientation and its relative inattention to long-term treatment or rehabilitation. Difficulties that arise in both cases are a consequence of the fact that in each, the employers (a small private employer and a small city's public library system) seek to reduce their insurance liabilities and select for their employees insurance policies that have many limits and exclusions. Further, if small employers' plans are experience-rated, so that subsequent premiums reflect past costs, such employers are less likely to insure for comprehensive services or to recruit and retain workers who have high personal health expenses.

Whomever the purchaser and whatever the system, health care will be rationed in some fashion. The U.S. system depends substantially on benefit design (restrictions, limitations, and caps on the services to be provided) and cost-sharing (coinsurance and deductibles). Other systems, such as the English National Health Service, purport to provide all necessary care with few restrictions, but they ration care by the unwillingness to expend the funds for needed facilities and specialists and maintain waiting lists for nonemergency services that typically extend for many months and sometimes years. Most systems have gatekeepers who can triage patients and avoid high-cost utilization that seems unnecessary or less critical.

All health systems must live within a finite budget. Beyond very expensive services (such as transplants), health programs typically give discretion to physicians to allocate services on the basis of their best professional judgment—that is, they use implicit rationing systems. Doctors in Jim's HMO probably had some clinical discretion in assessing whether a bilateral mastectomy was medically necessary, whatever the plan's limitations. Within the U.S. system, such discretion and advocacy for the best interests of patients is now affected by the personal income incentives that many HMOs use to keep physicians within specified utilization targets (Mechanic and Schlesinger 1996). Some modest incentives can be useful in inducing the physician to be more thoughtful and judicious and not necessarily give patients everything they demand. But when these incentives and other risk-sharing arrangements become too extensive, physician judgment becomes suspect. To the extent that this is the way American medicine will be practiced in the future, it seems prudent to provide appeals processes that allow outside experts to review whether good medical judgment is being exercised. Some believe the market will eventually drive out poor performers, but the market is a thin thread on which to base one's life.

These two cases also illustrate the need for a broader view of medical care that is sensitive to the needs of the whole person and not simply a narrowly defined medical condition. Competent treatment of Jim requires consideration of his developmental needs and how his problem affects his personal and social function, his relationships with peers, and his sense of competence and coping. To do anything less is to serve him badly.

Medicine also requires a longer-term perspective on the patient than is typical. Ruth Meyer may not have had a right to an electric wheelchair under her insurance contract, but a good medical service would assess both her immediate and her long-term needs carefully. The loss of her upper body strength and future difficulties were probably predictable and should have been taken into account. Such preventive care may or may not have saved money in the long run. What matters is that anticipating future needs and problems, and preventing future deterioration, is central to high-quality medical care. It is also ethically correct (Mechanic 1994).

References

Mechanic, D. 1994. *Inescapable Decisions: The Imperatives of Health Reform.* New Brunswick, N.J.: Transactions Publishers.
————. 1997a. "Muddling Through Elegantly: Finding the Proper Balance in Rationing." *Health Affairs* 16, no. 5:83–92.
————. 1997b. "Managed Care as a Target of Distrust." *Journal of the American Medical Association* 277, no. 22:1810–11.
Mechanic, D., and Schlesinger, M. 1996. "The Impact of Managed Care on Patients' Trust in Medical Care and Their Physicians." *Journal of the American Medical Association* 275, no. 21:1693–97.
Russell, L. B. 1986. *Is Prevention Better Than Cure?* Washington, D.C.: The Brookings Institution.

COMMENTARY

Kate T. Christensen, M.D., F.A.C.P.

Both cases under discussion challenge any easy definition of "medical necessity" and raise questions about the optimal process for resolving disputes over health care coverage. Benefit coverage disputes, as in the cases of Jim and Ms. Meyers, are usually handled through an administrative appeals process, which evaluates the fair application of the rules of the contract. However, a different approach using a multidisciplinary review board with community or patient members, either internal or external to the health care organization, could ensure greater flexibility and individualization to health plan coverage decisions. Explicit and publicly developed criteria for making coverage decisions in disputed cases would be more useful than the current, relatively stringent doctrine of fair application of the rules of the contract. Still, prevention is always better than cure. More resources should be invested in programs aimed at improving physicians' abilities to manage and resolve disagreements with patients over health care decisions in the medical office, before they reach the level of the appeals committee.

The Obligations of Health Care Organizations and Health Plans

What are the relevant obligations of health care organizations? They must treat their patients or members fairly, which means treating like cases similarly and avoiding the expenditure of resources on unnecessary, marginal, or frivolous treatments. They also are obligated to provide tests or treatments necessary for the patient's health, defined as "medically necessary care" in most contracts. An additional obligation is to avoid the harm of useless tests or treatments. These three obligations reflect the principles of justice, beneficence, and nonmaleficence.

In the appeals process, justice or fairness means applying the rules evenly, without preferential treatment. Beneficence means covering treatments that provide a health benefit, and nonmaleficence means not covering procedures that might harm the patient without a compensatory benefit.

Fitting specific cases into definitions of medical necessity is much more complicated than it seems. For example, who should decide whether a specific treatment is more helpful than harmful to a specific patient? According to what criteria? Public trust in physicians and health care organizations is at an all-time low. This lack of trust, coupled with the move toward treatment decisions based on research instead of individual opinion (called "evidence-based medical practice"), means that the physician's word alone is no longer reason enough to decide if a particular treatment would provide a tangible benefit to the patient. Even more troubling are questions about coverage for services not strictly defined as "medical." We can imagine many things that contribute to our health, such as good food and warm clothing, for which we would not expect our health plan to pay. There are other items, such as crutches, orthotics, corrective lenses, or wheelchairs that we would more readily define as "medical necessities." Yet most health plans do not provide coverage for all these items for all of their members. Until we come up with a new and better way to define the responsibilities of health care organizations, it will be necessary to consider each case individually, with some latitude for interpretation of the rules.

Two Conflicting Paradigms

Providing health care is a messy undertaking, one that resists clear definitions and simple yes/no choices. Who can unequivocally define "normal functioning" or "experimental treatment"? Coronary artery disease or hypertension should be treated, but how far should a health plan go in treating infertility, obesity, or short stature? This same ambiguity applies to ordering tests and prescribing medication or equipment. Discovering what a patient needs is very often a matter of trial and error, wait and see, or best guess. Given the inherent variability in individuals' response to disease and treatment, providers usually act on probabilities applied to their specific patients and rarely, if ever, on certainties. The overriding principle in this setting is beneficence, as the physician seeks the best treatment for each individual patient.

In contrast, health care delivery is becoming increasingly circumscribed by contracts and benefits language. Those who pay for health care in the United States, largely the government and employers, are calling for reduced costs and account-ability to ensure that medical dollars are going toward medically necessary care. The widespread adoption of practice guidelines and evidence-based practice is one way to accomplish this end. The benefits language in the health plan contract is another mechanism for excluding care not deemed medically necessary. However, if the contract tries to become too precise by specifically excluding certain services, the physician can be hindered in finding the right treatment for the patient.

When the patient perceives a medical need for something not covered in the contract, the result is often a power struggle between the patient and the health plan. On its side, the health plan has the power of the contract itself and the power to deny coverage. Patients have on their side the appeals process, the threat of litigation, the heat of the media and public opinion, and the ear of legislators. When the problem gets to this stage, there are very few winners on either side, as the patient's real health care needs get lost in the conflict over one particular test or treatment.

The Appeals Process

The ambiguities and uncertainties of medical practice undermine the neat divisions and definitions in the contract and create a steady flow of patient complaints and ap-peals for exceptions to the contract limitations. The parties involved are challenged to satisfy competing, and at times, mutually exclusive, values—the equitable applica-tion of the contract rules and the duty to provide for the patient's health care needs.

Once disagreement over treatment coverage reaches the appeals process, fairness can be hard to deliver, particularly when the facts are in dispute. Who should get the benefit of the doubt—the health plan, the physician, or the patient? The obligation to provide for the patient's health care needs is dependent on who defines these needs and how they are defined. A patient can maintain that a certain (noncovered) treatment results in better health, while medical research has shown no benefit and possible harm. Coverage decisions often are made on the basis of population studies, but individual responses to treatment can lie outside the norm.

Treating John's Gynecomastia

Let us look at our two cases to see how they may be handled differently in the legalistic appeals context and within the therapeutic relationship. Jim, the teenage boy with gynecomastia, had the condition for two to three years. His parents belonged to a health plan that excluded surgery for "correction of male breast enlargement." In fact, most health plans do not cover any type of cosmetic surgery. Armed with two out-of-plan surgeons' opinions, Jim's parents appealed the denial, arguing that the surgery would be "medically necessary care" and therefore a covered benefit. Implied in this story is the argument that the gynecomastia is causing Jim physical harm and not just embarrassment, because he is avoiding sports, has become depressed, and as a result of these two factors has become quite overweight.

As decided on the basis of the rules of the contract, Jim did not get the surgery, because it was specifically excluded. Looked at from a legalistic or contractual perspective, this approach would be fair, because the rules apply equally to everyone enrolled in the health plan. The fact that at the time of enrollment Jim's father most likely did not know about this exclusion, or did not think it would be relevant, makes this a misfortune for them but not a reason to extend coverage for the procedure. The health plan might also prevent harm to Jim if an unindicated surgery is prevented. However, the health care needs of the patient may not be well served in this case, because his needs are greater and more complex than a simple "surgery/no surgery" decision.

How could this conflict be better resolved within the therapeutic relationship? Instead of defining the problem as a conflict between two opposing interests (for and against surgery) we can redefine it as an ongoing issue that requires a more complex response. What are Jim's psychological needs, and possibly those of his family? How might diet and exercise impact his breast size? Is he taking any drugs, like marijuana, that might affect his breast size? How might his condition change over time? Jim and his family have waited two or three years, but they may need to wait a few more before deciding that surgery is their only recourse. The degree and nature of his gynecomastia also might influence the decision regarding surgery. For example, is Jim's condition very apparent or less so? Is the breast tissue made up more of fat or of fibrous tissue? Is the condition stable or still changing? There is no universal agreement among pediatricians and surgeons about the best treatment for teenage gynecomastia, and the best approach depends heavily on the particular facts of the case.

If the health plan recognized this uncertainty and the need for individualizing the treatment plans, and dropped this specific exclusion, the physician could offer to set a time frame and set of steps for deciding if surgery is truly the only option. This approach keeps the door open in case Jim's gynecomastia does not resolve. In the meantime, Jim and his family might benefit from contact with a support group for gynecomastia. He also should be referred to a weight management and exercise program. If Jim and his parents remain adamant that surgery is the best solution, a panel made up primarily of pediatricians and surgeons could review the case and help find a solution. Such a panel could be within the plan or independent of it. Ultimately, Jim's parents still could end up wanting a procedure that the plan would not cover, but the process for denial would have been more respectful of the particular facts and issues in this case, and ongoing help to Jim and his family would have been provided.

With this approach the physician, patient, and family have an opportunity to work together to find the best solution to Jim's problem. A trusting relationship between the physician and the patient and family is required for this process to be successful. Trust needs time to develop, as the physician demonstrates a commitment to finding a solution for the patient's problem, even if that solution is not immediately forthcoming. This sense of trust is entirely missing once the process becomes a struggle by the parents to get the surgery done and paid for by a health plan. In the context of this power struggle, there is only one treatment the parents see as helpful to their son, and the physician and health plan become simply obstacles to getting that treatment. By maintaining a flexible stand in areas where there is disagreement or uncertainty about the best treatment approach, the health plan might win in the long run by promoting trust, retaining loyal and happy patients, and avoiding conflict.

Ms. Meyer's Wheelchair

Ms. Meyer's situation is another example where the contract serves neither her medical needs nor the financial interests of the health plan. Her arms have become very weak from multiple sclerosis, too weak to push a standard wheelchair. The lack of an electric wheelchair has caused painful and expensive trauma to the tendons in her shoulders. Her health plan contract, however, excludes coverage for durable medical equipment costs of more than $2,000 per item, which would (we assume from the case) put the electric wheelchair out of her reach. On appeal, this conflict was approached from a contractual perspective. The principle of fairness was upheld by the even application of the rules regarding equipment coverage limitations, but her medical condition suffered as a consequence.

However, an exception to this rule came about through public pressure. Such ad hoc exceptions undermine the fairness of the contract rules by relying on subjective and inconsistently applied criteria. Fairness could be reclaimed by strictly adhering to the contract, denying medically necessary equipment to some but achieving consistent application of the rules. Alternatives include doing away with the limitation on durable medical equipment altogether (which could prove prohibitively expensive) or setting medical-need criteria for equipment coverage instead of dollar limits.

Another approach to achieving fairness, beneficence, and nonmaleficence in conflicts over coverage would involve the development of a generally agreed-upon process for considering exceptions to the contracted dollar limits. This process could include a multidisciplinary review group as previously mentioned, which should include representatives from providers, the health plan, members/patients, the broader community, and payers. Some appeals committees may already be composed of care providers and member representatives, as well as health plan representatives. Others may need to redefine their structure and role or contract with an independent body to provide such reviews. This review board could then develop explicit principles and criteria for considering exceptions to contractual benefits limitations or for resolving disputes over "medical necessity." Public discussion, participation, and input to this process, and joint development with multiple health plans, would promote a more trusting public environment for resolving conflicts.

Granted, acknowledging publicly that exceptions do occur could undermine the legitimacy and integrity of the contract limitations, and it potentially could generate a flood of appeals for exceptions to coverage limitations. On the other hand, applying this approach to all benefits issues could create an area of acknowledged ambiguity, which lies between the clearly covered (for example, treatment for high blood pressure or diabetes) and clearly noncovered services (for example, hair implants). This process might serve to mitigate the power struggle over benefits and create a more favorable context for problem solving between the patient and the physician.

In the case of Ms. Meyers, review by a multidisciplinary board that included member representatives could provide a better outcome. If the board applied a generally accepted set of criteria for deciding her case, it is likely her wheelchair expenses would be paid by the health plan, as her history has already demonstrated her medical need for the electric wheelchair. If they decided not to cover her wheelchair costs, the review, based on a publicly acknowledged and commonly adopted process, would have a far better chance of being perceived as fair and therefore more acceptable by Ms. Meyers.

Bolstering the Physician-Patient Relationship

Within the physician-patient relationship itself, we also can take steps to avoid showdowns with patients over benefits coverage. Some physicians need to polish their skills in problem solving with patients. Whether in private practice or in a managed care setting, the pressure to see many patients in a day creates a temptation to simply say no to a patient's request "because it is not covered" or "not indicated," without going more deeply into the problem and seeking a solution.

Establishing and maintaining rapport and trust with a patient is difficult; doing so when the patient and physician are at odds is even harder.

There are also many times when physicians must say no to requests for certain tests or treatments because the modalities in question simply would not provide any benefit. A very common example is the request for antibiotics to treat a viral infection, like a cold or the flu. Another is the request for a head scan or neurology referral for a headache. How the physician says no could mean the difference between an ongoing collaborative and therapeutic relationship and an antagonistic appeals process that serves no one. The conversation needs to include much more than a refusal. The physician needs to educate the patient on why the test or treatment would not answer his or her medical needs and attempt to understand the source of the patient's concern (perhaps a frightening family history, the experience of a friend, or a story seen on the news). The patient and physician can then decide on a plan aimed at addressing the patient's current concerns and real needs.

Accomplishing all this in the brief space of a clinic visit is asking a great deal, but these are skills that can be learned. There are a growing number of courses designed to help physicians improve their skills in brief negotiation, shared decision making, and managing conflict in the therapeutic relationship. These courses can be found at many medical meetings, through physician organizations, in hospital staff education departments, and on the Internet. Physician organizations also can promote programs that help physicians learn communication and brief negotiation skills and, in particular, how to say no without losing patients' trust. The physician-patient relationship at its best is the ideal context for resolving conflicts over treatment.

References

Eddy, D. 1996. "Benefit Language: Criteria That Will Improve Quality While Reducing Costs." *Journal of the American Medical Associaton* 275, no. 6:650–57.

Gallagher, T.; Lo, B.; Chesney, M.; and Christensen, K. 1997. "How Do Physicians Respond to Patients' Requests For Costly, Unindicated Services?" *Journal of General Internal Medicine* 12, no. 11:663–68.

Mechanic, D. 1996. "The Impact of Managed Care on Patients' Trust in Medical Care and Their Physicians." *Journal of the American Medical Association* 275, no. 21:1693–97.

Showstack, J.; Lurie, N.; Leatherman, S.; Fisher, E.; and Inui, T. 1996. "Health of the Public: The Private-Sector Challenge." *Journal of the American Medical Association* 276, no. 13:1071–74.

PART TWO

Incentives to Contain Costs and Improve Quality

6

Referral Practices Under Capitation

CASE STUDY

Mr. Carmen lived in a large gulf state city and had been an employee of Western Manufacturing, Inc. for many years. Western provided health care benefits to its employees by contracting with an HMO named Truman Health. Under the terms of the Truman Health policy, Mr. Carmen was required to select one of the HMO's authorized primary care physicians. This physician would act as a "gatekeeper" of Mr. Carmen's health care. In order to see a specialist and have the visit covered, Mr. Carmen would need to obtain a written referral from his primary care physician.

Mr. Carmen chose Dr. Albright as his primary care physician. He was a partner at the Parkside Family Medical Clinic and had been the family doctor for Mr. Carmen and his family for many years. At the outset of their relationship, Mr. Carmen informed Dr. Albright of a family history of heart disease and communicated his concern for his own health. Mr. Carmen's father had died of heart disease while in his mid-fifties, and his mother had died from conditions including heart disease while in her early sixties. Mr. Carmen's two half-brothers had both undergone coronary bypass surgery for heart disease in their early forties.

In February of 1993, Dr. Albright administered an echocardiogram and tested Mr. Carmen's cholesterol level. While the echocardiogram was normal, Mr. Carmen's cholesterol was significantly elevated. Mr. Carmen altered his diet, began exercising, and tried various medications to help control his cholesterol level. Over the course of the next three years, Mr. Carmen's cholesterol level continued to rise, and he began experiencing a tingling sensation and shortness of breath as well as intermittent dizzy spells. By the end of 1996, he was experiencing regular tightness in his chest, difficulty breathing, buzzing in his right ear, and continuous lower back pain.

Mr. Carmen and his wife visited Dr. Albright eleven times during this three-year period, repeatedly requesting a referral to a cardiologist. On each occasion, Dr. Albright considered the symptoms and concluded that they were stress-related and that a referral to a cardiologist was not medically indicated. In January of 1997, Dr. Albright did perform a treadmill test. The test showed no indication of heart disease, and again Dr. Albright advised against a cardiology referral.

Finally, in the summer of 1997, after a brief hospitalization for dizziness, tightness in his chest, and difficulty breathing, Dr. Albright agreed to refer Mr. Carmen to a cardiologist, Dr. Capulski, who was also a partner at Parkside Family Medical Clinic. The Carmens had never met Dr. Capulski. They preferred to consult with Dr. Brown, a cardiologist Mr. Carmen's brothers had used and the family knew. The Carmens consulted the physician network list for the Truman Health plan and were pleased to find that Dr. Brown was on the list. Truman Health covered specialty services only if provided by a physician in Truman Health's network. The Carmens conveyed their preference to Dr. Albright, who refused to refer to a specialist outside his clinic, explaining that it was clinic policy to provide only internal referrals and that this practice was wholly consistent with the coordination of patient care.

The Carmens proceeded to appeal this decision through Truman Health, arguing they should have a right to access any network provider on the list and that Dr. Albright was improperly motivated by financial reasons to keep the business within the Parkside Family Medical Clinic. Truman Health refused to require the clinic to alter its referral policy and suggested that Mr. Carmen should instead consider changing to a new primary care physician outside of the Parkside Family Medical Clinic who would be willing to refer to Dr. Brown. While in the process of changing primary care physicians for this purpose, Mr. Carmen died at the age of forty-two. The autopsy revealed that Mr. Carmen died of a cardiac condition as indicated by stenosis of the coronary arteries.

Unknown to the Carmens until much later, Truman Health's contracts with its network physicians created financial incentives that may have discouraged a primary care physician from making referrals to specialists. In particular, Parkside Family Medical Clinic was paid a capitated amount per member per month for each enrollee who chose a Parkside Family Medical Clinic primary care physician. The clinic was then obligated to provide all medically necessary primary and specialty care under the policy to that enrollee for that month. Any fees for specialty care had to be paid by the clinic. Any amount left over at the end of the month accrued to the clinic, and any amount owing was the liability of the clinic. The clinic, in turn, determined how individual physicians would be compensated.

In conjunction with her lawsuit against the physicians and the plan, Mrs. Carmen claimed that if her husband had known his doctor had financial incentives to not provide a referral, he would have sought a second opinion at his own expense. Furthermore, she claimed that Truman Health's complicity in the Parkside Family Medical Clinic's referral policy is a breach of her health plan contract.

Questions for Consideration

➤ How might physician financial incentives potentially interfere with the physician-patient relationship?

➤ Are some financial incentives less troublesome than others? Why?

➤ How does the financial incentive to undertreat in the HMO context compare with the incentive to overtreat in fee-for-service arrangements? Which is more powerful? More dangerous?

➤ If physician financial incentives are used, should they be disclosed to the enrollee as part of informed consent? If so, how detailed should such disclosures be? Who should make the disclosures and when?

➤ Should the use of physician financial incentives be governed by industry standards? Professional ethics? State or federal regulation?

➤ What arguments might a primary care physician make that it is his or her prerogative to provide a referral only to some specialists on the preferred provider list?

➤ What arguments might Mrs. Carmen make that she should have a right to access any provider on the preferred provider list?

➤ Should providers be permitted to share risk with the plan? Why might the use of physician financial incentives that create risk-sharing between plans and physicians be ethically defensible? Why not?

COMMENTARY

Gail J. Povar, M.D., M.P.H.

A doctor sitting on the peer review committee of Dr. Albright's clinic, reviewing the case of Mr. Carmen, might first ask whether Dr. Albright was paying attention to basic tenets of medical diagnosis. Given Mr. Carmen's risk factors, Dr. Albright should have insisted that Mr. Carmen consult the cardiologist as soon as symptoms suggestive of cardiovascular disease appeared. He should certainly not have repeatedly refused the request for referral over a three-year period! In such a patient, even a negative exercise stress test cannot be assumed to rule out significant coronary artery disease. Dr. Albright's care of Mr. Carmen, at least with the benefit of hindsight, is completely unjustifiable.

It is difficult to imagine a physician so utterly divorced from all sense of ethical propriety that he would fail to refer such a case on financial grounds alone. Were a moral compass lacking, surely the fear of malpractice litigation would spur a physician to refer a patient like Mr. Carmen for definitive evaluation. We must therefore surmise that Dr. Albright failed to recognize the situation before him. Assuming Dr. Albright to be reasonably competent, how could this have occurred?

Systemic Influences on Quality of Care

Financial considerations may have been influential, albeit indirectly, in Dr. Albright's failure to diagnose Mr. Carmen's symptoms properly. After all, financial incentives to limit referrals, especially outside the clinic, existed at two different levels. Dr. Albright's group had a general incentive to reduce its overall expenditures given its capitated contract with the managed care entity, *and* Dr. Albright's individual share of Parkside Family Medical Clinic's "profits" would probably reflect his particular practice patterns in some fashion. Capitated groups (groups that contract with the insurer to provide all the clinical care a patient needs, for a fixed monthly payment) typically enroll as many patients as possible, thereby "spreading risk" (the larger the group, the better the likely balance between those who need a lot of attention and those who do not) and increasing income (the more patients, the higher the monthly check from the insurer). Enrolling large groups of patients carries with it, however, increasing demand for appointments. If Dr. Albright and partners want to profit well from their capitation contract, they will each want to see as many patients as possible, rather than hire additional clinicians. More appointments per day may mean that some patients' charts are not reviewed before each visit, or that the history or the exam is truncated. Time to consider a case carefully may be lacking as well. In short, time pressures resulting from the doctors' desire to earn more money by enrolling as many patients as possible in their clinic could have *created the conditions* under which an otherwise competent physician missed the diagnosis of coronary artery disease.

Maximizing revenue by maximizing the numbers of patients seen per day is not unique to managed care. The fee-for-service system offers the physician economic incentives to do the same. Other factors also contribute to the pressure to see many patients per period of time, among them doctors' income expectations and the amount of money generated per visit. So-called Medicaid mills were fee-for-service situations in which many patients were "pushed through" in a given clinic day, in part because the reimbursement level per patient was disproportionately low compared to other insured patients. More patients had to be seen per unit of time to achieve an income equivalent to physicians in other settings. While in capitation arrangements, the managed care organization does not pay on a per-visit basis, the amount paid to the clinic per member enrolled per month may be so low that many patients must be enrolled if a doctor's income expectations are to be achieved. In either instance, the economic incentives influence the organization and delivery of care very directly. Both situations create a conflict of interest, for the payer (whether the Medicaid administration or the managed care organization) has created a payment mechanism in which physicians' economic self-interest is pitted against the ethical commitment to provide patients with appropriate care.

Unfortunately, there is no way to avoid this sort of conflict of interest in the practice of medicine so long as all clinicians must earn their livelihood by taking care of patients. Under a fee-for-service system, the doctor therefore has an incentive to do more of any service for which he or she is reimbursed. That is, the recommendation to test or to treat may be influenced by the desire to generate revenue. Since patients with adequate insurance have no reason to object to the physician's recommendations on economic grounds, the incentives present in fee-for-service can easily result in too much care. In particular, the physician has little incentive to desist from ordering tests that are relatively free of inherent risk, such as echocardiograms or most X-rays. Yet marginal or unnecessary tests can be dangerous. False positive tests (a stress test that is positive in a healthy young man) may lead to procedures with known risk of mortality (cardiac catheterization), not to mention anxiety and subsequent denials of insurability. Excess surgery clearly increases the risk of death in patients who need not have had the surgery in the first place (Franks, Clancy, and Nutting 1992). At the very least, the incentives present in the fee-for-service system do little to encourage consideration of the most cost-effective approach to care.

It comes as no surprise, then, that those interested in a more efficient, less costly health care delivery system—employers, patients, and the U.S. government among others—would look to systems of care that alter the incentives. Capitation contracts in managed care organizations like Truman Health create incentives to limit services, since physicians receive the same amount of money whether they see a patient two or twenty times a year, whether they order an echocardiogram or not, and whether they refer the patient to a specialist or not. Because every service provided costs a clinic like Dr. Albright's, the physicians have reason to think carefully before offering an additional appointment, ordering a test, or making a referral. The conflict of interest remains, but the incentive is to do less rather than more. In Dr. Albright's clinic, the incentives inherent in capitation may well have resulted in so little time with patients that Dr. Albright failed to think carefully about the symptoms Mr. Carmen described.

The failure to provide adequate time to properly assess patients represents a *systemic* problem arising in response to the capitation arrangement Dr. Albright's group entered into. Mr. Carmen's case thus may demonstrate the potential for disaster when entrepreneurial physicians take on more than they can reasonably handle in order to maximize their profit. Alternatively, it may demonstrate the potential for disaster when insurers pay physicians so little per patient that even a physician with modest income expectations must see patients at a pace that outstrips reasonable competence in order to pay the rent and staff salaries. Either way, the conflict of interest is not specific to the individual doctor-patient relationship—in this case, between Dr. Albright and Mr.Carmen—but generalizes to the implied commitment of the clinic to all those patients for whom it has assumed responsibility. The breach in ethical obligation occurs if the clinic's organizational efforts to maximize revenue result not only in more efficient care but in substandard care. Clearly, there is need for balance between a capitation system that encourages physicians not to see patients or to see them too briefly, thereby jeopardizing care, and a fee-for-service system that rewards unnecessary repeat patient visits and inefficiency without improved outcomes.

Incentives and the Physician-Patient Relationship

Let us assume for the moment that Dr. Albright *did* recognize Mr. Carmen's symptoms and risk factors as suggestive of coronary artery disease. Conservative management, justifiable perhaps at the outset, neither controlled rising cholesterol levels nor prevented escalating symptoms. Dr. Albright's failure to refer Mr. Carmen for cardiologic evaluation suggests that some other factor influenced the doctor's judgment. Perhaps the capitation arrangement with the Parkside Family Medical Clinic was structured internally through negotiated contracts with each individual physician so that clinical behavior and individual income were linked. Dr. Albright would suffer financially if he "overreferred," even within the clinic.

Contracts designed to influence an individual physician's decision making are common in both fee-for-service and managed care environments. In the fee-for-service setting, for instance, continued employment may be contingent on ordering a certain number of tests per month (Hemenway et al. 1990). In the managed care setting, it is common to withhold part of a physician's income pending evaluation of how much testing or referring he or she has done. Although there is general evidence that such incentives are associated with differences in practice, as yet there is little or no data on what level of "withhold" or, alternatively, "bonus" payment will consistently alter the behavior of individual clinicians. The dilemma about physician economic incentives arises because, in fact, some level of influence on physicians' clinical behavior is not only inevitable but desirable (Hall and Berenson 1998). Managed care organizations and the clinics with which they contract both seek to increase efficiency of care by reversing the economic incentives prevalent in fee-for-service practice. But the incentive to reduce unnecessary care risks becoming, as it did in Mr. Carmen's case, an incentive to provide substandard care.

Mr. Carmen's case highlights a critical difference in the implications of the conflict of interest between individual income and patient well-being that exist in both managed care and fee-for-service settings. In a fee-for-service setting, patients offered a test or treatment about which they are dubious have the option of seeking a second opinion. Patients therefore have greater potential to protect themselves against the excesses the fee-for-service system encourages. In the managed care setting, however, physicians may simply remain silent about the options they prefer patients not have. Unless patients are aware (as the Carmens apparently were) and can prevail upon their physicians to discuss and accede to alternative options (as the Carmens were not), there is a serious risk that the conflict of interest inherent in the individual physician's contract will result in inadequate care. Patients who are unaware that physicians are operating under such incentives are perhaps particularly vulnerable. To the extent that scenarios such as the Carmens' occur, one must conclude that some, and perhaps many, physicians are willing to rationalize inadequate care when their livelihood is at stake. Sadly, the physician's obligation to fidelity—to place the patient's interests ahead of one's own—is compromised.

The tragic outcome of the Carmens' case does not mean that all incentives to save money in health care are morally intolerable. Indeed, there is no system that is without perverse incentives. Even a salary-based system has been attacked on the grounds that physicians without a stake in their income will be disinclined to work as hard as they might. It is also worth noting that incentives designed to decrease inappropriate overuse of resources ultimately may allow managed care organizations to offer coverage not available as easily in the fee-for-service system, from preventive screening to prescription plans. For the Carmens, for physicians, and for policy makers, the problem then becomes one of discerning when resources are being used wisely and when they are being denied unfairly.

Preferences Are Not Necessarily Moral Claims

While Dr. Albright should have acted more expeditiously to evaluate and even to refer Mr. Carmen, and while financial considerations may have determined Dr. Albright's behavior, it does not follow that all decisions that economically favored Dr. Albright were morally wrong. For instance, Dr. Albright probably stood to gain financially by referring Mr. Carmen to Dr. Capulski, the clinic's cardiologist, but Dr. Albright nevertheless may also have been completely justified in insisting on this pattern of referral.

Dr. Albright is obligated to provide a reasonable standard of care to Mr. Carmen. Assuming that Dr. Capulski has proper credentials as well as the respect of her peers, there is no a priori reason to believe that the cardiologist the Carmens preferred was a better doctor. Furthermore, Dr. Albright may argue that he can more efficiently and effectively coordinate care with Dr. Capulski than with someone whose office is remote from the clinic and with whom he does not usually consult. If efficiency and effectiveness are served well by referral to Dr. Capulski, then Dr. Albright cannot be held responsible for the further delay in Mr. Carmen's care that resulted from the Carmens' decision to appeal the referral decision. A preference for a different doctor, assuming both to be of equal competence, does not translate into a moral claim on Dr. Albright to respect their choice.

Does Disclosure Matter?

Nonetheless, we feel that the Carmens have been wronged. But by whom? Here the issue of disclosure becomes important. The Carmens reasonably assumed that they could have access to anyone within their insurance plan, based on the information they received from Truman Health. The specific rules of Parkside Family Medical Clinic were unknown to them. Parkside was obligated to inform the Carmens about its unique procedures, because the more stringent limitation on referral options would have been material to the Carmens' decision to select Dr. Albright as their primary care physician.

Some might argue that Dr. Albright should personally have disclosed to the Carmens Parkside's arrangements with Truman Health and his own financial stake in that agreement. The practical problem is that most clinics and physician offices contract with many different insurance plans, each of which may have different terms. In larger group practices, individual physicians may even be totally unaware of the contract between their group and a particular payer. In addition, reimbursement formulas *within* clinics may be quite convoluted. Disclosure statements are therefore likely to be at best complicated and at worst misleading. Finally, the fact that a patient is primed by disclosure to suspect short shrift does not license managed care organizations or physicians to cut corners. The Hippocratic oath does not say, "Do no harm unless you can get away with it." Disclosure therefore cannot, at least by itself, address the problems inherent in incentives to underserve.

Managed care organizations like Truman Health, however, ought to disclose the methods that they employ to achieve savings in health care delivery. Disclosure by the organization differs from disclosure by the physician in two important ways. First, the individual who has a choice of insurance plans may find such information material to the decision regarding which plan to choose. The consumer choosing between insurance options is in a different position from the patient already in a particular insurance plan who visits a primary care physician for the first time. Second, disclosures by insurers may help consumers to understand that there are real trade-offs between the cost of insurance and freedom of choice. By and large, the more autonomy patients wish to exercise, the more out-of-pocket costs they will encounter, either in copayments or in premiums. Assuming reasonably comprehensible disclosure, the individual should then be expected to comply with the limitations on autonomy associated with the choice of a less costly health plan.

Towards "Morally Tolerable" Conflict of Interest

No reimbursement method can avoid altogether introducing conflict-of-interest issues into the physician-patient relationship, but there are approaches that are potentially less problematic than direct financial incentives to either do too much or too little. An acceptable system would reward care that is both effective and cost-conscious (American College of Physicians 1998), but the rewards would be remote from individual patient care decisions.

An ethically defensible cost-conscious system would also have to account for the variability in patient populations. Particularly when clinical groups share risk with the managed care organization, there is an incentive to enroll those patients least likely to need care—the young, the affluent, and the healthy—and to avoid attracting those most in need of help—the ill and the less affluent. Therefore, a managed care organization's contracts with clinicians must be adjusted for the "risk of utilization," so as not to penalize those who are willing to assume the care of the most frail or least affluent patients.

Finally, the worst excesses of both the fee-for-service and the managed care systems could be avoided if *appropriate care* as well as economic prudence were rewarded. Absent incentives to meet certain standards of quality, however, any reimbursement scheme inevitably emphasizes the fiscal implications rather than the clinical outcomes of care. Conflicts of interest inherent in physician reimbursement schemes must therefore be balanced by vigorous quality monitoring, outcome assessment, and quality improvement (American Medical Association 1995).

Public information about relative quality of care among clinical groups and managed care organizations could serve as a serious disincentive against abuses and create competition on the basis of quality rather than price alone. Unfortunately, currently available data primarily reflect patient satisfaction surveys, which provide important information about the service orientation of individual clinics or large managed care organizations, but little about the technical quality of care or the relative rates and duration of illness among enrollees (Povar 1995). Likewise, grievance patterns may provide insights into failed patient-provider relationships, but these patterns do not necessarily reflect the quality of medical judgments.

Managed care's computerized systems, designed to monitor costs, are enormous potential sources of information about actual medical care, from referral to prescribing patterns. Managed care organizations are thus already equipped to balance concerns about underservice by measuring and reporting publicly on quality of care. Managed care organizations would thereby actively support the ethical obligation of physicians to do good and to avoid harm. Confronted with evidence of economic incentives run amok, physicians could not rationalize away below-standard outcomes in their patient populations. Finally, measuring outcomes of care will permit comparisons of different processes of care in terms of the trade-offs between efficiency and quality.

The characteristics of a more ethically sound reimbursement system are as follows, and they apply equally to physician, clinic, and managed care organization, for all are engaged in a shared endeavor to provide efficient and appropriate care. Incentives should reflect (1) the global experience of a relatively large group of clinicians (to increase the personal distance between income and decision), (2) an annual (as opposed to monthly or quarterly) assessment of relative savings (or losses) to increase the temporal distance between income and clinical decisions, (3) a modest (so as not to overwhelm other variables) proportion of overall income, (4) health care utilization adjusted for the specifics of the physicians' patient populations, and (5) quality measures, ranging from relationship issues to appropriate use of screening tests to referral for specialist management of chronic illness, with regular feedback to individual physicians regarding their performance relative to professional norms. Had these conditions existed when the Carmens first sought care from Dr. Albright, Mr. Carmen might have lived to comment on the excellent care he received from his managed care plan.

References

American Medical Association, Council on Ethical and Judicial Affairs. 1995. "Ethical Issues in Managed Care." *Journal of the American Medical Association* 273, no. 4:330–35.
American College of Physicians, Ethics and Human Rights Committee. 1998. "Ethics Manual, Fourth Edition." *Annals of Internal Medicine* 128, no. 7:576–94.
Franks, P.; Clancy, C. M; and Nutting, P. A. 1992. "Gatekeeping Revisited—Protecting Patients from Overtreatment." *New England Journal of Medicine* 327, no. 6:424–27.
Hall, M. A., and Berenson, R. A. 1998. "Ethical Practice in Managed Care: A Dose of Realism." *Annals of Internal Medicine* 128, no. 5:395–402.
Hemenway, D.; Killen, A.; Cashman, S. B.; Parks, C. L.; and Bicknell, W. J. 1990. "Physicians' Responses to Financial Incentives: Evidence from a For-Profit Ambulatory Care Center." *New England Journal of Medicine* 322, no. 15:1059–63.

Povar, G. J. 1995. "Profiling and Performance Measures: What are the Ethical Issues?" *Medical Care* 33, no. 1:JS60–68.

COMMENTARY _____

Mark A. Hall, J.D.

Capitation or other financial incentives—such as bonuses or withholds—directed to physicians are *permissible*. They are not, however, ethically *ideal* since they create a financial conflict of interest between the patient's best medical interest and the physician's economic interest. Under these payment methods, physicians are rewarded for compromising optimal care. Fiduciary principles of both law and ethics frown on financial conflicts of interest (Rodwin 1993; Orentlicher 1996). A fiduciary relationship is one where one party confers great trust and power in another, creating a situation of vulnerability. Examples include lawyer-client, priest-penitent, trustee-beneficiary, and agent-principal relationships. The physician-patient relationship fits squarely within this model. However, fiduciary legal principles do not ban all financial conflicts of interest; they only insist that financial conflicts be reasonable, disclosed, and agreed to by those affected (Hall 1996).

To demand more than this is unrealistic, since conflicts of interest are ubiquitous in human affairs and permeate medical relationships under any payment system (Hall 1996). For instance, fee-for-service reimbursement also creates a conflict of interest by encouraging physicians to overtreat patients and to run up costs. Even straight salary is not beyond reproach, since this method of payment encourages doctors to slack off. The dangers of fee-for-service incentives may not be as serious as incentives to undertreat, but incentives to contain costs may also have virtuous aspects. Fee-for-service payment rewards doctors more the sicker their patients are, whereas capitation payment rewards doctors for keeping their patients healthy. The health promotion incentive can be seen here in the fact that Mr. Carmen received cholesterol screening and an echocardiogram even prior to having any symptoms; he also received dietary and lifestyle advice, as well as medication to reduce cholesterol.

In addition, capitation and other cost-containment incentives directed to physicians can be ethically defended by observing that the flaws of other forms of cost containment are even worse. Keeping health care and health insurance affordable is a legitimate social goal that can be achieved through a variety of means. One is to make patients pay more of the costs of their treatment. But this is not feasible for the poor, and it requires going without insurance to some extent and forces consideration of finances during the anxiety and vulnerability of illness. The second broad mechanism for rationing is for third parties such as insurers or government agencies to set explicit, rule-based limits on what treatments are unnecessary or not worth the cost. Many ethicists maintain that rule-based rationing is preferable to physician bedside rationing (Hall, 1997a), but some disagree. Although ideal democratic and deliberative institutions might be imagined for this role, such institutions do not presently exist and are difficult to create and maintain. Tough social problems usually cannot be solved in the real world by imagining ideal decision makers and then calling them into being. Even if this were not so, there are many reasons why setting rule-based limits on medical practice is not the best solution, all of which are captured in the insight that medicine is as much an art as it is science.

For bedside rationing to be justified, it is not necessary that everyone agree with this approach. It is ethically significant, however, that some substantial number of people agree. Public opinion polls confirm that this indeed is the case. In most such polls, people prefer by a wide margin that, in general, if limits must be imposed, they are best imposed through discretionary decisions made by physicians at the bedside, considering the alternatives. This is known as the logic of the second best or the least worst. As Winston Churchill might say, bedside rationing is the worst form of cost containment, except for all the others. If bedside rationing is the role that society assigns to physicians, medical ethics is not entitled to object. Medical ethics is a role-based ethic, one that responds to and implements the role that society assigns physicians rather than a more universal or absolutist ethic that defines the role itself (Hall 1994). Therefore, medical ethics can help articulate how bedside rationing should occur, but it is not entitled to prohibit it altogether.

Financial incentives are one among several possible mechanisms for implementing bedside rationing. Other mechanisms such as educating, cajoling, and advising physicians are also possible, but empirical studies show they have much less impact than we might hope. Financial motivation has been adopted because it works. It is not inherently suspect or evil, as long as it is kept within proper bounds (Hall 1994, 1997a).

As financial conflicts go, the one in this case is well within bounds. For the most part, the payment to the Parkside Family Medical Clinic targets its physicians' time and not their out-of-pocket expenses. We are not told precisely how the clinic in turn compensates Dr. Albright, but the incentive to him is probably pooled with the incentive to all physicians in the clinic. This dilutes the impact of the incentive on any single treatment decision, such as the denial of Mr. Carmen's request for a cardiac referral. Dr. Albright is also probably subject to different types of incentives from other fee-for-service and managed care payers, and he may not be immediately aware of which patient has which kind of insurance. Again, this serves to dilute the impact of the incentive of any individual treatment decision.

Although apparently not the case here, capitation payment is even more ethically acceptable if it occurs within a nonprofit salaried setting where all the patients come from a single insurer. Then, it can fairly be said that money saved on one patient goes to help another patient in the same insurance pool who the physician believes needs the resources more. Allocation within a group modifies but does not reject the traditional medical ethic that allows no form of allocation. Group-based allocation still allows physicians to strive for medically optimal care for all of their patients, given the resources at hand (Hall and Berenson 1998).

Regardless of the precise financial arrangements, there are several guidelines for maintaining ethical standards in the face of conflicting incentives. One is for physicians to exercise impartiality in their medical judgment, that is, to offer the same level of medical care for each of their patients, without regard to source or amount of payment (Hall and Berenson 1998). This might not always be realistic, however, if the sources and amounts of payment are widely divergent, for instance, ranging from no insurance to Medicaid to commercial HMO coverage to unlimited indemnity. An alternative approach, therefore, is treatment-specific disclosure. If Dr. Albright felt that Mr. Carmen's insurance did not allow him to offer the level of care he personally thought was acceptable in the circumstances, he could have told Mr. Carmen as much. "Gag clauses" in managed care contracts that would prevent such communications are widely considered unethical and are now illegal in most jurisdictions (Morreim 1997; Sage 1997). Dr. Albright could also have made sure that Mr. Carmen knew about the financial incentives that potentially affected Dr. Albright's medical decisions.

Disclosure of physician financial incentives presents additional issues meriting discussion: Who should disclose? When? And at what level of specificity? For reasons already discussed, physicians should certainly be free to make bedside disclosures of financial conflicts of interest as part of the process of informed consent, but is this mandatory? In general, this is not currently required by informed consent law, and there are pragmatic reasons for removing this onus from the bedside doctor. The primary ethical obligation should rest with Truman Health at or before the point of enrollment, with periodic reminders during each renewal period. It is Truman Health that created the first layer of incentives that filtered down to Dr. Albright. Although the clinic creates the second layer of incentives in the manner in which they paid Dr. Albright, it would be best if Mr. Carmen had had this information prior to enrollment or prior to seeking treatment, when it might have been relevant to his choice of insurance or primary care physician. Requiring Dr. Albright to make this disclosure at each treatment encounter not only would be unrealistic and formalistic, it would be counterproductive since it would require him to focus on the very incentives that we hope operate only as background or subliminal influences. A preference would be the "transparency standard" for informed consent, which would require Dr. Albright to disclose only his actual thought processes and deliberations and not to constantly make self-deprecating confessions of potential fallibility (Brody 1992). The latter obviously threatens to undermine patients' trust.

Truman Health's disclosure of financial incentives could take many forms. Haavi Morreim (1997) has crafted a plain language description of each of the major incentive methods, including capitation, salary, and fee withholds. Alternatively, Truman Health might choose to define capitation and put the consumer on more specific notice of possible effects, including the extent to which various categories of providers bear risk and the potential disincentives to render or refer care. It is difficult to know which of several approaches is preferable without some period of experimentation and study. We do not know very much about what information patients are interested in or capable of absorbing and how they will react to this information.

Until we know more about these issues, it is difficult to formulate a legal requirement for disclosure of financial incentives. As of 1998, only a few states have made disclosure mandatory through statutory law. One federal appellate court has imposed a disclosure obligation as a matter of fiduciary law under Employee Retirement Income Security Act (ERISA) (*Shea v. Esensten* 107 F. 3d 625 [8th Cir. 1998]). In other cases, the issue is pending whether disclosure is required by common law tort doctrine in order to avoid medical malpractice or informed consent liability. Still elsewhere, a few HMOs have undertaken disclosure voluntarily, and this trend is likely to accelerate.

Despite these uncertainties, some legal mandate for disclosure is desirable and probably inevitable. Purely voluntary disclosure might be sufficient for a short time, as a way to experiment with different approaches and gain valuable practical experience. But HMOs' competitive concerns over corporate image make them reluctant to be the first to undertake disclosure, and antitrust concerns may keep them from doing so in concert. Legal pressure is probably necessary to make disclosure happen on a widespread basis. The source of law should be federal rather than state, since state law may not reach self-insured employers and state requirements will undoubtedly be inconsistent. The federal law should be regulatory/statutory in nature, rather than being imposed by the courts. The risk of inconsistent directives is even greater coming from juries, and it is too easy for juries to second-guess the inadequacies of disclosure after the fact and thereby impose disclosure requirements that are unattainable or excessive. If HMOs fail to make the required disclosures, however, it is certainly appropriate for juries to assess liability and damages where injury results.

Mr. Carmen's case is one such instance where disclosure was not made. What should the legal consequences be? Mrs. Carmen's lawsuit alleges that the incentives caused Dr. Albright to make bad medical decisions, which led to her husband's preventable death. If these allegations are true, should liability be imposed on Truman Health? The law on this matter is not settled, but reasoned analysis is possible based on analogy from legal precedent.

If Dr. Albright's decisions fell below the prevailing standard of medical care, not only is Dr. Albright responsible, but in all likelihood so is Truman Health under theories of vicarious institutional liability for medical malpractice. This is not primarily because of the financial incentives, however. It is simply because we are assuming for the moment that medical malpractice occurred and because of Truman Health's relationship with Dr. Albright (which in part is a financial relationship). The suit against Truman Health would likely be preempted by ERISA. To avoid ERISA preemption, Mrs. Carmen would have to sue Dr. Albright directly. In a suit against Truman Health, under ERISA, she could receive damages from Truman Health only for the promised benefit, namely the cost of treatment, but not for personal injury or punitive damages. This is because ERISA was written with pension plans in mind, which affect only financial affairs. This thoughtless and accidental legal scheme cries out for reform, but so far Congress has failed to act, largely because of the intense web of vested interests that surround existing ERISA law.

If we assume, on the other hand, that Dr. Albright's care was not substandard, then we reach a series of different legal conclusions. Although Dr. Albright could not then be sued personally for medical negligence, Mrs. Carmen still might sue either him or Truman Health or the clinic, claiming that Dr. Albright's decisions would have been different if Truman Health and the clinic had not created the financial conflict of interest. This raises the issue of whether Truman Health's and the clinic's payment methods, in and of themselves, constitute an independent, actionable legal wrong. Existing law says almost nothing on this issue. One federal court held that capitation payment may constitute a breach of fiduciary duty by an HMO if the payment method is not disclosed (Shea v. Esensten), but here the case states that Mr. Carmen knew that Truman Health's payment methods discouraged referrals outside his group. All that he failed to realize is that the payment method discouraged a referral at all, but that is largely moot since the decision to make a referral had been made. At most, the referral was delayed. Even if this gives rise to a claim against Truman Health, it would likely be preempted by ERISA, which severely limits damage recoveries.

Another legal basis for suit, one that might be brought against Dr. Albright even if his care was not substandard, is failure to obtain informed consent. However, informed consent actions are usually not brought when treatment is foregone. Moreover, there is only scant legal support for recognizing informed refusal liability when the patient realizes the medical risks but fails only to understand the financial factors affecting the physician's decision. In addition, as noted, Mr. Carmen already knew some of the financial factors.

Should the law evolve to embrace new or expanded theories of liability related to the use of financial incentives? If a payment incentive is otherwise legal and has been adequately disclosed by the HMO, it should not, standing alone, serve as the basis for liability. If negligent treatment occurs, then the payment incentive might be found to be a contributing factor, helping to expose the HMO to liability for the physician's medical malpractice. As noted, however, there may be no adequate remedy against the HMO due to ERISA preemption, which is a serious flaw that should be corrected.

One further possibility exists: A financial conflict of interest might be used to heighten the damages against a negligent physician by awarding punitive as well as compensatory damages. Plaintiffs' lawyers can encourage a jury to find that, in light of the financial conflict, what might otherwise be viewed as an ordinary medical mistake is instead willful or wanton misconduct deserving severe punishment. The few courts that have spoken on this point have ruled that, if the financial incentive is otherwise legal and appropriate, it should not be introduced into evidence for this purpose since it is not relevant to liability and will likely inflame the jury (Hall 1997b). Other courts will undoubtedly differ.

To summarize, the financial incentives that Truman Health and the clinic used to encourage Dr. Albright to minimize treatment costs are ethically and legally permissible, but they should have been disclosed to patients. Mr. Carmen knew something about these incentives; how much more he should be told, when, and by whom are issues on which reasonable minds can differ and on which we require more study and experimentation. If an inadequate disclosure is made, the legal result is unsettled. The clearest case is one that assumes Dr. Albright's care was negligent. Then, liability turns on simple medical malpractice law subject to ERISA preemption, but not so much on the financial incentives. If care was not substandard, Mrs. Carmen still might sue either Dr. Albright or Truman Health and the clinic based on breach of fiduciary duty and lack of informed consent, but this legal theory has not yet been established in legal precedents and its factual basis in this case is not strong, considering what Mr. Carmen apparently knew about his medical condition and the way in which Truman Health operates.

References

Brody, H. 1992. *The Healer's Power*. New Haven, Conn.: Yale University Press, pp. 115–18.

Hall, M. A. 1994. "Rationing Health Care at the Bedside." *New York University Law Review* 69, no. 4-5:693–780.

———. 1996. "Physician Rationing and Agency Cost Theory." In *Conflicts of Interest in*

Clinical Practice and Research. Edited by R. Spece, D. S. Shimm, and A. E. Buchanan. New York: Oxford University Press.

———. 1997a. *Making Medical Spending Decisions: The Law, Ethics and Economics of Rationing*. New York: Oxford University Press.

———. 1997b. "A Theory of Economic Informed Consent." *Georgia Law Review* 31:511.

Hall, M. A., and Berenson, R. 1998. "Ethical Practice in Managed Care: A Dose of Realism." *Annals of Internal Medicine* 128, no. 5:395–402.

Morreim, E. H. 1997. "To Tell the Truth: Disclosing the Incentives and Limits of Managed Care." *American Journal of Managed Care* 3, no. 1:35–43.

Orentlicher, D. 1996. "Paying Physicians More to Do Less: Financial Incentives to Limit Care." *University of Richmond Law Review* 30:155.

Rodwin, M. 1993. *Medicine, Money and Morals: Physicians' Conflicts of Interest*. New York: Oxford University Press.

Sage, W. M. 1997. "Mandatory Public Disclosure in Managed Care: Lessons From the Securities Industry." In *Achieving Quality in Managed Care: The Role of Law*. Edited by J. Blum. Chicago: Health Law Section of the American Bar Association, monograph 5.

7

Shifting Costs and Care to Public Programs

CASE STUDY

Seven-year-old Anna was diagnosed with a brainstem glioma that was treated with radiation five months ago. During the course of radiation therapy, Anna had difficulty with recurrent aspiration pneumonia and a feeding tube was placed so that the therapy could be completed. At the conclusion of her radiation therapy, an MRI showed some decrease in the size of the tumor, and Anna was discharged from the hospital to her home. She received daily visits from nurses and a physical therapist from Redwood Home Care.

One month later, Anna began to have seizures and was rehospitalized. She was placed on a ventilator to assist with breathing, and a CT scan showed severe damage to the brainstem. A care conference was held. In response to information about the devastation to her brainstem and the physician's prediction that Anna would likely die within two weeks, Anna's family chose to have her extubated, signed DNR/DNI (do not resusitate/do not intubate) and DNH (do not hospitalize) orders, and took her home with comfort care measures in place. Anna's feeding tube was discontinued, and she was placed on intravenous fluids and medications for pain, agitation, and anxiety. At home, she received twenty-four-hour nursing care provided by Redwood Home Care.

Redwood is a for-profit home care agency located in a northwestern state. Redwood contracts with individuals, provides services to patients within its parent health system, and contracts with health plans like Anna's HMO. Anna is enrolled in a staff model HMO (that is, an HMO whose physicians are salaried employees) that purchases home care from Redwood on a discounted fee-for-service basis. Anna's physician is a salaried employee of the HMO and becomes eligible for bonuses when his capitated clinic meets quarterly financial targets.

Three weeks after being home, Anna moved slightly to touch, responded to pain but not to verbal commands, and held her body stiff with her back arched when her temperature was elevated. Since Anna had survived longer than expected, her family began to question whether Anna's situation was as hopeless as the physician had indicated. Anna's mother began to express concern that they may not have given her an adequate chance to live. Despite Anna's episodes of hyperventilation and agonal breathing, Anna's physician agreed to the parents' request to reverse the DNR/DNI and DNH orders and resume tube-feeding.

The HMO case manager considered these steps tantamount to adopting a "maintenance" approach to Anna's care, a benefit that was excluded from the HMO's contract with its enrollees. She called a care conference to arrange for the initiation of an application for the transfer of coverage responsibility for Anna from the HMO to Medicaid, which would entail a transfer of her care from Redwood Home Care to the state's contracted home care agency.

Anna's primary nurse from Redwood was very concerned about whether the mother's decision making was adequately informed. It seemed that Anna's best interests were not the focus in discussions about her care plan and that her family needed more assistance with their adjustment to her continued grave situation. The care conference disturbed her more. After the physician reviewed Anna's medical condition, he concluded that Anna was not "actively dying" but was in a "steady state." He said that it was not clear what had happened in her brainstem. When Anna's nurse asked if he had changed his view that Anna's diagnosis was terminal, he responded that they had been fooled many times before.

The case manager explained that because Anna was not actively dying, and her family was choosing to discontinue her DNR/DNI and DNH orders, start tube feedings, and if necessary, hospitalize her and treat her with antibiotics, her care would be classified as maintenance care and would no longer be covered by the HMO. She explained that the costs of Anna's care would be assumed by Medicaid and that her care would be transferred to another agency after a two-week transition. If, however, the family were to choose to end the feedings, the HMO would then consider Anna terminal and cover comfort care for her.

The home care nurse was disturbed by the failure of the physician and the case manager to discuss Anna's care plan in terms of goals that could reasonably be held for Anna, or to discuss the nature of each of the options open to the family. The desires of the HMO and the HMO-employed physician to be free of financial responsibility for a very costly client were obvious to her. Anna's parents were told details of the transition to the new coverage arrangement only if they asked. They were not told that the state would cover less care than Anna had been receiving, despite her extensive reliance on technological supports and constant medical monitoring. Because Medicaid would also be using the "maintenance" classification, a licensed practical nurse or a personal care attendant would be covered but not the specialist nurse who had been caring for Anna. Anna's family would have to manage more and more of her care, although they were not being informed of this.

Indeed, it became clear to Anna's mother only late in the care conference that the care team would soon be replaced by an entirely new team of nurses and that coverage "might not be" provided by the state for the same level of care Anna had been receiving. Since the HMO also held the Medicaid contract for the county in which Anna lived, the HMO would continue to provide case management and medical services to Anna after the state became responsible for coverage. The payer and the home care personnel would change, and the HMO would begin to receive reimbursement for the health care and case management services it would continue to provide for Anna.

Just before the transition to the other home care agency was to take place, Anna had another severe seizure and was rehospitalized. The family then requested that the DNR/DNI and DNH orders be reinstated. Anna's home care remained with Redwood until she died two months later. The family continued to have difficulties coping with Anna's dying, but no support system was made available to them.

Questions for Consideration

➤ Should a managed care organization cover end-of-life care but not maintenance home care? What effect might a policy permitting coverage of one but not the other have on a capitated physician's or a capitated plan's approach to end-of-life decision making?

➤ What should the Redwood Home Care nurse do if she feels that her professional obligations are being compromised by either the actions of HMO representatives or the HMO's benefit exclusions?

➤ How should conflicts of interest that arise from risk-sharing arrangements be addressed in situations like Anna's?

➤ As home care becomes more prevalent, and health plans control care options, how can clients, families, and contracting entities be guaranteed access to effective ethics consultation services? Whose ethics resources should be involved? Redwood Home Care's? The HMO's? The state's? All of them? Some other source?

COMMENTARY

Joel E. Frader, M.D., M.A.

The case involving Anna and home care raises a number of important ethical issues, although it is quite possible that some of the same concerns would have arisen under a more traditional indemnity insurance program. In this case, the problems revolve around (1) clinical issues, including the value of home care, uncertainty about prognosis in fatal illnesses in childhood, and difficulties professionals and family members have acknowledging and communicating clearly about end-of-life care in pediatrics; and (2) the recent drive to reduce spending in health care.

Managed care, especially when it involves capitation, has increased the pressure on institutions and individuals by attaching financial penalties to the use of health care resources. Any insurance mechanism, whether for-profit or nonprofit, in which clinicians and/or administrators perceive systemwide demands to reduce spending (and therefore to contract with providers that "discount" their services) risks a tendency to provide inadequate services for the members of the plan.

Clinical Concerns

The case illustrates a recent trend in medical care in the United States that has received little analysis by those in bioethics or health policy. After radiation therapy, Anna's care shifts from the hospital to her home without much fanfare. We know only that she received (presumably because she required) daily nursing attention and physical therapy. The assumption here is that home care is appropriate in the first place. The drive to provide more in-home medical treatment has two distinct origins (Okun 1995). The first, which emerged from pediatrics and geriatrics, developed out of the recognition that patients and families often prefer a more homelike environment than has typically been available in the hospital. With chronically ill children, especially those with chronic respiratory failure, whose care was otherwise not especially complex, home care became desirable, in part, because of the focus on cognitive and emotional development. Clinicians and parents believed that stimulation and consistency of care were more likely to be achieved at home than in the hospital, despite good efforts from skilled nurses, child life specialists, and others. Elderly patients were often much more comfortable, more oriented, and more cooperative in familiar surroundings, especially their own homes. The push to increase home care has also been economically motivated. Under many circumstances, home care is less expensive than hospital care, given the large fixed costs of running hospitals, which are inevitably reflected in patient charges.

So what could be better? Children develop more quickly at home; older patients prefer the psychological advantages of surroundings they know well. There are many fewer institutionally acquired infections; and it costs less. However, the last claim is problematic. What a managed care plan has to pay out for home care may be less, but the overall economic and psychosocial costs have yet to be fully tallied. Home care arrangements rarely provide twenty-four-hour nursing care or home health aide assistance. Family members and other loved ones typically make up the difference. The opportunity costs of the time devoted by parents, children of the elderly, friends, and others are rarely counted when the true costs of home care are calculated. The time spent by others could be measured in dollars per hour to provide care equivalent to that provided in institutional settings. Moreover, when loved ones must themselves give up income-generating activities in order to provide care in the home, these too are real costs of the in-home services (Sevick et al. 1996).

Over and above these costs, home care can engender significant emotional and social stress. How shall we account for the anxiety of having responsibility for medical and nursing care felt by those without professional training or supervision or for the lost sleep, diminution in opportunity to engage in social activities, and reduction in the capacity to spend time with other family members? All of these things change when we shift care from hospitals and nursing homes to family dwellings.

Some families readily and willingly adapt. Others do not. Yet today we rarely take the time to think about these imposed costs and even more rarely hesitate to send patients home. As a society we have not looked seriously at the question of how great a burden—financial, social, psychological—we can reasonably ask families to assume. In the case of Anna, one might well wonder whether there is an unexplored subtext that involves the difficult disruptions associated with home care. Perhaps Anna's family members are reacting, even unconsciously, to the weight of Anna's care that has been shifted to them.

After Anna's rehospitalization and the demonstration of progressive brain damage, the clinicians predict that Anna will die within two weeks. Physicians are notoriously bad at predicting the time until death, and predictions about dying children appear to be more elusive than prognostications about dying adults. In any case, most providers of pediatric palliative care urge caution in attempting firm statements about how long it will be before the child dies. It is hard to imagine that capitated care arrangements would alter the likelihood that providers could make more accurate prognostic judgments. While it seems clear that patients whose deaths occur quickly will cost a health care system less money than whose who have a prolonged course, this should not affect how well clinicians predict survival time. In this case, it appears that the expected short time until death probably contributed to Anna's parents' willingness to agree to limitations for her treatment. When the prediction failed to come true, Anna's family lost some degree of confidence and trust in what the doctors had told them.

The case does not detail what the physicians did or did not say to Anna's family about her expected clinical course. One would hope that what they said revealed the large element of medical uncertainty in prognostic pronouncements. One can also hope that part of the ongoing interaction—this discussion is likely to need much more than a single, all-inclusive "care conference"—between the clinicians and the family would include making sure the parents understand what they have been told. In addition, the clinicians should attempt to appraise the family members' emotional response to the developments surrounding Anna's deterioration. Under capitated arrangements, clinicians generally have no way to seek compensation for the time and effort required for explanatory and supportive communication aimed at helping families and patients. Thus, the professionals have at least an implicit incentive to minimize their interaction with the family. To be fair, however, even in a fee-for-service system, clinicians could rarely obtain reasonable payment for counseling and support under similar circumstances.

We can only speculate about Anna's mother's guilt. Guilt does constitute one element of grief. Perhaps forthright, repeated, compassionate acknowledgement of how difficult it must be for the parents to lose their daughter, to experience some loss of trust in their doctors, and to watch Anna's loss of capacity might have helped reduce the family distress and avert their request to reverse the limits on rescue attempts.

Issues in Case Management

The struggle over who should provide (and pay for) home care seems to have arisen from a rather legalistic (or perhaps merely bureaucratic) approach to whether Anna's care amounted to "maintenance" services or palliative care and hospice services. From the HMO case manager's perspective, Anna's home care, without the DNR/DNI and DNH (or other) limitations, was not part of what the HMO was obligated to provide under the terms of the contract. We presume that the contract requires maintenance care to come from the state's Medicaid program because care of chronically ill, severely disabled persons is expensive and often goes on for a long time. What disturbs the primary care nurse and us is that the case manager seems concerned only with contractual matters and shifting costs to another entity. The values of good patient care appear to be abandoned.

With the switch from Redwood Home Care to Medicaid, continuity of care is lost. The relationships built between the Redwood nursing staff and the family apparently mean little to the HMO. Clearly, the HMO does not seem troubled by the reduction in the amount (hours per day) or skill level (registered nurse versus licensed practical nurse or patient care assistant) of the care Anna will receive when Redwood departs. Contracts and dollars take precedence over clarifying the goals of care and designing interventions intended to meet those goals.

Falling back on artificial, if not bizarre, distinctions between the patient's condition as "steady state" versus "actively dying" seems to miss the point. The clinicians had an obligation (1) to understand the impact of Anna's condition on her family, especially in light of the failed prediction as to the timing of her death; (2) to assess the patient's and the family's need for physical care and psychosocial support; and (3) to design, with appropriate family participation, a plan of care designed to meet mutually agreed-upon goals. Whatever financial and other constraints might arise as to how to achieve the goals, those constraints do not diminish the professional obligation to attempt to provide treatment consistent with some sense of fidelity toward the family. That is to say, while managed care contracts may specify the conditions of care, they must not ignore the underlying goal: provision of a reasonable level of health care services for the members. To do otherwise—to see the contract as simply a series of limitations on what the company has to provide—ignores the clinical duty doctors and nurses have to try to meet the needs of their patients. Service beyond mere contractual relations is constitutive of the very notion of professionalism, at least in a traditional sense.

The "flexibility" displayed by the case manager in "offering" to continue Redwood's involvement contingent on the family's acceptance of limits on rescue efforts seems coercive. Few insurance programs of any sort provide for specific hospice services for children. Indeed, there are few hospice programs in the United States designed especially for children. Most efforts to provide pediatric palliative and hospice care in the United States have gone forward only with an understanding that the "usual" (Medicare-driven) rules of forgoing "heroic" life-sustaining therapy and a firm prediction of death within six months simply will not work for parents and children. Many parents cannot, for emotional reasons, agree to put aside continued rescue efforts. If insurers maintain a "no resuscitation" requirement for children to qualify for palliative and hospice care, many families who could benefit from these services would not be permitted to do so. It does no good to call this common parental response to the plight of their dying child "denial." The term refers to a normal and normally healthy psychological mechanism to defend against terribly painful thoughts and feelings. Denying the value of denial, while common enough, often gets health care professionals who work with dying children in trouble when they use confrontational tactics to get parents to "accept reality."

Managed care plans should, of course, include adequate arrangements for home care, including palliative and hospice care, designed to meet the needs of children. But given the statistically small likelihood of a plan needing to contract for pediatric hospice services in any given year and given the substantial cost of providing high-quality end-of-life home care, we should not be surprised that

HMOs and others have largely ignored this issue and approach it on a haphazard, case-by-case basis.

All of this raises the question of what staff members or families should do when conflicts about the adequacy of care emerge. Most managed care systems as well as indemnity insurance programs have appeals processes. Professionals have a duty to use these systems. If a clinician perceives that the services being provided to a patient (or family) fall below some reasonable standard, the professional has an obligation to bring the deficiency to the attention of the appropriate authorities. This duty presumably includes the need to appeal to the patient representative, if any, to a corporate ombudsperson or similar agent, or eventually to the medical and/or nursing director, if previous steps fail. Families should have access to the same appeals process. Some experts in home care for children go so far as to say that the families "should have the central role in determining what outcomes are important for them and their child and whether those outcomes are being achieved" (Perrin, Shayne, and Bloom 1993).

Whether or not ethics consultants or ethics committees have a place in these sorts of disputes seems far from clear. Ethics consultants either volunteer their time (that is, they have another role in the system and take on the consultative functions as an extra activity) or receive some compensation specifically related to their institutional ethics function. In either case, the consultant's fortunes are tied (sometimes literally) to those of the organization. No matter how well intentioned or virtuous, it seems quite unlikely that an ethics consultant could survive for long by squarely opposing policies and procedures designed to save money. Insiders who consistently demand more spending "just" for the sake of serving patients' or families' interests will find that they are expendable because their actions contradict institutional interests.

If this is true of consultants, it is probably even truer of committees. Committees will likely have administrative representatives in the group. Not only will such individuals directly defend organizational policy and mission, their presence may inhibit others from dissent (Lo 1987). One worries that ethics committees organized to react to troubles with managed care cases will become institutional window dressing designed to demonstrate the appearance rather than the substance of fair and effective systems for responding to perceived ethical violations. The matter turns on the actual independence of the ethics process—whether structured as consultation by individuals or as committee review.

One theoretical possibility for insulating the ethics investigative mechanism would involve review of cases, stripped of identifying information about patient, family, and providers, by individuals or groups without a direct financial tie to the managed care organization. This could be done by local universities with ethics programs, by accrediting bodies, or by voluntary organizations that provide educational and policy support and review to the industry. Of course, such arrangements could create bureaucratic and legal obstacles rendering them impractical, but they have the advantage of reducing potential conflicts of interest.

The Organization of Anna's Care

Care conferences notwithstanding, Anna's care did not seem efficiently or effectively organized. In theory, managed care fosters "care coordination." Here, we have coordination only in the most bureaucratic sense. The managers arranged ("coordinated") care by shifting it to a new set of in-home health care personnel, providing less service, because the rigid definitions of the type of care to which the patient was entitled under a contract so dictated. However, successful end-of-life care, including palliative and hospice care, arises from careful interdisciplinary planning and continuity of service. We do not know who participated in the conferences regarding Anna and her family. One hopes that a compassionate team of physicians, nurses, social workers, chaplains, therapists, and others who routinely participate in the delivery of home care, especially palliative and hospice care, would prevent the development of problems like those illustrated by this case. Sensitive team members focus their attention on the overall situation of the patient and family, rather than concentrate on purely technical aspects of physical care or the limits of the managed care organization's contract. They would attend to the problem of uncertainty in prognostication and communicate with families about the feelings patients and loved ones may experience (including anger with the professionals, guilt about decisions they reached, and so forth) while they await death. These same compassionate clinicians would remain in frequent communication with one another and with the family to assess developments and to provide new interventions as necessary.

The main ethical problem in Anna's case has to do with the change in the locus of authority for directing care. In managed care, decisions more and more rest with administrators (even if dressed in clinical clothes, as with some case managers) who focus on institutional interests, not on the interests of those served by the institution. While these interests do not *necessarily* conflict, they appear to conflict with alarming regularity. Conflicts of interest did and continue to exist in fee-for-service medicine. Under that system, clinicians and institutions benefited by excessive intervention. Most of the time excess resulted from fear of liability associated with leaving some stone unturned or from inadequate thought. Doctors and hospitals typically believed they were serving their patients, if somewhat naively accepting the notion of "more is better."

With the commodification of health services and the stress on relative scarcity and the need to conserve resources (if only to hold down costs), we have systems *designed* to reward clinicians and institutions for offering and providing less. We have become unbalanced. Major shifts in policy and economic behavior have had unforeseen and unintended (negative) consequences. Many barriers exist to providing satisfying home care for the medically complex child, including loss of privacy for family members when strangers invade their home, exhaustion associated with providing care when paid staff is not available, and guilt associated with the child's underlying condition and any perception of unmet needs under the circumstances of home care (Kohrman 1991). When managed care creates incentives for those responsible for providing the care to minimize assistance and maximize the family's hardship, we have to wonder whether we really want the "efficiencies" created by capitation.

References

Kohrman, A. F. 1991. "Medical Technology: Implications for Health and Social Providers." In *The Medically Complex Child: The Transition to Home Care*, pp. 3–13. Edited by N. J. Hochstadt and D. M. Yost. Chur, Switzerland: Harwood Academic Publishers.

Lo, B. 1987. "Behind Closed Doors: Promises and Pitfalls of Ethics Committees." *New England Journal of Medicine* 317, no. 1:45–50.

Okun, A. 1995. "The History of Respirators and Total Parenteral Nutrition in the Home and Their Use in Children Today." In *Bringing the Hospital Home: Ethical and Social Implications of High-Tech Home Care*, pp. 35–52. Edited by J. D. Arras. Baltimore: Johns Hopkins University Press.

Perrin, J. M.; Shayne, M. W.; and Bloom, S. R. 1993. *Home and Community Care for Chronically Ill Children*. New York: Oxford University Press.

Sevick M. A.; Kamlet M. S.; Hoffman L. A.; and Rawson I. 1996. "Economic Cost of Home-Based Care for Ventilator-Assisted Individuals." *Chest* 109, no. 6:1597–1606.

COMMENTARY _____

Ronald E. Cranford, M.D.
Karen G. Gervais, Ph.D.

Changing organizational arrangements and payment systems are creating new ethical dilemmas in American health care settings. When multiple payers, health systems, institutions, and providers, associated by diverse contractual and reimbursement arrangements, are involved in the care of an individual patient, impediments to effective communication and decision making, as well as to the continuity of care, may arise. Anna's case raises the question of whether traditional clinical ethics resources are adequate to address the ethical tensions in managed care arrangements, tensions arising from the impingement of clinical, financial, and organizational interests upon each other.

Anna's case illustrates the need to distinguish among clinical ethics, organizational ethics, and even interorganizational ethics. It suggests that an organizational ethics resource (for example, an individual or group skilled in conducting ethics consultations addressing dilemmas fueled by the clash of clinical, financial, and organizational interests) could have helped the health care professionals and organizations caring for this child, as well as her family. Further, the fact that there were multiple organizations involved in this case suggests that an independent, interorganizational ethics resource may sometimes be better than the ethics resources internal to any one of the organizations involved.

A Clinical Ethics Perspective

It is important to distinguish between ethical dilemmas unrelated to managed care and those that are generated or exacerbated by managed care arrangements. Many of the clinical issues in Anna's case are not unique to managed care. Until the first care conference, everything seems to have been handled well by the health care professionals and institutions involved. But when the physician wrote orders for the child's treatment and care at home, he made a serious error. He stopped the tube feedings but, for some unexplained reason, continued intravenous fluids. This decision triggered a series of adverse consequences for all the major participants in this case but particularly for the family. Many of these problems could have been avoided, or at least minimized, had the physician explained to the family the implications of stopping both artificial nutrition and hydration.

Had all medical treatment except palliative care measures been discontinued, Anna would have died within two weeks, as her physician predicted. But especially in cases involving children, while family, physicians, and nurses may be willing to stop artificial feedings, they cannot bring themselves to stop artificial hydration. The physician should have known, and he should have told the family, that with continued intravenous fluids the child could live longer than expected.

The physician should also have been clearer about Anna's prognosis. In caring for patients with serious neurologic conditions, physicians need to be very precise and explicit when distinguishing between a "poor prognosis" for recovery of neurologic functions, such as consciousness and other voluntary functions, and the prognosis for life itself. Anna's prognosis for neurologic function was extraordinarily poor when her brainstem glioma was first diagnosed and treated with radiation. Generally, children do very poorly with this type of tumor—with or without aggressive medical treatment—as the glioma continues to infiltrate the brainstem over a period of months or years. However, with vigorous treatment and artificial means to sustain vital functions of breathing, heart beat, blood pressure, eating, and drinking the prognosis for continued life can be quite variable.

During the care conference held before Anna's parents took her home, and during the following days and weeks, the family and the nurses should have been fully informed and educated about what to expect during the dying process. That Anna "moved slightly to touch, responded to pain but not to verbal commands, and held her body stiff with back arched when her temperature was elevated" did not mean that she was improving. It therefore represented no significant change in the overall prognosis for the recovery of meaningful neurologic functions. Of all life's tragedies, none is worse than losing a child. It is not surprising to learn that Anna's mother began to lose confidence in the physician's predictive abilities and recommendations for care and treatment and to express guilt about treatment decisions she and her husband had previously made. And it appears that there was no adequate support system for these parents, psychologically and in other respects. If a home hospice team had been involved, or if the patient had been placed in an institutional hospice, such support would very likely have been available.

It is hard to understand why the physician or other knowledgeable and experienced members of the health care team did not call another care conference to review the appropriateness of the treatment plan. At such a conference they could have explained to the family that Anna's outlook had not changed. They also could have explained why reinstituting aggressive treatment would only prolong Anna's suffering (in the unlikely event that she were conscious). Anna's episodes of hyperventilation and agonal respiration suggest that there was no good reason to restart aggressive treatment.

The physician's inaccurate description of Anna as not "actively dying" but in a "steady state," as well as his vagueness about the neurologic prognosis for recovery and his comments—that "they" (presumably doctors) had been fooled many times before—were not just bad ethics and bad economics but most of all bad medicine, and wholly insensitive to the emotional well-being of the family. The family's denial of their daughter's dying could only have been made worse by the physician's inaccurate and intemperate comments. Similarly, when Anna's care was classified as "maintenance care" by the HMO case manager, and thus no longer covered by the HMO, the family was offered a completely untenable choice. Already reeling with grief, guilt, and emotional pain, they were given a choice by the HMO: stop the feedings, let their daughter die now, and have the HMO pay for her care; or do not stop the feedings, let her live, and a new set of nurses would provide a potentially lower level of home care covered by Medicaid. If the family was feeling guilt before, imagine how they must have felt after being presented with this alternative.

Were there no neurologists, neurosurgeons, pediatric neurologists, or any physician with some degree of neurological expertise involved with this case who could have clarified the prognostic facts and helped the family to cope with the reality of their daughter's hopeless condition? There was no indication that any further neurological assessment of Anna's condition was sought when the family began to doubt the treatment plan that had been in place for several weeks. Would this not have been a justified expenditure, serving the interests of all concerned, in response to the family's deepening confusion?

Why did the physician and case manager conduct the care conference as they did? Why did the home care nurse not take a more active role in advocating for her patient, given her concerns? The explanation must lie in the organizational and financing arrangements surrounding Anna's care.

An Organizational Ethics Perspective

Until the HMO case manager considered reinstitution of aggressive treatment (reversal of DNR/DNI and DNH orders and surgical insertion of a feeding tube) as a "maintenance" approach to Anna's care, most of the ethical dilemmas and responses to them could be regarded as unrelated to organizational or financial arrangements. At this point, however, the ethical dilemmas were made much more complex and less amenable to humane resolution, apparently because of features of the organizational relationships involved, the employer/employee arrangement between the HMO and the physician, the purchaser of coverage and the HMO, and Redwood Home Care and the HMO.

Anna's case signals financial and organizational dilemmas that require ethics resources beyond those of a standard institutional ethics committee. She and her family were not served by a single health care organization alone. Multiple individuals and organizations with diverse interests, incentives, and commitments were involved. In Anna's case, the organizational participants included the hospital, the HMO-owned physician clinic, the HMO, and two home care organizations (one contracted to the HMO, the other to the state Medicaid program). The individual participants included specialists, the primary care physician, home care nurses, the case manager, and the patient's family.

Both the case manager's and physician's approach to the care conference are difficult to understand unless they can be attributed to the financial arrangements and organizational options affecting the providers and insurers in this case. The HMO, as well as the physician's clinic, is capitated for Anna's care, making her an enormously expensive patient for them both. The HMO apparently has the loophole of refusing coverage for maintenance care, even though the patient has a terminal diagnosis. Thus, the HMO has the cost-shifting option of enrolling Anna in a state-funded Medicaid program, which entails a change in home care provider. The physician and case manager seem to be more interested in the option to shift the cost of Anna's care to the state and its taxpayers than to promote ethically informed decision making on the part of her parents at this important juncture. The failure of Redwood Home Care's nurse to advocate on behalf of her patient may be attributable to the importance of her agency's maintaining its larger contractual relationship with the HMO.

The decision that was most financially beneficial to the staff model HMO and the physician in Anna's case—stopping treatment earlier rather than later, and also stopping treatment in such a way that death would occur within a shorter period of time—also happened to be the most humane and caring way of treating this child dying of a brainstem tumor. A decision to stop both nutrition and hydration, however, could easily be viewed as a serious conflict of interest for the HMO. This is unfortunate because of the chilling effect this perception might have on the responsible development of end-of-life care plans by providers and patients or their agents. When perceived or real conflicts of interest exist between what is in the best interest of the patient and family and what is in the best interest of the HMO, the managed care organization should have an organizational ethics resource with clearly defined access rules, an accountable process, and thorough medical records documentation.

Whose responsibility is it to call an ethics consultation? What might prevent a representative of the HMO or the home care organization from doing so? Whose ethics resources (assuming each organization represented at the table had one) should have been called? All of them? What ethics process could the family have accessed if it wished to? Anna's case focuses us on the question of how, in our increasingly complex health system, a safe haven for ethical reflection and decision making can be secured. It also raises the issue of how managed care organizations can avoid the charge of conflict of interest when they raise the issue of termination of treatment to patients and families. To eliminate costly end-of-life care is certainly in the financial interest of the HMO. So how can the HMO ensure that it provides adequate processes for decision makers that are not compromised by the HMO's financial interests?

Clinical Ethics Resources

Institutional ethics committees have proliferated throughout hospitals and long-term care facilities in the United States. These clinical ethics committees have developed a successful track record in the facilities they serve. However, they do not work nearly as well for health care organizations involved in managed care. A traditional hospital ethics committee would not, for example, have been of much value in Anna's case since once she went home, the committee no longer had any standing in the case. Furthermore, clinical ethics committees have not focused their attention on policies and activities having to do with organizational issues such as continuity of care and financing arrangements that involve issues such as risk-sharing on the part of physicians, cost-shifting, and resource allocation. They have little experience in addressing ethical issues arising out of the combination of the care delivery and financing roles that characterizes managed care.

Clinical ethicists have frequently emphasized the "three Cs" of ethical dilemmas—caring, communication, and common sense. Many apparent "ethical" dilemmas are in fact problems that stem from the need for a more caring and sensitive attitude toward patients, from a lack of communication between the physician (or various physicians, in the era of multispecialties and high technology) and the patient and loved ones, or from a lack of just plain common sense in making clinical decisions. Perhaps continuity should now be the fourth "C" of clinical ethics. Discontinuity of care is widespread and prevalent in U.S. medical care today. The discontinuity of care in Anna's case was exacerbated by the lack of coordination among the numerous health care organizations, individual providers, and payment systems that Anna's parents faced throughout their ordeal, which included acute care hospitalization, Redwood Home Care, the state's home care agency, the HMO, many specialists, the primary care physician, and the case manager; potential transfer to a new team of nurses financed by Medicaid; potential transfer to home hospice nurses or a hospice; then rehospitalization after a seizure. When continuity of care is threatened, and when complex organizational needs encroach unfavorably on patient care, ethics consultation becomes particularly important, but the best method of providing it becomes particularly unclear, when, as in Anna's case, multiple, contractually linked organizations are involved in caring for the patient.

Organizational Ethics Resources

The emergence nationwide of organizational ethics resources is still in the early stages of development; their development to this point corresponds roughly with the development of institutional ethics committees in the early 1970s. In the broadest sense, the overall mission of organizational ethics committees and organizational ethics consultants is to assist an organization and its individual components in addressing organizational issues of an ethical nature (in contrast to strictly clinical issues) by educating, advising on policies, and providing consultation services.

An organizational ethics resource could help those involved in Anna's case overcome the barriers to good decision making and to providing the full range of appropriate services for this patient and her family, including psychological and spiritual support for the parents. It could, for example, recommend (1) having a neurological specialist present at the care conferences to ensure that the family is fully informed of the neurologic condition and prognosis; (2) encouraging accurate and consistent communications with decision makers and avoiding confusing and contradictory terms to refer to Anna's situation (which in this case included: likely to die within two weeks; terminal diagnosis; terminal; terminal, if a decision is made to end tube feedings; imminently dying; hopeless; fooled many times before; maintenance approach; steady state; and not actively dying); and (3) reducing if not eliminating financial conflicts of interest on the part of Redwood Home Care's nurse, the physician, and the HMO.

An Interorganizational Ethics Resource

Which of the organizations involved should provide the organizational ethics resource in Anna's case? Clearly, a concern might arise about the potential bias of the ethics resource if it represents just one of the many organizations involved. Increasingly, as multiple organizations are involved in a patient's care, an independent organizational ethics resource may become important for ensuring unbiased and trusted ethical reflection and advice. Thus, in a case like Anna's, an interorganizational ethics resource, contractually agreed to in advance by the organizations involved, may be preferable when multiple organizations with conflicting interests require ethics resources.

The unfortunate way Anna's case was managed and the unnecessary harm this mismanagement brought to so many people illustrate the complex ethical issues that may arise in managed care settings. The ethical dilemmas in Anna's case occurred in stages, suggesting that effective clinical ethics consultation will play an essential preventive ethics role in our changing health care system. Preventive clinical ethics may resolve conflicts that would otherwise escalate into classic managed care ethical dilemmas, namely, clashes among the clinical, financial, and organizational interests at stake in the case. The multiorganizational conflicts that arose around the proper care of Anna also show why managed care organizations should create mechanisms to approach ethical issues in a systematic and comprehensive manner, as well as why contractual arrangements among care delivery organizations and health plans should include explicit provisions about the manner in which ethics consultation will be handled when ethically problematic situations arise.

8

Choice of Venue and Provider Under Capitation

CASE STUDY

Enrollee Request to Change Primary Care Clinic

Six weeks ago, Chris Cataldo, a nineteen-year-old college student, was critically injured when a van running a red light broadsided the car she was riding in. The drivers of both vehicles were killed. Ms. Cataldo suffered severe head and neck injuries, including the fracture of two cervical vertebrae, and was taken by ambulance to Mercy Hospital, the closest trauma center.

The night of the accident Ms. Cataldo underwent six hours of emergency brain surgery and a shunt was placed to drain excess fluid in her skull. A large portion of her skull was removed, to be replaced as the swelling in her brain decreased. Four weeks after the accident, she was transferred to a skilled nursing facility that is adjacent to and a division of Mercy Hospital. Now, six weeks after the accident, she is awake but nonverbal and paralyzed on her right side but able to follow movement commands on her left side. Since she remains unable to swallow, she is fed through a jejunostomy tube. She receives intensive rehabilitation services, including physical therapy and speech therapy, twice daily for half-hour sessions. In the near future, she will need surgery to complete the cranioplasty.

Ms. Cataldo's family (parents and two younger sisters) lives twenty miles from Mercy Hospital. At least one family member visits her daily. Her mother reports that only in the past week has Ms. Cataldo been able to distinguish her family from her nurses and other caregivers. She notes that Ms. Cataldo is particularly responsive to and cooperative with her regular physical therapist and markedly less cooperative with the replacement staff on the therapist's days off. The family, too, has developed a rapport with Ms. Cataldo's caregivers, particularly the neurosurgical team. They are also very pleased with the care provided to their daughter and the support offered to family members.

Ms. Cataldo has insurance coverage as a dependent on her father's group policy through CAP Health Maintenance Organization, a network HMO. CAP HMO is the largest single insurer in the state and has contracts with about half of the multispecialty clinics in the metropolitan area where Ms. Cataldo and her family live. CAP HMO uses capitation as its primary method of provider payment. It pays a lump sum per enrollee per month to each multispecialty clinic with which it has a contract. This capitated payment is meant to cover the costs of all professional and ancillary services provided to plan enrollees (including primary care, specialty care, pharmacy, lab, and care in skilled nursing facilities). If the actual cost of care is less than the capitated amount, the clinic gets to keep the surplus; on the other hand, if the actual cost exceeds the capitated amount, the clinic is responsible for the difference. This payment arrangement thus shifts financial risk from CAP HMO to the clinics. CAP HMO's payments to its affiliated hospitals, which are also made through capitated payment arrangements, are separate from its payments to the clinics.

Ms. Cataldo's family joined CAP HMO about six months ago, when the plan was first offered as an option by her father's employer. Upon joining the plan, enrollees must select a primary care clinic from the list of clinics with which CAP HMO has contracts. The family selected Valley Clinic, which is closest to their home. Since enrolling in the plan, however, no family member has ever received care at Valley Clinic.

For the rehabilitation phase of Ms. Cataldo's care, Valley Clinic requested that Ms. Cataldo be transferred to a skilled nursing facility with which it is affiliated (Valley Clinic has no affiliation with Mercy Hospital). With this transfer, Valley Clinic would assume responsibility for managing Ms. Cataldo's care and, according to its administrators, enable the clinic to coordinate her care more effectively and efficiently.

Ms. Cataldo's family points out that there are no services at the new skilled nursing facility that are not also available at Mercy Hospital and its skilled nursing facility. They also note that the proposed transfer would require a change in the neurosurgical team for their daughter's care and a change in all therapists. Instead of the hospital transfer, they request a change in their primary care clinic—from Valley Clinic to Park Clinic, which has a long-standing affiliation with Mercy Hospital. Most important to Ms. Cataldo's family, switching to Park Clinic would allow Ms. Cataldo to stay with her current caregivers.

CAP HMO has denied the family's request. While CAP HMO generally permits a change in an enrollee's primary care clinic if the enrollee gives timely notice to the plan, it prohibits such changes during a hospitalization or other acute confinement. CAP HMO cites this policy in its denial, explaining that the family's request to change clinics could not occur while Ms. Cataldo was hospitalized since it would be "financially unfair" to the capitated clinic receiving the enrollee. During the past two weeks, Ms. Cataldo's care at Mercy's skilled nursing facility has cost Valley Clinic approximately $5,000 a week.

Transfer for Rehabilitation Care

Aside from infrequent colds and other common ailments, Mary Stevens was a fit, active, and remarkably healthy woman. But six weeks ago, just two weeks after her seventy-second birthday, Ms. Stevens suffered a major stroke. After the stroke, her speech was impaired and she was partially paralyzed on her left side. Following a short hospital inpatient stay, she was transferred to the hospital's acute rehabilitation facility for an initial seven- to ten-day evaluation period. A few days into this period, Ms. Stevens's medical team, including her long-term internist, Dr. Kennedy, determined that she was an appropriate candidate for the facility's intensive rehabilitation program and that she would require a total stay of about three weeks. Ms. Stevens and her family agreed with this plan.

Ms. Stevens's rehabilitation program at the facility included a total of three hours per day of physical therapy, occupational therapy, and rehabilitation nursing (to educate the patient regarding self-medication and other skills she would need once she returned home). This level of rehabilitation services reflected the prevailing community standard in rehabilitation facilities but exceeded the level provided to similar patients in nursing homes.

Ms. Stevens had Medicare coverage through a managed care plan. She had joined this plan two years ago and had selected the Walnut Grove Clinic (part of the same health care system as the rehabilitation facility where she was now a patient) as her primary care clinic. Since Dr. Kennedy practices at Walnut Grove Clinic and is included in her managed care plan's physician network, this arrangement would enable Ms. Stevens to keep Dr. Kennedy as her primary physician. The managed care plan pays the clinic a monthly capitated payment intended to cover the costs of all professional and ancillary services provided to Medicare enrollees assigned to the clinic.

A few days after Ms. Stevens's stroke, her clinic assigned her a case manager, as required by its policy for any case that exceeds a certain threshold in expenditures. Typically, the hospital would notify the case manager of any patient transfer to a rehabilitation facility. During the first week of Ms. Stevens's rehabilitation, however, the social worker discovered that the hospital had not notified the case manager of the transfer. When the case manager was then told of the transfer, he consulted with Dr. Kennedy and they decided to order discharge from the rehabilitation facility to a nursing home after the first week. According to the case manager, Ms. Stevens could be more appropriately and efficiently cared for in the less intensive nursing home setting. The case manager informed the patient's social worker of the proposed transfer; the social worker then informed the attending rehabilitation physician and rehabilitation team.

Ms. Stevens and her family disagreed with the proposed discharge to a nursing home and requested that the social worker seek a longer stay in an acute rehabilitation setting. The social worker had several discussions with the case manager, a nurse with little rehabilitation training or experience, regarding the patient's excellent rehabilitation potential. She stressed that based on the facility's experience with similar patients, Ms. Stevens would likely be discharged to her home faster if she remained in the intensive rehabilitation program at the facility than if she were transferred to a nursing home. During these conversations, the case manager reminded the social worker that by advocating for the patient to remain in a more expensive acute rehabilitation setting, she was spending her employer's money from the capitated funds.

Questions for Consideration

➤ Whose request—the clinic's request to transfer Ms. Cataldo to another facility or the family's request to change primary care clinic—should be honored? Why?

➤ In what way is a transfer of a patient during a hospitalization "financially unfair" to the clinic receiving the patient?

➤ What payment arrangement(s) would best meet the interests of Ms. Cataldo and Ms. Stevens? The clinic's interests? The HMO's interests? How should these interests be balanced?

➤ What priority should patient choice regarding location and level of treatment have in capitated care?

➤ How should the Cataldo family's preference for continuity of care be balanced against the HMO's contractual obligations with the clinics?

➤ How should the HMO inform enrollees about its policies regarding transfers between clinics?

➤ Under what circumstances should the social worker take financial considerations into account when making decisions regarding Ms. Stevens's care? What about the case manager and the internist?

➤ How should the responsibilities to advocate for the patient differ, if at all, among the social worker, the case manager, and the internist regarding Ms. Stevens's care?

COMMENTARY _____

Susan B. Rubin, Ph.D.
Laurie Zoloth-Dorfman, Ph.D.

Cases of limitation in managed health care delivery systems fill the popular imagination because they resonate with the darkest fears of the American psyche—when you need it, the help you count on will not be there. What will be at stake will be not your individual worth, potency of need, or essential human rights but only whether your care can be delivered within externally imposed, marketplace-driven constraints. But the specter of abandonment is not distinctive to managed care. It can arise any time the interests of the individual and the collective must be balanced. The challenge to fairly distribute resources raises issues of justice for all societies. Fairly distributing health care resources, invariably limited and emotionally freighted, only heightens the challenge.

These two representative cases of rehabilitation and chronic care compel us to consider whether it is fair to grant every patient unlimited access to rehabilitation resources of their choosing.

How ought societies pay for the care of their injured? Given that decisions about the resources spent on rehabilitation have an aggregate effect beyond individual patients, should these decisions be viewed as primarily personal or social? In light of different needs and disparate coverage, what should the standards for such benefits be? Should there be any limit to rehabilitation? Raising these questions draws attention to the limits of the marketplace in adjudicating the claims of justice, the vulnerable, and the social commons. All health care systems must respond to these competing claims and invariably, distinct ethical problems arise—justice, consent, and the accessibility of an appeals process.

Justice Broadly Considered

Attending to broad concerns of justice at the societal level involves identifying our needs, defining our priorities, and establishing standards for distributing the goods and services we value. The dominance of the "rule of rescue" and the establishment of an acute care system built around its assumptions demonstrate how difficult it has been for Americans to face these questions prospectively. We have come to rely on a system of care based on reactive rather than preventative medicine. Until recently, medical attention has devolved primarily to hospital admittance, the presumed social location of choice for all effective care, and care delivered outside that venue has been largely makeshift, unregulated, and private.

Lacking consensus on the appropriate parameters of health care benefits, we have responded erratically to concerns of justice. Cases that seem the most tragic, the most unusual, or even the most familiar pull us toward a sympathetic response. In structuring and funding particular services, like rehabilitation, we are conflicted over how much to credit "quality of life," age, or social worth, yet we routinely fund a system driven by overt political constituencies. Similarly, we establish legal entitlements for the disabled but fail to make the necessary investment of resources over time to fund long-term rehabilitation.

TRIAGE AND TRANSFER

Justice is not only about assigning services in a minimally fair way. It is also about implementation of the technical details that divide actual services among competing individuals within a capitated system. Should our relationships to each embodied patient, a relationship that all health care providers are taught to honor, be trumped by larger social contracts with others who stand just outside of the immediate clinical world?

Capitation can allow for rational, equitable, and open allocation of services, economies of scale, and robust discourse on the needs of community. Unlike fee-for-service plans, capitation allows all to plan, justify, and openly appeal for resources. The moral weight of competing factors can be adjudicated, and theoretically, the temptation to overtreat can be avoided. The needs one anticipates in purchasing capitated health benefits may turn out to be inaccurate, but this is a feature of temporality and our imperfect prognostic ability (even season theater tickets might disappoint us). The difference is that health care decisions are both necessarily social and far more painful: capitation acknowledges that resources for any individual are limited and proceeds from there to make decisions about allocating shared goods within the system, including decisions about where care will be provided and to what degree.

In an important respect, though, decisions about triage and transfer that arise in such a context might have little to do with capitation or managed care itself. The phenomena of accidents at foreign venues and of premature births in unexpected places have always necessitated awkward transfers, with resultant changes in caregivers, even in fee-for-service systems. In reflecting on the importance of venue, we are reminded of the classic case of Larry McAfee. After he used up all of his lifetime health care benefits (capped at $1 million), McAfee was transferred out of a premier rehabilitation setting in his community to a large center in a distant state. On Medicaid, isolated from his family and friends, and existing in a large and impersonal setting engendered a despair so deep that McAfee initiated legal proceedings to withdraw his ventilatory support and die. McAfee had good private fee-for-service insurance: it just had limits, like all contracts. Even a robust plan and a strong family were not able to meet the significant challenge of ongoing care without a responsive community.

Given this history and reality, it is curious therefore to frame the case of Ms. Cataldo as an ethical problem of managed care. Ms. Cataldo's story is unsettling because of the starkness of her tragedy and our empathic sense that a moral community that cannot undo her fate at least might try to make her family happier in the face of such loss. But this does not make her insurer's insistence on transfer unethical. At issue is how far any HMO must go to accommodate the desires of such families. Ms. Cataldo's family had thought about the best venue for their health care and signed a contract with the closest clinic in their area, surely a defensible and reasonable choice at the time. In the context of their decision, refusing to try the place they chose in advance is asking more than their share.

Triage and transfer decisions are not automatic cause for ethical concern. If a caring medical team makes a decision to transfer, it can be a measure of trust in mutuality and collegiality rather than a sinister manipulation. Triage of the best resources to the ones most able to benefit is not an aberration of managed care. In all acute care medicine, one treats according to a system of justice based not on status, gender, race, or class but only on acuity and efficacy in the use of scarce resources. In the chronic care setting the same principle can offer a sense of order to an otherwise fallen and unfair world.

CAREGIVERS AND VENUE

Ms. Cataldo had access to the rehabilitation treatment she needed. At issue was her family's preference for particular caregivers and their sense that familiarity breeds compassion in the healing profession. For Ms. Stevens, the issue was access to an appropriate level of rehabilitation. Unlike the case of Ms. Cataldo, the argument against the managed care organization in Ms. Stevens's case rests on a stronger claim. The two rehabilitation settings offered measurably different quality of care—a difference that could matter a great deal in her recovery and survival. The social worker who raised this concern in Ms. Stevens's case confronts a team seemingly united in approving the transfer. Is the social worker's intuition correct that this unanimity is based on a coerced consensus? Is the long-time physician talked into approving a diminished level of care out of a vague fear, or is the team somehow blinded to the possibility of recovery for the patient because of her age? Does the assessment, triage, and transfer simply fall into place as an appropriate response to outcome studies that show poor results in this population? To what degree do our biases generate biased outcomes data, that is, could we achieve better outcomes if we were committed to the most intensive (and most costly) rehabilitation care at the outset? These are the questions that call for further discussion.

THE QUESTION OF THE GOOD

In a world in which health care providers are increasingly asked about the bottom line, we must remain focused on the "basic decent minimum" that ought to be provided in a just system. In the cases described, the assumption that lies beneath the surface is that autonomous choice is itself the ultimate good, and any denial of choice is an unfair restraint on medical care. Autonomy can serve well in many instances, but it will leave us unable to address the rationing choices that arise in any social contract when scarce resources are at stake. Choice itself is not the strongest or the trumping appeal. It is the gesture of solidarity and care, rather than the gesture of liberty, that ought to compel our attention in these cases. From this perspective, it may be more justified ethically to transfer, change teams, and send patients to venues with the best concentration of resources.

Informed Consent and the Responsible Dialogue

What processes can legitimate decisions in managed care? The informed consent/informed refusal standard provides direction. As patients are faced with consumer contracts, in which health care is bought in advance of need, more is being asked of them than in the standard-issue physician-patient relationship.

As the families and the patients in these cases signed their health care "contracts," how much did they know and when did they know it? Were they aware of what might befall them if these tragic scenarios ever came to pass? Did Ms. Cataldo's family, for example, understand the implications of signing on for care at the closest clinic? Informed families often choose to pay for additional services to maximize their children's chances for a better future, for example, by choosing to send their children to private colleges rather than public universities. While we allow for such preferences, we certainly do not think it is our social responsibility to provide them. Like all choices made in anticipation of an imagined future, choosing a health plan will carry an element of risk. But it is the same sort of choice parents must make all of the time: choosing one set of goods over another and hoping it will be good enough and safe enough.

The case of Ms. Stevens is different in kind and quality. The managed care organization's approach appears to be "bait and switch." "We will promise," says the health care plan to the elderly client, "to figure out what you need and make sure that you get it." But just when the patient is most in need, the plan changes the terms, offering only the cheapest and most minimal rehabilitation. If cost will be the major factor in the determination of the context of care, then Ms. Stevens should know this prior to agreeing to this plan, when she is in a position to make other arrangements. What is most worrisome in every case of this type is not only the short-range problem of this patient and this social worker but of every patient and every social worker in the system. Who, we are led to ask, is guarding the chicken coop if the physicians in the plan are unable to fight for access to the care that their patients need and have been led to expect? Members of a plan, and American citizens involved as both participants and witnesses to the care of the most vulnerable, have a stake in creating and ensuring a system where moral agency is not a matter of luck or caprice but is embedded in the institution.

A Just Process

But how to structure such a system? Ms. Stevens's case raises problematic concerns about power and advocacy if her need for intensive, expensive rehabilitation is at odds with the financial goals of her insurance company. Is this in fact the case? Her long-term internist seems caught between concerns about the best interests of his patients, unspoken concerns with cost, and perhaps a covert dread of discipline from the insurance plan. If the physician with the deepest relationship to the fragile patient is not the one to make the assessment about best interests, but rather a disinterested and distant party, then at the very least, we need safeguards to protect the integrity of the choice that is finally made.

What ought to be the role of the social worker or case manager? If a decision is made to reduce a level of care, a compelling justification must be provided that goes beyond the pursuit of profit. We need a sense that the health care professionals are competent, actually care about particular patients, and have thoughtfully considered all alternate paths without fear or pressure. This is not so remarkable a requirement. It is a categorical imperative that finds its roots in both a Kantian and a biblically based promise of social reciprocity.

In our work we stress the centrality of regular reflection on the value of care, the need for a credible appeals process, and the creation of a larger moral community that struggles openly and transparently with the nature of the contract itself. How best to accomplish this task? There are many practical routes. First, we urge consistent and regular ethical reflection within an accessible ethics committee. We advocate the development of systemwide ethics committees that include community members and actual members of the health plan as active participants. And finally, we urge ethicists and health care professionals to take the lead in the development of wider national standards.

BUSINESS AND CONTRACTS IN HEALTH CARE

Calling for such a thoroughgoing reflective process raises the issue of the role of business and contracts in health care. Business allows for the single-minded pursuit of profit. Business praxis allows for secrecy surrounding proprietary information, just at the juncture that ethicists in health care call for open discourse. As bioethicists, we are on new terrain. As we construct a system frankly rooted in the competitive marketplace, what ought be the role of competition? Who decides? Ought it be the traditional corporate leadership? Or is there a necessary task for the medical expert? How ought we credit the voice of the vulnerable patient herself? And, hopefully not last, what is the role for the "prophetic voice" of ethics and moral philosophy?

When the question is a fair contract between the vulnerable and the powerful, and the issue is life and death, we need to pay particular attention to the process of reflection and decision making. A contractual relationship allows for little na-iveté—something all American consumers understand. Increasingly, the delivery of health care services is like any industry. But can we justify the proposition that health care can be made and sold like pencils in the free market? If health care is different, we will have to identify and defend the *caritas* aspect of our delivery system and find su-pererogatory ways to fund care not only for the vocal but also for the voiceless.

Although health care contracts may have binding features, they are not "just like any contract." As ethicists we are called to look not only at the specifics of each case but to find a language that can allow justice to have a voice over the siren song of profit. In this, we are aware that our attention to any one case ought to set a conversational, casuistic norm for the rest. If we allow for changes based on yearning, the yearning of each must be credited. We are asked to enter the case as the "last best hope" for the vulnerable patient, but we must recall our responsibility to the not-yetness of other hopes, the call of the future patients on shared resources. It is a trust that must be taken quite seriously. In the case of Ms. Stevens, when a disempowered social worker must stand alone, it is our task to set the basic standards for a substantive appeals process. We must insist that the "processing" of the patient be stopped in its efficient tracks long enough to ask the question of ethics—the question of the good. And when that question is raised, we need to celebrate and protect the moral agent who raises it.

What of the deeper issues reshaping health care itself? Allowing the restructuring of the American health care delivery system to be carried out solely in the rough-and-tumble of the market ignores primary commitments to the marginalized and vulnerable. It is a discredit to our vision of democracy to not allow for the fullest and most participatory debate on our shared future. The cases described emerge after the deals have been struck and hence are seen as issues of exception. But they are not exceptional; they are ordinary. While it is valuable to seek just solutions for these families, ultimately this is a limited response to the deeper issues of accountability and authority raised by the nature of the contracts themselves.

Medicine cannot promise salvation from tragedies. Setting limits to the compassionate response are not new. What can be new is a determination to link that compassionate response to a larger narrative of justice that can be made tangible in the clinical world if we allow our cases to teach us what will be necessary for health care reform.

References

Holmes, S. 1990. "Disabled People Say Homecare is Needed to Use New Rights." *New York Times* Oct. 14, p. 22.

COMMENTARY

Arthur L. Caplan, Ph.D.

Capitation and fixed forms of reimbursement characteristic of managed care are frequently cited today by health care professionals as the only obstacles to their efforts to advocate for the best interests of patients. But money and the way it is paid to health care providers, health systems, and health institutions is not the root of all that is evil in the cases of Chris Cataldo and Mary Stevens. This is especially so in the area of access to rehabilitation care.

Both Ms. Cataldo and Ms. Stevens require intensive rehabilitation care. A key part of rehabilitation for patient and family is to receive care from experienced, competent personnel in comfortable surroundings that are easily accessible by the patient, family, and friends. Both Ms. Cataldo and Ms. Stevens are encountering very real problems in getting the quality of care they need in the settings that would be optimal for them and their loved ones. It looks as if they are having problems because managed care companies are balking at incurring the costs and the hassle involved in giving these patients what they want and their health care providers think they need.

Ms. Cataldo's HMO is refusing reassignment of her primary care clinic from Valley Clinic to Park Clinic in order to protect the financial interest that Valley has in receiving reimbursement for her care and to protect Park from financial loss from enrolling, midyear, a known high-cost patient. For her part, Ms. Stevens is being sent to a cheaper alternative for rehabilitation care consequent to a stroke, even though her doctor, her social worker, her family, and she herself believe that intensive rehabilitation care in a hospital would be in her best interest and might even result in a faster discharge home for her. Money and the way it is used in managed care is surely a factor in the limitation of covered rehabiliation options for these patients, but it is not the only moral culprit in these cases.

A quick look back at the not so distant days of fee-for-service medicine reveals that access to rehabilitation care after accidents and strokes has always been a major problem in American health care. At no time since World War II have all those who needed rehabilitation care been able to get it (Caplan, Haas, and Callahan 1988; Caplan 1992, 1998). During the 1970s and 1980s—long before anyone even thought of the term "managed care"—patients receiving care in the Veterans Administration system, through Medicaid, Medicare, or private insurance, found themselves facing the same sorts of problems of access and inconvenience and lack of choice as today confront patients such as Ms. Cataldo and Ms. Stevens. Those who had no health insurance were simply not admitted anywhere other than to short-term acute rehabilitation, no matter how much benefit they might have derived from more sustained forms of rehabilitation services (Caplan, Haas, and Callahan 1987; Caplan, Jennings, and Callahan 1988; Caplan 1989; Kane and Caplan 1990). Advocacy from physicians, nurses, and administrators was in very short supply.

The American health care system and its providers have long had a strong orientation toward the provision of acute care in hospital settings. Long-term care, chronic care, and rehabilitation have for decades been marginal. Few who worked in hospitals would take any time or spend any energy for those who could not afford services, much less for those who could not get those services where they would have preferred to receive them.

This nation has never had a mechanism for the payment of long-term and chronic care that would ensure universal access to those in need (Caplan, Jennings, and Callahan, 1988; Caplan 1998). For many Americans, access to rehabilitation services after a stroke, a traumatic brain injury, or a severely disabling spinal cord injury has been contingent on their ability to pay out-of-pocket for such services or to spend their assets down to poverty levels to qualify, and then only in some states with relatively generous coverage, for services to be given through Medicaid (Kane and Caplan 1990; Caplan 1992).

The problem with access to high-quality rehabilitation care is that our society has not been willing to share the cost of it. So rehabilitation services, which are often costly, have been and remain far more available to those with the means to pay for them directly or to purchase private coverage than they are to others. Those who can pay more have always had more choice.

Ironically, managed care plans, in trying to manage a full range of services for their enrollees, find themselves struggling with issues of coverage for rehabilitation that would not have arisen ten or twenty years ago because the ability to pay or not to pay would have ended all discussion about access (Caplan, Haas, and Callahan 1987, 1988). Doctors and administrators left to social workers the problem of advocating for patients and their families who could not pay. Social workers could rarely offer any help, and the poor and underinsured were turned aside with little remorse or hesitation. Battles such as those faced by Ms. Cataldo or Ms. Stevens might have ended without so much as a whimper ten years earlier because no one was on the line to make sure that patients like these, or others who had little or no insurance, actually got any rehabilitation services.

When individual physicians, nurses, and social workers did choose to argue for the Ms. Stevenses and Ms. Cataldoes of a decade ago, they would have made their appeals not to managed care companies but to private and often for-profit rehabilitation companies. They would have tried to persuade these private firms to extend generosity toward patients who might benefit from speech therapy, occupational therapy, or physical therapy but who could not pay for it. Often the answer was simply no (Caplan, Haas, and Callahan 1988). Many private companies refused even to consider patients covered by Medicaid. Others would not accept any clients other than those covered by private insurance.

Now that patients are enrolled in managed care plans that contract to provide them with all "needed" services, it is likely that more persons will gain access to rehabilitation services than was true in the world of fee-for-service medicine. Of course, managed care companies need not contract for these services. Some have found them too costly to provide and have dropped coverage. Not every state requires managed care companies to cover rehabilitation services, and no state mandates that they be covered with some degree of patient choice of setting and location, as Ms. Cataldo and Ms. Stevens seek. But the problem of access did not begin with managed care, and in some ways managed care has shouldered more of the burden for worrying about patient access to rehabilitation than was true before capitation came to health care.

Still, Ms. Stevens and Ms. Cataldo do face problems of access and choice. Whatever the cause of the continuing inability to gain access to convenient, high-quality rehabilitation might be, they face obstacles now to getting the care they want. Should their interests dominate decisions by their managed care companies or should corporate interests predominate?

In the case of Ms. Cataldo the answer seems obvious. She should be able to get reassignment of her primary care provider to get the rehabilitation she needs in the setting of her choice, where she can receive continuity of care. Since the primary stumbling block is compensation, the managed care organization should adopt policies that permit patients facing long-term care needs to reassign themselves. This should not prove all that difficult: the number of people who will want to do what Ms. Cataldo seeks to do is small, and the organization can simply adjust the overall income levels of primary care clinics at the end of each year to account for such reassignments. Patient self-interest should not be sacrificed to the bureaucratic needs of a system that can find other ways to make sure that all primary care providers get a fair shake with respect to the income they earn. Good business ethics requires some flexibility in the case of a request such as Ms. Cataldo's.

The case for Ms. Stevens is a bit more difficult. The claim is that in a hospital setting she can get better care that will make a difference to her. The real question is whether there is any data or information to support her belief.

Many people think that the hospital is the best place to be for any form of care, but that is not always true. For example, many families are loathe to see their loved ones discharged from intensive care units for any reason. They fear that they will not get the same quality of care if they are moved to other parts of the hospital or to a nursing home. But, it is not always best for the patient to receive care in an intensive care unit. Nor is it fair to allow someone to consume intensive resources that could be used in the care of other patients who would be better able to benefit from them. For services such as rehabilitation a hospital may not prove to be the optimal setting in terms of outcome or cost for delivering care.

Ms. Stevens has every right to know exactly why her case manager thinks she can do just as well outside the hospital setting. She also has every right to request a transfer to that setting if her rehabilitation does not progress after a few weeks inside the hospital rehabilitation setting. Both such requests should be responded to with full, complete, and understandable information—about the choice of setting or the right to change settings if progress is not forthcoming.

Managed care has many, many flaws. Capitation can certainly lead to situations in which patient interests are sacrificed to the bottom line. But the bitter truth about American health care is that money has always been allowed to drive access to the system. The rich always do better than the poor. Those who know how to work the system do better than those who do not. Those who are lucky enough to be able to enlist the active support and advocacy of family and care providers fare better than those who cannot. Managed care and capitation do not change any of these facts. It will take systematic reform of our health care insurance and delivery systems to do that.

References

Caplan, A. L. 1989. "Ethical Issues in the Care of the Elderly." In *Improving the Health of Older People*, pp. 667–81. Edited by R. Kane, G. Evans, and D. Macfadyen. New York: Oxford University Press.

————. 1992. *If I Were a Rich Man Could I Buy a Pancreas? and Other Essays on the Ethics of Health Care*. Bloomington, Ind.: Indiana University Press.

————. 1998. *Am I My Brother's Keeper? The Ethical Frontiers of Biomedicine*. Bloomington, Ind.: Indiana University Press.

Caplan, A. L.; Haas, J.; and Callahan, D. 1987. "Ethical and Policy Issues in Rehabilitation Medicine." *Hastings Center Report* 17, no. 4:1–20.

————. 1988. *Case Studies in Ethics and Medical Rehabilitation*. Hastings-on-Hudson, N.Y.: Hastings Center.

Caplan, A. L.; Jennings, B.; and Callahan, D. 1988. "Ethical Challenges of Chronic Illness." *Hastings Center Report* 18, no. 1:1–16.

Kane, R. A., and Caplan, A. L., eds. 1990. *Everyday Ethics: Resolving Dilemmas in Nursing Home Life*. New York: Springer Publishing.

PART THREE

Quality Care in a Competitive Market

9

Credentialing Standards and Quality Care

CASE STUDY

Nebraska Partners, an integrated health care system based in a large city in Nebraska, would like to expand its service area to a number of rural counties in order to participate in the Medicaid program. Federal Medicaid law requires that a managed care plan have an adequate provider network, defined to mean a primary care provider within thirty minutes or thirty miles and specialty providers within sixty minutes or sixty miles, of every enrollee. If Nebraska Partners cannot arrange for a complete network in these rural areas, it will not be able to obtain a Medicaid managed care contract.

In one rural town in particular, there is only one clinic made up of three physicians—two family practitioners and a surgeon. One of the family practitioners has a greater-than-average disciplinary history and an unusually high number of medical malpractice cases and was also recently denied coverage by his professional liability carrier. The other family practitioner is board certified only as a pathologist but has practiced and represents himself as a family practitioner. Finally, the surgeon never completed his surgery residency due to a family crisis and has never been board certified in surgery, but he has no disciplinary or medical malpractice history.

If this clinic were in the metropolitan area, Nebraska Partners would not contract with any of these providers because they would not meet the company's credentialing standards, and there are other providers who would. The credentialing standards require that every provider must have completed an accredited residency and be board certified in their stated area of practice. The standards also require that network providers have no significant disciplinary or medical malpractice history. If an applicant has one or two isolated incidents, the plan will solicit additional information and make a case-by-case determination. But in no case is a provider with a significant disciplinary history or history of medical malpractice credentialed. In fact, the credentialing standards automatically exclude a provider who has been denied liability coverage. Nebraska Partners has established and consistently implemented these standards as part of its quality-improvement program.

Despite the evident shortcomings of these providers, Nebraska Partners is considering making a business exception and contracting with this rural clinic. First, the managed care contract would improve access to comprehensive, affordable care in this rural area. Many current Medicaid enrollees in this rural area drive over sixty miles to the metropolitan area to obtain covered care. As a result, they often forego necessary care. Other Medicaid enrollees pay out-of-pocket for services closer to home or use the emergency department. A contract with this clinic would maintain existing physician–patient relationships and significantly reduce costs, in time and money, to these Medicaid participants. Second, Nebraska Partners feels that the risk is manageable and that the quality of services at the clinic could improve with oversight and education of the providers. Finally, from a business perspective, the Medicaid contract is very lucrative. In order to secure the contract, the plan must contract with this clinic because it is not economically feasible for the plan to build or support a new clinic in this area. Besides, the community is loyal to the physicians at this clinic. A contract excluding these providers would be unpopular and detrimental to Nebraska Partners' reputation in this and other outstate areas.

The contract unit has asked the credentialing committee to make an exception to the standards for all three providers, arguing that it is a defensible business decision and that access is more important than quality in this rural area.

Questions for Consideration

➤ Should Nebraska Partners forego the Medicaid contract? Why?
➤ Should Nebraska Partners include all, some, or none of the providers in its provider network? How could a plan justify different credentialing standards for certain rural providers than those applied elsewhere in the system? When, if ever, is some provider better than no provider?
➤ Why might completion of a residency and board certification be inappropriate credentialing criteria?
➤ If Nebraska Partners does contract with this clinic, what might the plan do to monitor and improve quality?
➤ How else might the plan improve access without compromising quality? Would it be preferable for a plan to cover transportation costs to the nearest credentialed provider?

COMMENTARY

Ruth A. Mickelsen, J.D.

The heart and soul of most managed care organizations is the physician network. Managed care organizations undertake legal and ethical obligations to both deliver and finance health care. Since health care is not deliverable without an adequate provider network, the selection and retention of a provider network is a fundamental and necessary organizational task. The appropriate selection of a provider network requires Nebraska Partners to evaluate geographic accessibility and the quality of health care services. In an ideal world, geographically accessible providers are also high-quality providers. In the real world faced by managed care organizations such as Nebraska Partners, the best-quality providers are not always geographically dispersed in an ideal, uniform manner or in accordance with regulatory access requirements. In addition, accessible providers are not always of the highest caliber when evaluated against objective credentialing standards. As a result, Nebraska Partners must balance geographic accessibility with application of credentialing standards designed to facilitate good patient care.

Nebraska Partners seeks to provide geographic accessibility and facilitate good patient care in the context of a rural service area expansion. Nebraska Partners is considering expanding its service area in order to participate in the Medicaid managed care program. Significant questions remain unanswered regarding whether the managed care model fits the Medicaid program and the population it serves (Manski, Peddicord, and Hyman 1997). Nebraska Partners is no doubt aware that geographic and cultural barriers are generally more acute with the Medicaid population than the commercial population enrolled through employers, unions, or labor trusts. Lack of transportation frequently impedes access to services for an economically disadvantaged population. This population will likely have a higher-than-average incidence of chronic conditions and poor health. Finally, continuity of care and close geographic proximity are likely to be quite important to this population.

Despite these challenges, managed care arrangements may be beneficial for this population due to the enhanced capacity of a managed care organization to monitor and direct care. Those organizations generally track physician visits, immunization rates, well child care visits, and other indices of medical care delivery. They also have the capacity to assist in the management of chronic conditions such as asthma and diabetes through development and use of disease management guidelines. Managed care organizations are also formally and publicly "accountable" to government payers for the quality of care provided to Medicaid members.

State laws and national accreditation standards impose various standards on managed care organizations for the selection of providers for their networks (Joint

Commission on the Accreditation of Healthcare Organizations 1997). These standards require Nebraska Partners to establish detailed written selection standards and to apply such standards in a fair and reasonable manner. In addition, many state regulatory schemes require that providers be "accessible," frequently defining accessibility in terms of number of miles or driving time. However, neither the law nor accreditation standards dictate a decision-making process that requires a "balancing" or "trade-off" between geographic access and quality-based criteria. Nebraska Partners is organizationally responsible for evaluating this trade-off on behalf of its future members.

This case presents organizational challenges that are not focused exclusively on the traditional health care dilemmas of clinical bedside ethics but rather on regulation and policy at an organizational or system level. A system ethic must balance the importance of the physician-patient relationship with the interests and needs of the entire managed care population and the business and commercial goals of the organization. This area constitutes the type of "real-world" dilemma faced by organizations in determining what is the "right" thing to do and how the organization should function. The goal for Nebraska Partners should be to make principled trade-offs grounded in organizational rules and procedures that will lead to overall satisfaction for all organizational stakeholders.

The "Doing Good" Standard

In making principled trade-offs, the fundamental ethical question is: Will inclusion of this clinic in the Nebraska Partners provider network likely "do good" by improving member health? Nebraska Partners' mission is to finance and provide quality medical care to its members. The primary value underlying its provider selection policies and practices should be good patient care that improves the health of its members.

A variety of measures may be used to assess health improvement and quality of care for these potential members. One critical component of quality health care is a strong physician-patient relationship characterized by choice, competence, continuity, and honesty (Emanuel and Dubler 1995). These four attributes provide a useful structure to analyze the trade-offs faced by Nebraska Partners in this case.

Choice is a critical factor in patient satisfaction and expression of a patient's autonomy (Dworkin 1998). Patients want to be able to choose the provider from whom they will receive medical care. This rural Nebraska community is presumably already loyal to the physicians at the clinic in question. The clinic is already serving some members of the Medicaid population on a fee-for-service basis. As a result, some members have established a physician-patient relationship with these practitioners. Although the practitioners in question have a greater-than-average disciplinary history, a history of medical malpractice, and an incidence of denial of coverage by a professional liability carrier, Nebraska Partners is not aware that the local community is dissatisfied with the clinic.

Patients also value professional competence. Nebraska Partners may be legally accountable if it knowingly credentials incompetent practitioners (Dorros and Stone 1995). Competence encompasses numerous elements including technical competence, good clinical judgment, an understanding of one's limitations and a willingness to consult with other providers and specialists as required, and a good fund of current knowledge (Emanuel and Dubler 1995). The facts in this case indicate among the clinicians a greater-than-average disciplinary history and history of medical malpractice, a recent denial of coverage by a professional liability carrier, a lack of board certification, and failure to complete a residency. Each of these facts may be an indication of an incompetent provider, but they do not automatically warrant that conclusion.

Nebraska Partners will likely need additional information in order to accurately assess the professional competence of these clinicians. The evaluation of disciplinary and malpractice history is not an algorithmic exercise. Competent providers make mistakes that can result in malpractice actions. Competent providers are also the subjects of disciplinary actions. The facts do not provide any indication of what type of behavior was at issue or the length of time since the disciplinary case was closed. Nor do the facts indicate the seriousness of the medical malpractice cases reported, their dates, or the practice setting in which the untoward events occurred. Denial of professional liability insurance may be an indicator of past incompetence or it may reflect overly strict underwriting criteria.

The critical question is whether a history of malpractice or disciplinary action is a reliable predictor of future poor-quality care. This is a subjective and difficult judgment that often requires a complex, multidisciplinary evaluation. A poor practitioner is often difficult to identify. Academic studies have noted the lack of correlation between malpractice history, disciplinary history, and quality of care.

Other factors noted by Nebraska Partners as an indicator of future incompetency include failure of the surgeon to complete a residency in surgery and to obtain board certification in surgery. Board certification is a commonly used factor in assessing physician competence (Summer 1995). Although board certification and completion of residency requirements are not unreasonable or arbitrary criteria, they are also not absolute predictors of quality care or future skill levels. The case does not note the number of years this surgeon has been in practice. The surgeon may have been in practice for many years and acquired an acceptable skill level. It is certainly true that poorly trained physicians can harm patients. However, this surgeon has no disciplinary or medical malpractice history. As a result, there is no indication that, in this particular case, lack of formal training or board certification is a good predictor of likely incompetence and poor-quality care.

None of these practitioners satisfies the credentialing criteria developed by Nebraska Partners for its urban business. Managed care organizations are inherently conservative and cautious in the development of provider selection criteria. Credentialing criteria are generic and developed for multiple purposes. Among them is the enhancement of the quality of medical care delivery. A secondary purpose is the limitation of managed care liability under various legal theories that have found a managed care organization liable for the malpractice of a negligently credentialed provider.

The use of practitioners whose history strongly suggests that they are dangerous is unacceptable under traditional principles of nonmaleficence and beneficence. However, the use of practitioners who may be below average is ethically justifiable when other alternatives are not available and oversight mechanisms are available to monitor and potentially improve the quality of care. This is particularly true when a physician shortage means no alternate physician care is easily accessible for a population.

Although the clinic practitioners in this case do not satisfy the generic criteria, the facts do not necessarily lead to the conclusion they are incompetent or dangerous. Clinic participation in managed care quality-improvement processes has the potential for actually improving the care provided at the clinic. If this clinic is included in the network, Nebraska Partners presumably has the operational capacity to engage in quality oversight through chart audits, focused quality studies, and provider education. Patient satisfaction surveys may also be useful in identifying practitioners with whom members are dissatisfied. National accreditation criteria require recredentialing every two years. Managed care organizations frequently consider the results of provider-specific quality-assessment studies and satisfaction surveys in their recredentialing process. Any emerging evidence of incompetence and poor-quality care can therefore be regularly evaluated.

In addition to competency, patients value continuity in a physician-patient relationship. At least some of the patients have already established a relationship with these practitioners. Continuity of care is particularly important with patients who have chronic conditions and the vulnerable, young, and disabled populations that often constitute a disproportionate share of a state's Medicaid population. A good physician-patient relationship requires a significant investment of time by both parties. Managed care organizations are frequently criticized for disrupting continuity of care by establishing small networks. Nebraska Partners should be sensitive to member dissatisfaction created by disruption of existing caregiver relationships and recognize that continuity of care and the preservation of a trusting physician-patient relationship are important aspects of quality health care.

Nebraska Partners may also entertain the option of contracting with some but not all of the providers in this clinic. However, in a rural area with a limited number of physicians able to share "call" arrangements, such an option may be ineffective and difficult to administer. Selective contracting within a clinic disrupts the continuity of care established by the clinic with its patient base. If a Medicaid member sees the noncredentialed provider in an emergency situation, Nebraska Partners will be required to pay for the care, without the benefits of a prior physician-patient relationship or any quality oversight. On a practical level, the clinic may find a selective contract arrangement so burdensome that the other providers will be unwilling to contract with Nebraska Partners.

Honesty is often discussed in the context of full disclosure of the terms and conditions of the managed care contract and financial arrangements with providers (Rodwin 1996). Honesty is also relevant to the disclosure of qualifications and provider performance information (Sharrott 1992). In support of full disclosure and the related concept of informed consent, Nebraska Partners should disclose to its members provider- and clinic-specific quality data, provider performance data—for example, process measurements related to immunization and mammogram rates—and member satisfaction survey information. Nebraska Partners possesses a large database of information relating to its credentialed providers. Some of this information may have been provided by network physicians under a contractual promise of confidentiality in the clinic's contract with Nebraska Partners. For example, it is common for malpractice histories to be considered peer review information—a special category of information that is not discoverable by courts or otherwise disclosable in order to facilitate honest peer review by other providers. However, disciplinary data (for example, license suspension, license revocation, or fines paid), board certification, satisfaction survey information, and other process-based performance data are not generally classified as peer review data or subject to confidentiality restrictions.

If these rural providers are included in the Nebraska Partners physician network, results of satisfaction surveys and performance criteria should be made available to members in order to facilitate more informed and autonomous choice by members. The provision of such information may also facilitate enhanced communication between the provider and the patient. From an ethics perspective, the primary goal of enhanced communication is the preservation of patient trust in the physician. Trust should be based on demonstrated physician competence, not simply a naive belief in physician competence. From a market perspective, disclosure of satisfaction and performance measurements should assist consumers in choosing the provider who best satisfies their individual needs and desires.

The disclosure of provider-specific data allows individual members to make their own individual decisions regarding the "principled trade-off" between provider competence and access. It is true that the lack of immediate alternatives to these practitioners will constrain easy member exit from the clinic in question. However, the lack of easy exit does not provide an ethically justifiable reason to refrain from providing the same level of detail on provider competence and performance as would be provided in an urban setting, where exit is a more viable option. The principle of choice also supports individual patient evaluation of the trade-off between quality and access. Nebraska Partners should facilitate and enhance patient choice through disclosure of provider-specific information.

Although Nebraska Partners may not be able to disclose every type of information it possesses because of confidentiality restrictions, disclosure is no less necessary simply because all the information possessed by Nebraska Partners may not be shared. In a perfect marketplace, consumers possess perfect information about the services and commodities they use. The health care marketplace is far from perfect, and imperfect information is often better than no information.

Absent clear identification of a dangerous or incompetent provider, Nebraska Partners is not ethically or legally prohibited from making a global trade-off between quality and access on behalf of all its prospective Medicaid members. The decision to contract with a less-than-perfect provider may permit Nebraska partners to "do good" through use of its standard quality and health-improvement processes. Nebraska Partners may also be able to enhance patients' understanding of a particular provider's strength and weaknesses, thus enabling individual patients to more realistically perform their own principled trade-off evaluation.

The Business and Organizational Realities

The ultimate ethical question of what Nebraska Partners should do as an organization must also be evaluated in the context of what is practically possible. In the new era of organizational health care, ethical issues are bounded by fundamental design questions of what is and is not possible (Feldstein and Ogle 1997). Systemic weaknesses in the current health care system—in this case, the lack of abundance of providers in rural communities—cannot be remedied by a single managed care organization. Nebraska Partners has some organizational ability to improve the quality of care delivered, provided that it effectively partners and cooperates with the providers who are already practicing in that area. If Nebraska Partners can contribute to measurable improvements in various quality indicators, it will be "doing good" for its member population. The fact that access and quality vary from one geographic region to another may be poor public health policy and may be unfair. It is a fact that rural health care communities are not structured or staffed in the same manner or with the same number and types of practitioners as urban medical communities. However, as a single managed care organization, Nebraska

Partners can only work with the community as it finds it. What counts as "doing good" is, in part, determined by organizational structures, technological possibilities, regulatory requirements, and the realities of the rural health care marketplace.

As a competitive business organization, Nebraska Partners must continuously improve its practices and products. This requires market expansion, new product development, and member growth. Nebraska Partners has a strong business incentive to start this product line before its competitors. The state has structured its managed care contracts to be profitable precisely to encourage managed care organizations like Nebraska Partners to offer a Medicaid product. Nebraska Partners arguably has a fiduciary duty to its other members and possible shareholders to seek and obtain new profitable lines of business, provided that such business opportunities contribute to member health improvement. There is no clear evidence that inclusion of these providers will constitute a danger to member health. In fact, it is more probable that Nebraska Partners will improve health care processes and outcomes through quality-improvement programs and effective partnering with these local physicians.

It is important to recognize that this is not a "once and for all" decision. Satisfaction and performance data may later demonstrate that health care quality would be improved by use of physician extenders, patient use of a distant clinic, or services received via a tele-medicine link. Inclusion of these providers in the network does not preclude removal from the network at a later time or the subsequent adoption of other approaches to the delivery of quality care in this community.

The ethical issues inherent in this case are driven in large part by the disparity in health care services between urban and rural communities. These are issues of applied public policy that must be ultimately resolved by the market, regulatory mechanisms, and political debate. The principled trade-offs inherent in this decision will not disappear once a decision is made. They will simply evolve, requiring constant and careful vigilance and reexamination. Nebraska Partners' primary ethical obligation is to continuously examine its business decisions using a framework that prioritizes improving the health of the population it serves. By electing to prioritize population health improvement in its business decisions, it will be "doing good."

References

Dorros, T., and Stone, H. 1995. "Implications of Negligent Selection and Retention of Physicians in the age of ERISA." *American Journal of Law & Medicine* 21, no. 4:383–418.
Dworkin, G. 1988. *The Theory and Practice of Autonomy.* New York: Cambridge University Press.
Emanuel, E. J., and Dubler N. N. 1995. "Preserving the Physician Patient Relationship in the Era of Managed Care." *Journal of the American Medical Association* 273, no. 4:323–29.
Feldstein, B., and Ogle, R. 1997. "Satisfaction, Managed Ethics and the Duty to Design." *HEC Forum* 9, no. 4:333.
Joint Commission on the Accreditation of Healthcare Organizations (JCAHO). 1997.

Accreditation Manual for Health Care Networks; National Committee on Quality Accreditation (NCQA). 1997. *Standards for Accreditation*; Utilization Review Accreditation Commission (URAC). 1997. Standards for *American Accreditation Healthcare Commission* (formally known as URAC). 1997.

Manski, R.J.; Peddicord, D.; and Hyman, D. 1997. "Medicaid, Managed Care and American's Safety Net." *Journal of Law, Medicine, and Ethics* 25, no. 1:30.

Rodwin, M. 1996. "Consumer Protection and Managed Care: Issues, Reform Proposals and Trade-offs." *Houston Law Review* 32:1319.

Sharrott, D. 1992. "Provider-Specific Quality-of-Care Data: A Proposal for Limited Mandatory Disclosure." *Brooklyn Law Review* 58:85.

Summer, S. 1995. "Medical Staff Credentialing: Physician Challenges to Board Certification Criteria." *American Journal of Trial Advocacy* 18:673.

COMMENTARY

Matthew K. Wynia, M.D., M.P.H.
Linda L. Emanuel, M.D., Ph.D.

Can access to care be in competition with quality of care? Since each is an ethical good, such a competition would pose an ethical dilemma. However, even before addressing this potential ethical dilemma, the reader may wonder whether business considerations are really what is at stake. Thus we shall briefly consider some relevant business considerations, which may have ethical ramifications for Nebraska Partners. We will then discuss access and quality, including the appropriate use of structural quality indicators such as credentialing standards. Finally, we will consider the use of absolute minimum standards and consider how to build such a floor on a solid foundation that is most likely to promote quality care.

Business Considerations

Though the contracting unit at Nebraska Partners professes concern for improving this community's access to health care, the case suggests they may be more concerned with the plan's own access—to a "very lucrative" statewide Medicaid contract. They urge dropping the plan's credentialing standards in this community as a "business exception." And it is not immediately clear whether Nebraska Partners will even bring significantly improved access to this community. The

Statement of authorship contribution: Dr. Wynia codeveloped and corefined the concepts in this commentary, and was responsible for drafting several early versions of the manuscript, as well as the final manuscript. Dr. Emanuel codeveloped and corefined the concepts in this commentary, and provided editorial comments on early drafts, as well as the final manuscript.

physicians in question already practice in the community, and the case suggests that they already care for at least some Medicaid patients.

Gaining a lucrative statewide contract for Nebraska Partners does, however, have ethical implications. An improved market position could mean improved quality and access, and lower costs, to the plan's subscribers across the state. Even if the local community's access is unchanged, the plan might justify contracting with these local physicians if doing so could improve care for subscribers elsewhere. Would this constitute the instrumental use of this community to benefit others? Perhaps. Especially so if the local community is worse off. The plan as a whole, and especially the credentialing committee and others involved in this decision—for example, the ethics committee—ought to start by asking itself what its primary purpose is in developing the network in this area. Is it to improve health care for this community? Is it to improve the plan's market share? What does the plan's mission statement say? Is access to Nebraska Partners' plan the only, or best, route to improved health care for this community? Early and consistent attention to motivation can help prevent purely self-serving considerations from overwhelming an appropriate level of concern for this community.

A second business consideration with potential ethical implications is that developing managed care networks in rural areas is notoriously difficult. It requires strong commitments from local practitioners, who may rightly feel they can be picky when choosing contracts. The plan may need to make concessions to these physicians, in addition to lowering its credentialing standards, to entice them to join its network (Kongstvedt and Plocher 1996). The nature of these concessions could impair quality and raise costs for the plan's subscribers.

Finally, the plan must consider state and federal regulatory requirements, as well as network accreditation requirements, that may preclude contracting with one or more of these physicians. If the plan does not consistently uphold credentialing standards it could be liable in future malpractice awards for this negligence or for misrepresenting its credentialing process to the public.

For our remaining discussion, we will set aside the apparent strong financial motivation for Nebraska Partners and focus on its local ethical obligations. We will assume that Nebraska Partners' intentions are centered on improving health care for this community.

Access and Quality

Problems of health care access cover a broad swath. For example, patients in rural Nebraska who must drive over sixty miles to see a specialist have a barrier to access (physical inaccessibility), and so do Portuguese immigrants in downtown Omaha who cannot find a family physician who speaks their language (cultural inaccessibility). In Lincoln, a businessperson may want "access" to a leading specialist at the Mayo Clinic for knee surgery, and a Native American might want "access" to the use of traditional healers. Both people would mean that they need insurance to reimburse the costs of obtaining these services (financial access). Combinations of access problems are common among the rural poor.

The arguments in favor of improving access to health care in this rural community are compelling (Bindman et al. 1995). The case states that patients in this area are foregoing necessary care because of the time and expense of traveling to the city for covered care. Poor patients are also paying out-of-pocket for uncovered services nearer home and are using suboptimal sites for receiving medical care, such as emergency departments. We are told that a Nebraska Partners contract with the rural clinic will allow existing "loyal" patient-physician relationships to remain intact, a potentially significant medical and community benefit. For Medicaid patients in this rural community, it appears that easier access to the clinic and doctors in question might mean the difference between some medical care and none at all. So how could this improved "access" be bad for health care "quality"?

For purposes of discussion, we shall adopt the definition of health care quality produced by the Institute of Medicine: "[Quality is] the degree to which health services for individuals and populations increase the likelihood of desired health outcomes and are consistent with current professional knowledge" (Schuster, McGlynn, and Brook 1997). Note that in this definition, health care quality makes sense only in the context of the actual provision of health services because it is based in part on outcomes. The health services in question must be *used*: services that are inaccessible are by definition not being properly used, so one cannot meaningfully discuss their quality.

With this definition of quality then, it makes sense to understand access as a component of and a necessary prerequisite to quality medical care. That is, access and quality are closely interrelated (and usually complementary) goods. But access, though necessary to quality health care, is not sufficient to guarantee high quality. After all, patients may have unfettered access to otherwise poor-quality care. Access is only one (the first) of many measurable components of quality. Other measurable components of quality include health care structures, processes, and outcomes (Donabedian 1980; Brook, McGlynn, and Cleary 1996). Of these, outcomes are of particular relevance initially because to pursue health care quality, one must develop some understanding of what "desired" health outcomes are (Cleary and Edgman-Levitan 1997).

Determination of health care quality, especially as measured by outcomes, involves value judgments on the part of the recipients of health care. Because quality is value-based, it is ever changing and infinitely multifaceted. What quality *is* and how it is measured must include a spectrum of health care access, structures, processes, and outcomes; the measures of which will develop varying roles and interpretations over time and across locales. Hence quality measurement cannot guarantee quality, it can only make quality more likely. It is best, therefore, to view quality measurement as a probabilistic exercise.

Measuring Quality and Setting Standards

For this case, structural measures of quality are also important. Structural aspects of a health plan's quality are quantifiable plan characteristics that are believed to lead to improved health outcomes for patients (Donabedian 1980). The credentials of a plan's physician staff are structural indicators of the plan's quality. Nebraska Partners has at least three structural quality standards for physicians, relating to training, board certification, and malpractice experience. These are the measures of quality that Nebraska Partners will breach if they contract with the physicians in question.

The question is whether these three structural quality indicators related to credentialing are good ones. One might hope that they would be quite good. After all, it is inexpensive and not very complicated to determine whether physicians are board certified, have completed residency training, and have few malpractice claims. Moreover, because they are inexpensive, common, and have a long history, such measures of structural quality remain cornerstone measures for health plan accreditation (National Committee for Quality Assurance 1997). Unfortunately, data on these measures may also be complicated to interpret and poorly correlated with health outcomes. Whether a physician has passed a certifying examination may say more about his or her age and specialty than it does about the quality of care that physician can deliver. In at least one study, board certification was actually associated with higher malpractice claims experience (Sloan et al. 1989).

Malpractice lawsuits are correlated with numerous factors, but studies have not shown a reliable correlation between malpractice history and poor quality of care (Entman et al. 1994; Taragin et al. 1994). In this case, for example, a family physician who delivers the babies of women with poor health and social status, in a rural area with few facilities or colleague specialists, might well develop a higher-than-average claims history, and find it difficult to retain malpractice coverage, yet still be providing the best possible quality care. Risk-adjustment of malpractice data eventually might provide assistance in interpreting malpractice rates, but current risk-adjustment in this area is poor (Kravitz, Rolph, and McGuigan 1991; Taragin et al. 1994).

Residency training holds perhaps the strongest relationship to providing high-quality care because many features of training programs have been shown to affect quality of care. Nevertheless, no studies are known that have compared the quality of family practice-trained physicians with that of generalists who entered the field before the advent of family practice as a specialty. In sum, weaknesses in correlating adherence to any one of these three structural quality measures with quality of care should make Nebraska Partners reluctant to base a decision on any one of these factors alone, or perhaps even all three.

Since no one factor can provide an adequate screening mechanism to ensure good quality (and each physician in question apparently fails on only one point), ideally Nebraska Partners will look to additional measures of quality before making a decision to contract (or not) with this group. It could look to additional structural indicators (for example, the condition of the clinic facilities or the number and training of the nursing staff) or to process measures of quality (for example, vaccination or mammography rates at the clinic), or to direct measures of patient satisfaction and health outcomes. A decision could then be made based on the broadest available set of quality indicators.

If no additional measures of quality are available and Nebraska Partners intends to contract with these physicians "for business reasons," then additional options should be considered. For example, the physicians might be asked to practice under some form of supervision for a time to ensure their level of quality. The physicians could be required to adhere to strict requirements for processes of care, and Nebraska Partners could prospectively set outcomes targets to help ensure quality of care. Ideally, the physicians would prove over time that their performance is up to par. If not, the plan could choose not to renew the contract in the future.

But what if all available additional measures of quality only demonstrate that the physicians in question actually are substandard practitioners? May a plan accept lower standards for quality in areas with a smaller physician supply? Consciously accepting a lower standard in rural areas appears to constitute discrimination toward patients living there. Uniform standards for safety are highly appealing. Society would not knowingly reduce standards for food safety in rural areas or reduce the requirements of the building codes in these areas, so why should we accept substandard medical care in rural America?

First, there may be no choice. Failing a move to lure or conscript high-quality physicians into practice in rural areas, policymakers may have to decide whether lower standard care is better than no care. This has sometimes driven decisions to expand the role of lesser-trained health care practitioners in rural areas. For example, Medicaid has contracted with nurse practitioners, at physician rates, to provide primary care in areas of physician shortage but generally has not done so in other areas (Warshaw 1998).

Second, consider whether a plan may set *more* stringent criteria for physician quality in areas of *greater* physician supply. Plans can and do just this, justified by their desire to offer to their members the highest quality health care possible.

Considered in reverse, the unacceptability of reducing standards where physician supply is low is not so obvious. Setting aside whether the standards are reliable and relevant, there is no doubt that plans have an obligation to provide their members the best medical care available.

Third, people who live in rural areas make sacrifices in the availability of numerous services. In part, they may consciously trade increased tranquility, safety, and so on for decreases in other amenities. For example, rural fire and police departments may have relatively longer response times. To the extent these trade-offs are recognized and accepted, they may be ethically justifiable as autonomous choices.

Finally, for members of this community, the important issue is whether they will be better off with access to Nebraska Partners' Medicaid plan compared to their other options. The quality of their health care relative to that of metropolitan residents is of much less importance. From the case, it appears they may be better off. Easier access, even if only to the same mediocre physicians, would be of benefit. The other appealing option to recruit new and better clinicians to the area is, we are told, not "economically feasible." Recognition that this community would be better off if Nebraska Partners contracts with these physicians is ethically relevant to Nebraska Partners. As the philosopher John Rawls (1971) has persuasively argued, the best determinant of a just decision is not that it produces absolute equality but that it produces relative improvement for at least some concerned parties, and that no others are harmed. That is, Nebraska Partners may be ethically justified in moving into this community, even with lowered standards, so long as the community's situation is at least improved over its baseline and no other party is hurt.

Is There a Minimum Floor?

If these considerations hold, then the only remaining issues are how much care in this community would be improved, and how much disparity in quality is ultimately acceptable. Let us assume that the improvement is substantial. If this is so, then Nebraska Partners must finally consider, for itself and its other members, whether strict and uniform adherence to the plan's structural quality standards is more important than the local benefits that will accrue if the standards are dropped in this community. That is, the final issue is whether there should be a floor below which the plan will not go even in areas of very low physician supply.

One option would be to set such an absolute floor at the point where receiving *no* care would likely be better than receiving even a little care from the contracting physicians (or other clinicians). Given the failings of structural quality measures already noted, this might require following the physicians over time to document that their care is hazardous. However, setting such a minimalist floor might not be wise. Public feedback could be severe. The liability risk is high. Preexisting professional norms and national standards set through accrediting organizations might not allow it. From a policy perspective, a very low floor could encourage a "rush to the bottom" mentality among competing health plans, mitigating against such a minimalist floor. Finally, for Nebraska Partners, there may even be marketing value in setting relatively high standards and sticking to them.

Wherever the floor is set it should be based on the largest feasible, best available set of quality indicators, recognizing that no single indicator or small set of indicators will provide enough information to make reliable decisions about quality. A floor made up of a few unreliable quality standards will be capricious and will discriminate against those providing otherwise high-quality care who do not happen to meet these standards. In addition, plans must recognize that using even an excellent set of quality standards will not be a perfect screen. Predicting quality is like measuring it: at best, a set of quality standards is a probabilistic tool that will improve the plan's odds of not contracting with a poor-quality clinician or group. The more valid and reliable the variables taken into account, the more likely it is that poor-quality clinicians will be screened out, but the tool will never be perfect.

In the end, Nebraska Partners will need to weigh the relative value of local access to its plan, through these physicians, against the risk that these physicians are worse than mediocre: the weighing must take into account the value to the plan (and possibly society) of having absolute minimum quality standards. In making this assessment, Nebraska Partners should understand that access to its plan might not be the only, or best, route to health care for this community. Nebraska Partners should avoid a self-serving confusion between its own access to a statewide market and this community's access to health care. The plan should be aware that reliance on a few, fallible structural quality indicators (such as malpractice and training history) to determine physicians' quality of care may pose problems. Seeking additional information on quality and working with the community to determine whether access to Nebraska Partners' plan will help them to achieve desired health outcomes are necessary steps in these considerations. Should Nebraska Partners choose to enter this community, despite a belief that the local practitioners are of poor quality, then establishing mechanisms to provide oversight and encourage quality improvement will be critical, as will continuous monitoring for evolving quality concerns.

Finally, Nebraska Partners may be forced to concede that its rural customers will receive inferior medical care in some respects, compared to their urban counterparts. This being the likely case, close attention to defining a floor below which the plan is never willing to fall will be necessary. Ethical, medical, and political concerns will rightly influence where this floor is set, and the relevant parties from Nebraska Partners must be involved in setting the floor and monitoring its effects. As far as possible, such a floor should be built on a solid foundation of valid and reliable measures of quality.

References

Bindman, A. B.; Grumbach, K.; Osmond, D.; Komaromy, M.; Vranizan, K.; Lurie, N.; Billings, J.; and Stewart, A. 1995. "Preventable Hospitalizations and Access to Health Care." *Journal of the American Medical Association* 274, no. 4:305–11.

Brook, R. H.; McGlynn, E. A.; and Cleary, P. D. 1996. "Measuring Quality of Care." *New England Journal of Medicine* 335, no. 13:966–70.

Cleary, P. D., and Edgman-Levitan, S. 1997. "Health Care Quality: Incorporating Consumer Perspectives." *Journal of the American Medical Association* 278, no. 19:1608–12.

Donabedian, A. 1980. *Explorations in Quality Assessment and Monitoring, Volume 1: The Definition of Quality and Approaches to its Assessment.* Ann Arbor, Mich.: Health Administration Press.

Entman, S. S.; Glass, C. A.; Hickson, G. B.; Githens, P. B.; Whetton-Goldstein, K.; and Sloan, F. A. 1994. "The Relationship Between Malpractice Claims History and Subsequent Obstetrics Care." *Journal of the American Medical Association* 272, no. 20:1588–91.

Kongstvedt, P. R., and Plocher, D. W. 1996. "Acquisitions, Joint Ventures, and Partnerships Between Providers and Managed Care Organizations." In *The Managed Health-Care Handbook*, 3rd ed. Edited by P. R. Kongstvedt. Gaithersburg, Md.: Aspen Publishers.

Kravitz, R. L.; Rolph, J. E.; and McGuigan, K. 1991. "Malpractice Claims Data as a Quality Improvement Tool: 1. Epidemiology of Error in Four Specialties." *Journal of the American Medical Association* 266, no. 15:2087–92.

National Committee for Quality Assurance. 1997. *Standards for Accreditation of Managed Care Organizations.* Washington, D.C.: National Committee for Quality Assurance.

Rawls, J. 1971. *A Theory of Justice.* Cambridge, Mass.: Harvard University Press.

Schuster, M. A.; McGlynn, E. A.; and Brook, R. H. 1997. *Why the Quality of US Health Care Must be Improved.* Santa Monica, Calif.: RAND.

Sloan, F. A.; Mergenhagen, P. M.; Burfield, W. B.; Bovbjerg, R. R.; and Hassan, M. 1989. "Medical Malpractice Experience of Physicians: Predictable or Haphazard?" *Journal of the American Medical Association* 262, no. 23:3291–97.

Taragin, M. I.; Sonnenberg, F. A.; Karns, M. E.; Trout, R.; Shapiro, S.; and Carson, J. L. 1994. "Does Physician Performance Explain Interspecialty Differences in Malpractice Claim Rates?" *Medical Care* 32, no. 7:661–67.

Warshaw, R. 1998. "Too Much Independence for NPs?" *ACP Observer* (January):1.

10

CEO Salaries in For-Profit and Nonprofit Health Plans

CASE STUDY

Philip Lancet is the CEO of MedOne, a nonprofit HMO in the Midwest that is part of an integrated health system including the HMO, three hospitals, and a number of large physician clinics. MedOne enrolls approximately 500,000 members. During Mr. Lancet's five-year tenure, MedOne has experienced tremendous growth and success both in financial terms and in terms of consumer perception and satisfaction. MedOne has consistently held its medical loss ratio—the ratio between health care costs incurred and premiums earned during a given period—at about 93 percent. This means that $93 of every $100 went to health care costs, and $7 went to administration of the product. Administration includes compensation paid to CEOs and others. In a for-profit setting, administration would also include any shareholder distributions. The last two years are the first years in which MedOne has not met its financial targets. Mr. Lancet has been instrumental in reacting to and leading MedOne into the next stage of managed care designed to stem these financial losses.

Mr. Lancet, who has an M.B.A. from Duke and a J.D. from Stanford, is paid $170,000 per year in salary and typically receives an annual performance-based bonus of approximately $70,000. He worked as a health lawyer for eight years before rising through the ranks at MedOne to become the CEO.

A large, for-profit Northeast HMO, Assure Health, is attempting to recruit Mr. Lancet to become its CEO. Assure Health has offered Mr. Lancet a base salary of $350,000 and a targeted bonus of 35 percent of base salary for the first year. Assure Health is a for-profit HMO and has historically had medical loss ratios of about 73 percent.

As a spokesman for MedOne over the past few years, Mr. Lancet has repeatedly pointed to its nonprofit status and high medical loss ratios as virtues of the corporation and as advantages to the consumer. Mr. Lancet now wonders whether Assure Health's for-profit status and lower medical loss ratios would adversely affect his ability to represent and lead the organization.

The board of directors of MedOne must consider whether it should respond to Assure Health's offer by raising Mr. Lancet's compensation. Advocates for this approach point out that the average base salary for managed care executives is approximately $210,000 with a bonus of about 38 percent. They argue that, as in any other business, in order to attract and retain quality leadership, it is necessary to offer competitive compensation packages. In fact, advocates point specifically to the fact that a CEO of a large medical supply company in the same city makes substantially more than Mr. Lancet, yet Mr. Lancet has comparable responsibilities at a much larger, more profitable company. Opponents on the board respond that executive salaries for local HMOs have already been the subject of broad criticism in the press and have contributed to the anti–managed care sentiment in the state. They predict that raising Mr. Lancet's salary is sure to lead to bad press and strong public criticism.

Questions for Consideration

➤ From an ethical perspective, should Mr. Lancet accept the position with Assure Health? Should the board of MedOne counteroffer with more money?
➤ How might for-profit and nonprofit HMOs differ from a member's perspective? A provider's perspective? A CEO's perspective? A community perspective?
➤ How might the for-profit status of an HMO affect quality of care?
➤ How does a for-profit HMO's obligation to its shareholders relate to its obligations to members, purchasers, providers, and the community?
➤ Some states require HMOs to be nonprofit. What might be the policy reasons for such a regulation? What are the arguments against such a limitation?
➤ At what point does a medical loss ratio become unacceptably low? Why?
➤ Should legislation limit HMO salaries? Why?
➤ Is health care a commodity morally distinguishable from other commodities and therefore deserving of different treatment?

COMMENTARY

Bradford H. Gray, Ph.D.

The case of Mr. Lancet and MedOne asks whether salaries and administrative costs in HMOs can be too high in absolute terms or as a percentage of premium dollars. The case links this question to the larger topic of for-profit ownership and asks whether operating health services organizations on a profit-making basis may be ethically suspect.

Let us begin with the narrow issue. The board of this nonprofit HMO must decide whether to increase the CEO's compensation from $240,000 (including bonus) in hopes of convincing him not to accept a competing offer that will pay him $472,500 (including bonus). The board is presumably contemplating an increase of between $50,000 (to reach what it believes to be the industry average) and $250,000 (to top the competing offer). The board believes that Mr. Lancet has been a very effective CEO, as indicated by the organization's "tremendous growth and success both in financial terms and in terms of consumer perception and satisfaction." Deciding whether to increase an executive's salary is clearly a business decision. Is it also an ethical decision?

Executive compensation packages might be considered in ethical terms from several standpoints. First is the question of whether giving Mr. Lancet more money is compatible with the duties of trustees. Rich executive compensation packages are often seen as a failure of corporate governance. In the for-profit world, cozy relationships between boards and top executives can result in huge compensation packages paid at the expense of shareholders. In response to this concern, the law limits executive salaries (as a tax-deductible business expense) to $1 million unless tied to performance-related incentives. In the nonprofit world, concerns about high executive compensation are usually framed in terms of impact on the organization's mission. Because of their ethos and fears of violating legal prohibitions on distribution of profits, nonprofits use performance-related incentives less than do for-profits. However, MedOne ties over 40 percent of its CEO's compensation to performance-based incentives, which attenuates the governance-failure concern about a larger compensation package. Moreover, Mr. Lancet is now underpaid, in comparison both to his market value and to prevailing salaries. So, a violation of the board's duty because of lack of deservedness does not seem to be an issue.

Second, the board might be concerned about widening the compensation gap between the CEO and other employees, since it would not be feasible to increase all employees' salaries proportionally. The growing disparity between the wealthy and poor in our society is seen by many as a matter of social justice that should be corrected. This could be a reason to oppose a large increase for Mr. Lancet, but there is no indication that MedOne's board sees the issue either in such terms or in terms of the more mundane danger that a big salary increase for Mr. Lancet would create jealousy and morale problems within the HMO.

Third, the board might worry whether a large salary increase might force premium increases that would damage MedOne's competitive position (a business concern) or reduce the affordability of its premiums (possibly an ethical concern regarding access). This does not appear to be a serious issue. A $50,000 increase spread across 500,000 members equates to $.10 per member per year; even an increase of $250,000 would amount to only $.50 per member per year.

Fourth, the board might also be concerned about increasing the plan's administrative costs and diverting premium dollars to administration. If MedOne's premiums are $1,800 per member per year (the national average according to the American Association of Health Plans), its total premiums are $900 million per year and its 7 percent administrative costs are $63 million per year. The contemplated increase for Mr. Lancet would raise that percentage nominally, between about .01 and .04 percent.

These numbers perhaps explain why the board does not focus on the impact on plan costs of the salary increase needed to retain Mr. Lancet. Their worry is about bad press and public criticism. Since some increase could be justified in terms of fairness to Mr. Lancet—why should MedOne expect him to accept far less than he can command elsewhere—and since the impact on premiums is minimal, the issue appears to be largely symbolic.

When do symbolic issues become ethical ones? Is there a salary/bonus threshold that is unethical to cross in health care? The executives of several large for-profit HMO companies have received salaries and stock options worth tens of millions of dollars in recent years. These have been criticized as unrelated to performance and for their alleged impact on services or costs. In one case, a regulator (the insurance commissioner of New York state) refused to approve a premium increase by Oxford Health Plans because of a multimillion-dollar severance package with the stricken company's CEO. Diversion of premiums to executive compensation was the issue. But our case does not involve Oxford-like compensation ($112 million for the CEO in 1996).

So, the MedOne board may replace an effective CEO because of public relations concerns. But is it ethical for a board to be more concerned about some letters to the editor from people who do not know what health care executives are paid today than about having an effective CEO for its HMO? And would it be responsible to seek a new CEO who is willing to take $240,000 to run an almost billion-dollar company?

What about the matter of the medical loss ratio? The extent to which premium dollars go to administrative costs and profits rather than to medical service providers has become controversial. Administrative costs are much higher in the American health care system than in countries that have government-administered universal health insurance, a point emphasized by advocates of universal health insurance. But the MedOne case is not about health system reform. HMOs' medical loss ratios have become attached to the debate about for-profit health care for two reasons. First, although nonprofit plans, like for-profits, must generate profits if they are to survive and grow, there is some evidence that medical loss ratios have been lower in for-profit plans than in nonprofits in recent years. Second, some publicly traded companies have touted their low medical loss ratios to attract investors, while some nonprofits have sought to make a virtue of their high medical loss ratios.

Loss ratios have long been one basis on which the economic health of insurance companies is judged. For regulators and investors, rising loss ratios may signal that an insurer or HMO is getting into financial trouble, with expenses rising in relationship to premiums. For-profit HMOs that have a low medical loss ratio seek to make a virtue out of it because it is a signal that they are doing well.

Health care providers, of course, prefer that as much of the premium dollar as possible finds its way into their own pockets. Not surprisingly, many of the organizations that have made an issue of medical loss ratios have been provider groups, such as the California Medical Association, which has used medical loss ratio data to argue that HMOs' administrative costs, not medical expenses, were driving up increasing insurance premiums. The California Medical Association has issued reports showing that for-profit HMOs in California have on average lower medical loss ratios, and higher administrative costs, than do nonprofits. Provider and consumer groups have called for legislation to set minimum allowable medical loss ratios.

To be sure, there is something perverse about HMOs making a virtue of spending only 60 or 70 percent of premium dollars on medical services. But a high medical loss ratio does not necessarily signal moral high ground. The interpretation of medical loss ratios can be very tricky (Robinson 1997) and may not tell us very much about whether a plan is wasteful or prone to deny needed care.

First, plan-to-plan differences in loss ratios can be due to differences in the size of premiums, not differences in administrative costs. Since medical loss ratios can be lowered by raising premiums, low medical loss ratios may signal that a given market is not very competitive.

Second, administrative expenses may be high if HMOs make serious efforts to minimize wasteful services and improve quality. Conversely, administrative costs are lowest if premium dollars are passed without impediment from purchasers to providers. But we know from experience that a system in which third-party payers simply pay for whatever is billed is the recipe for untenable cost increases, wide variations in patterns of care, uneven quality, and waste—the well-documented state of affairs to which managed care was a response.

Third, the lack of accounting standardization makes it hazardous to compare medical loss ratios across HMOs that have different organizational forms. To control their costs, HMOs can either have active cost-containment programs (with their attendant administrative costs) or they can use capitation to shift the economic risk to other organizational entities (for example, multispecialty medical groups) that provide medical care. In the latter instance, administrative costs borne by the medical groups may be accounted for by the health plan as medical expenses, and a high medical loss ratio may be an accounting artifact.

Fourth, the case perhaps suggests that the differences in loss ratios are due to ownership form—nonprofit or for-profit. However, neither the case study nor the critics of for-profit health care have supplied a reason why for-profit plans should have higher administrative costs than do nonprofits. Since profitability goals reward their keeping *both* medical and administrative costs under control, there is no incentive for for-profits to have higher administrative costs than do nonprofits. Perhaps they spend more on marketing (that is not documented) and perhaps they make greater use of cost-containment methods that boost administrative costs (again, not documented). Ownership-related differences seem to be small, and some for-profit plans have higher medical loss ratios than do some nonprofit plans. We cannot safely attribute the differences in loss ratios in our case to the HMOs' ownership form.

Finally, the size of an HMO's medical loss ratio is only partly under its control. If insurers could control costs perfectly and set prices with impunity, all insurers (including HMOs) would be profitable every year. Of course, this is not the case. Forty percent of plans reported losing money in 1997. A plan whose expenses exceed revenues is an unhealthy HMO, not necessarily a highly ethical one. The case posits a world in which loss ratios are stable from year to year—with the nonprofit MedOne being consistently high and the for-profit Assure Health being consistently low. But, real-world insurers are subject to the "underwriting cycle," a well-documented phenomenon in which three years of improving results are followed by three years of losses (Gabel et al. 1991).

In deciding whether to leave MedOne, should Mr. Lancet be influenced by the loss ratio information? The preceding analysis suggests that he may want to determine what lies behind the reported difference. As an experienced HMO administrator, he may worry that MedOne's loss ratio is too high. What happens if price competition or medical costs increase in his market? And if he believes that Assure Health's administrative costs are out of line, that might enhance the attractiveness of a position there. As a highly competent HMO executive, he could address the problem and the company's profitability would soar.

Both of the issues presented in this case have considerable polemical value, but neither lends itself to resolution by drawing a bright line on either policy or ethical grounds. The case does raise the question, What factors limit HMOs' pay to executives and their consumption of an excessive share of the health care dollar on operations and profit rather than services for enrollees? What mechanisms exercise restraint?

In a competitive field, market forces penalize organizations that do not deliver the services that are paid for or that spend too much money doing so. Organizations that have unusually high salaries or administrative expenses generally find themselves at a competitive disadvantage. The market discourages their behaving in this way. This is true for most services, but is it true for health care? If not, why not? Does the market fail?

In a classic article, the economist Kenneth Arrow (1963) observed that in fields (such as medical care) in which the seller of services knows much more about the need for and quality of those services than does the purchaser, the market may not do a good job of mediating price and quality. The seller can skimp on quality or charge more than the service is worth and the purchaser will not necessarily know. This bears on one of the great worries about managed care—that HMOs might without impunity put their financial interests ahead of patients' interests. This fear lies behind concerns that HMOs' physician payment and utilization review methods may compromise the physician's agency role vis-à-vis patients.

Might a low medical loss ratio signal that an HMO is skimping on services needed by patients, perhaps getting away with it because neither the patient nor the purchaser (a corporation or governmental program) can tell? There is no known evidence that links loss ratios and quality of care, but the connection has some plausibility, as does concern that for-profits might be particularly prone to exploit the contract failure problem of which Arrow wrote.

Worries that HMOs might take their premium dollars and provide fewer services than are needed (and paid for) has caused purchasers, led by large corporations, to insist that the HMO industry develop performance measurement standards, measures of enrollee satisfaction, and an accreditation system. Performance reports are now made regularly by a growing number of HMOs and by the National Committee for Quality Assurance (NCQA). The Health Plan Employer Data and Information Set (HEDIS) performance measures developed by NCQA are not perfect, but they have been rapidly improved through successive iterations over the last several years. HEDIS has been widely adopted by health plans and is certainly a better indicator of the quality of care provided by an HMO than is its CEO's salary or medical loss ratio.

What about the larger question of the ethics of for-profit health care? For many critics of the American health care system, for-profit health care symbolizes the view of health care as a private rather than a social good. Health care as a market commodity is anathema for some, the antithesis of the concept, rooted in social justice, of health care as a right. Yet it would be quite possible in principle to have a for-profit sector in a health care system that has universal health insurance. And, although nonprofit plans have developed subsidized premium programs for low-income populations, there is little evidence that nonprofit HMOs do very much to mitigate the problem of the uninsured.

The ownership of health care organizations by for-profit corporations has also been opposed for fear that the control of medical decision making by parties bound by the ethic of business rather than the fiduciary ethic of medicine would result in exploitation of vulnerable patients for personal gain. For much of this century, medical licensure laws were interpreted in many states as prohibiting employment of doctors by corporations, although exceptions were always made for public and nonprofit employers. These corporate practice laws have become ineffective in recent years, because they can be circumvented via various contracting arrangements.

For-profit ownership of hospitals and HMOs is not new. Indeed, half of hospitals were for-profit early in the century (Rosen 1983), as were many of the prepaid health plans that were precursors of HMOs, a term coined in the early 1970s (Durso 1992). Corporate ownership of *multiple* hospitals and HMOs is a phenomenon of recent decades, as is research on their comparative performance. A full summary of this literature is beyond the scope of this commentary, but several broad generalizations can be made (Gray 1991, 1997a, 1997b).

First, both for-profits and nonprofits in health care depend on the sale of services for their revenues, and both rely heavily on private sources of capital. The lenders who provide capital to nonprofits want financially sound investments, as do investors of equity capital in for-profit organizations. Thus, good financial performance is essential for access to needed capital for both for-profits and nonprofits. Second, studies mostly show that ownership-related differences in performance are small. However, the differences that have been found primarily show nonprofits to be better from a social point of view—more responsive to local needs, and more likely to provide public goods. (It can be argued that they should be held accountable for behaving in this way since they benefit from tax exemptions. The evidence suggests that performance in this regard is quite uneven.) Third, there seem to be no dimensions on which nonprofits and for-profits do not overlap. Differences are matters of degree, not of kind.

Properly functioning nonprofit organizations with effective governance and management structures mitigate some of the dangers of for-profit ownership regarding public goods and the exploitation of the vulnerabilities of patients and payment systems. Because for-profits can make greater use of financial incentives to encourage behavior that serves the organization's economic interests, for-profits may be more prone to the kinds of problems of which Arrow warned more than thirty-five years ago. However, in deciding whether to take the new position, Mr. Lancet should be sure to appreciate that the behavior of any particular organization is undoubtedly influenced by more factors than their form of ownership.

References

Arrow, K. 1963. "Uncertainty and the Welfare Economics of Medical Care." *American Economic Review* 53, no. 5:941–73.

Durso, K. A. 1992. "Profit Status in the Early History of Health Maintenance Organizations." Ph.D. Diss., Yale University.

Gabel, J.; Formisano, R.; Lohr, B.; and DiCarlo, S. 1991. "Tracing the Cycle of Health Insurance." *Health Affairs* 10, no. 4:48–61.

Gray, B. H. 1991. *The Profit Motive and Patient Care: The Changing Accountability of Doctors and Hospitals.* Cambridge, Mass.: Harvard University Press.

———. 1997a. "Conversion of HMOs and Hospitals: What's at Stake?" *Program on Nonprofit Organizations Working Paper,* no. 238.

———. 1997b. "Trust and Trustworthy Care in the Managed Care Era." *Health Affairs* 16, no. 1:34–49.

Robinson, J. C. 1997. "Use and Abuse of the Medical Loss Ratio to Measure Health Plan Performance." *Health Affairs* 16, no. 4:176–87.

Rosen, G. 1983. *The Structure of American Medical Practice 1876–1941.* Philadelphia: University of Pennsylvania Press.

COMMENTARY

David A. Hyman, M.D., J.D.

The Teachers Insurance and Annuity Association/College Retirement Equities Fund (TIAA/CREF) is a massive pension system for academics. Like many financial services providers, TIAA/CREF sends its participants a variety of marketing and promotional materials, including a quarterly magazine. In one issue of the magazine a letter from a participant pointed out the substantial disparity between the modest sums the writer earned as an academic (and the still more modest sums he was able to save for retirement) and the magnificent amounts paid to those who were making investment decisions for the funds entrusted to TIAA/CREF. The editors briefly sympathized with the writer, but quite sensibly responded that TIAA/CREF was required to pay "market rates" to attract and retain employees with the necessary expertise. Had the editors been less diplomatic, they might have added that the populist appeal of paying less than market rates would disappear the moment that strategy compromised the return earned by TIAA/CREF on the funds it held for its participants.

MedOne and TIAA/CREF face similar situations. If MedOne wants to retain Mr. Lancet's services, it will need to meet the going rate for doing so. It is possible that raising Mr. Lancet's salary may prompt some bad press and public criticism, but that reaction should not decide the matter. The correct question for the board of directors is whether the value added by Mr. Lancet to MedOne exceeds the cost of securing his services, and not whether their decision to pay a market rate for Mr. Lancet will prompt criticism from those who are less well informed about such matters. The board of directors should not be indifferent to the cost of the "inputs" (like Mr. Lancet) into MedOne's operations, but it would be better served by focusing its concern on the "outputs" that result from having Mr. Lancet around.

If Mr. Lancet is really "instrumental in reacting to and leading MedOne into the next stage of managed care," then a few pennies per member per month seems a small price to pay to keep him as the CEO of MedOne.

To be sure, MedOne is currently paying Mr. Lancet a princely sum—but Assure Health would not be offering to double it unless it believed that MedOne was significantly underpaying Mr. Lancet for his talents. Although the case is framed to suggest that nonprofit HMOs are the virtuous baseline, and for-profit HMOs are ethically problematic, the simple fact that Assure Health is willing to double Mr. Lancet's salary is some evidence that it is the "virtuous" nonprofit that is exploiting Mr. Lancet by paying him much less than he is worth. The fact that the CEO of a smaller and less valuable medical supply company makes more than Mr. Lancet confirms the point.

And what of Mr. Lancet's enviable situation? As noted, Assure Health obviously believes Mr. Lancet is woefully underpaid in his current position—and the organization is prepared to pay handsomely for his management skills, not his soul. Although there might well be some ethical issues if there were something unsavory about Assure Health, the case provides no evidence that Mr. Lancet's potential employer is anything other than an exemplary HMO. The case study does suggest that Mr. Lancet is concerned he cannot effectively "represent and lead" Assure Health, in light of its for-profit status and lower medical loss ratios. If so, he should certainly not take the job, although his prospects for career advancement and mobility are likely to be dim, since for-profit enterprise is now the rule in the HMO market (Claxton et al. 1997). It may be that Mr. Lancet is somewhat uninformed. As outlined next, nonprofit status simply does not neatly correlate with organizational virtue.

If Mr. Lancet believes in nonprofit health care, perhaps he should stay at MedOne at half his true market salary. However, MedOne should probably not count on all of its personnel demonstrating such refined sensibilities. If the board of directors of MedOne wants to put the issue to the test, it should cut the salary of all MedOne personnel by 50 percent and explain that participating in a virtuous nonprofit health care entity is its own reward. If the board of directors of MedOne follows that course, an employee-led insurrection would occur—followed by a mad search for employers who have a better understanding of the realities of supply and demand in the labor market. The net result will be a rapid (and deserved) deterioration in the quality of services offered by MedOne. Like TIAA/CREF, MedOne must pay market rates if it wants to attract and retain qualified personnel.

The more general issues raised by this case are the role of nonprofit enterprise in health care and whether the organizational status (for-profit versus nonprofit) of an entity that provides health care services should be an issue of concern to health plan employees, consumers, and policymakers. Viewed from a regulatory perspective, the issue is whether for-profit health care requires additional oversight because of quality concerns, low "medical loss ratios," or conflicts of interest between shareholders and patients.

Although these issues have been frequently debated over the past decade, they have drawn increased attention in connection with the conversion of a number of nonprofit hospitals to for-profit status (Hyman 1998). The debate about the merits of for-profit health care now rages in the mainstream news media, medical and policy journals, state capitols, and Washington, D.C. Unfortunately, much of the debate has been long on sloganeering and short on evidence. As was observed by one author, "Perhaps no health system change arouses more emotion and less rational policy discussion than the conversion of hospitals and health plans from not-for-profit to for-profit status" (Claxton et al. 1997). One gets a sense for the depth of feeling surrounding these issues from a document available on the Internet that purports to be a physician recruitment prequalification form for a prominent for-profit hospital chain. Applicants are disqualified if they received a grade higher than C+ in biomedical ethics, consider factors other than a patient's credit rating and insurance status in deciding whether hospital admission is required, or cannot see at least sixty patients per hour.

More concrete criticism of for-profit health care has focused on four interrelated concerns: cream-skimming, diversion, exploitation, and lack of community benefit. The charge of cream-skimming is based on the claim that for-profit firms focus on providing high-profit medical product lines to those who can pay and avoid less profitable but necessary services (Miller 1997). The charge of diversion results from the fact that for-profit firms sometimes have higher overheads and pay taxes and dividends, removing from the health care "pot" funds that would have otherwise been available to pay providers and cross-subsidize needed services (Nudelman and Andrews 1996; Christianson and Miles 1997). The charge of exploitation is based on the assertion that for-profit firms cannot be trusted to provide something as important as health care, and the nonprofit form is essential to protect patients from price-gouging, "bait and switch," and quackery (Gray 1997). The charge that for-profit firms do not provide sufficient "community benefit" is based on the claim that they do not shoulder their "fair share" of such public goods as charity care, medical education, and clinical research (Claxton et al. 1997).

Proponents of for-profit health care respond with a variety of arguments. The most basic claim is that the charges of cream-skimming, diversion, and community benefit largely miss the point (Hyman 1990). For-profit firms satisfy their civic responsibility by paying taxes. It is nonprofit firms that must justify the benefits and subsidies they receive. An extensive body of health services research has made clear that although there are some differences between for-profit and nonprofit firms, the differences are small and the overlap is substantial. Nonprofit status is a poor predictor of conduct, and it is conduct that health plan employees, consumers, and policymakers should be concerned with.

As for the exploitation of patients, if for-profit enterprise is so hazardous, why is it the rule in virtually every other sector of the economy? Most entities in the health care industry (physicians, nurses, medical equipment manufacturers, pharmaceutical companies, and nursing homes) have long been for-profit. A number of widely publicized incidents make clear that the nonprofit form is no guarantee of virtuous conduct (Brody 1997). One is left with the suspicion that the issue is not really trustworthiness but prestige and professional autonomy.

For all the articles that have been written on these issues, it is striking that much of "the debate about for-profit health care is fueled as much by values as by evidence" (Gray and McInerney 1986). Advocates have made extravagant claims for the merits of the nonprofit form, but "Americans are mostly unaware of which health plans are for-profit and which are nonprofit, and even when they know, they do not care" (Herbert 1997). Given the findings of health services researchers on the actual performance of nonprofit and for-profit firms, there is no particular reason why health plan employees, consumers, and policymakers should care about the institutional status of health plans.

The final issue is the significance of the medical loss ratio. Mr. Lancet is proud of MedOne's high medical loss ratio and has suggested that it is a virtue of the corporation and an advantage to the consumer. A medical loss ratio represents the percentage of premium dollars that are spent on purposes other than the direct provision of health care services. Health care providers obviously prefer a health plan that spends most of its premiums purchasing health care, since every dollar of "medical loss" is a dollar of income for them. Should consumers and regulators feel the same way?

There are good grounds for being cautious about relying on medical loss ratios in assessing the merits of a health plan. The comparison of medical loss ratios between health care plans is a complicated business, given predictable differences in accounting conventions, allocation methodologies, premiums, marketing strategies, and the like (Robinson 1997). Even if these differences could be ironed out, if a marginal dollar spent on administration saves more than a dollar of inappropriate health care expenses, then why should anyone complain about that fact (Altman and Shactman 1997)? Regardless, the medical loss ratio is at best a "process" measure, which bears no necessary correlation to the quality of care provided by the health plan and those with whom it contracts. Finally, since for-profit firms must generally pay taxes and dividends, they will typically have lower medical loss ratios than nonprofit health plans, all other things being equal. Condemning them for that structural reality is rather like saying one would like zebras better if they only got rid of their stripes.

The debate over the place of for-profit health care mirrors the inconsistent foundations of American health policy—a communitarian/egalitarian desire to ensure access for those in need, but simultaneous (and increasingly tough-minded) concern about incentives, efficiency, cost, and the trade-offs between public good, public goods, and private advantage. Some of the issues that arise from this intersection of conflicting values raise difficult problems of implementation and regulatory oversight. Thankfully, the situation faced by MedOne and Mr. Lancet is not one of them.

References

Altman, S. H., and Shactman, D. 1997. "Should We Worry About Hospital's High Administrative Costs?" *New England Journal of Medicine* 336, no. 11:798–99.

Brody, E. 1996. "Institutional Dissonance in the Nonprofit Sector." *Villanova Law Review* 41:433–504.

Christensen, C., and Miles, S. H. 1997. "The Ethical Importance of Differences Between Managed Care Systems." *HEC Forum* 9, no. 4:313–22.

Claxton, G.; Feder, J.; Shactman, D.; and Altman, S. 1997. "Public Policy Issues in Nonprofit Conversions: An Overview." *Health Affairs* 16, no. 2:9–28.

Gray, B. H. 1997. "Conversion of HMOs and Hospitals: What's at Stake?" *Health Affairs* 16, no. 2:29–36.

Gray, B. H., and McNerney, W. 1986. "For-Profit Enterprise in Health Care: The Institute of Medicine Study." *New England Journal of Medicine* 314, no. 23:1523–24.

Herbert, M. E. 1997. "A For-Profit Health Plan's Experience and Strategy." *Health Affairs* 16, no. 2:121–24.

Hyman, D. A. 1990. "The Conundrum of Charitability: Reassessing Tax Exemption for Hospitals." *American Journal of Law & Medicine* 16, no. 3:317–80.

———. 1998. "Hospital Conversions: Fact, Fantasy, and Regulatory Follies." *Journal of Corporation Law* 23, no. 4 (forthcoming).

Miller, L. 1997. "The Conversion Game: High Stakes, Few Rules." *Health Affairs* 16, no. 2:112–17.

Nudelman, P. M and Andrews, L. M. 1996. "The 'Value Added' of Not for Profit." *New England Journal of Medicine* 334, no. 16:1057–59.

Robinson, J. C. 1997. "Use and Abuse of the Medical Loss Ratio to Measure Health Plan Performance." *Health Affairs* 16, no. 4:176–87.

11

Hospital Staffing Levels

CASE STUDY

Robert Nelson suffered his first heart attack two years ago, when he was sixty-four years old. The father of eight children (and now the grandfather of twelve), Mr. Nelson had retired three years earlier from his position as a foreman at a large construction firm. Since retiring, Mr. Nelson and his wife have divided their time between their cabin in northern Wisconsin and their condo in the Southwest, spending about six months a year at each location. The couple was in the Southwest for the winter when Mr. Nelson had the attack.

As soon as Mr. Nelson complained of severe back and shoulder pain, his wife brought him to the hospital. He was admitted to the cardiac intensive care unit. Tests indicated a myocardial infarction, and further tests revealed moderate blockage in one of Mr. Nelson's arteries. He underwent angioplasty to remove the blockage and was released two days after the surgery. His total hospital stay was seven days.

Both Mr. and Mrs. Nelson were impressed with the care Mr. Nelson received while at the hospital. They remembered one nurse in particular, Julie Cohen, who was his day nurse after he had been transferred from the intensive care unit to cardiac special care, the hospital's intermediate-level cardiac unit. Ms. Cohen had worked as a cardiac care nurse since she received her registered nurse's degree twelve years before. As she tried to do with all her patients, Ms. Cohen took time to explain to Mr. Nelson and his wife the reasons for various tests and what their results meant. She informed them what to expect during the recovery period and was adept at responding to their fears and anxiety. She worked hard to give Mrs. Nelson both the information and confidence needed to care for her husband after he was discharged.

Mr. Nelson's recovery progressed well. Soon after leaving the hospital he initiated an aggressive exercise regimen (gradually building up to a daily five-mile walk).

He quickly adjusted to the recommended diet and other lifestyle changes that were designed to reduce the risk of future heart attacks. Three months later, the couple returned to northern Wisconsin in time for the opening of the fishing season.

Almost exactly two years later, when the couple was once again in the Southwest for the winter, Mr. Nelson suffered a second heart attack. He was rushed to the same hospital and admitted to the intensive care unit. As soon as he was stable, but before the extent of any damage to his heart was known, Mr. Nelson was transferred to the same special cardiac care unit as before. And once again, Julie Cohen was one of his nurses. But in the past two years, much had changed at the hospital and on this unit.

The hospital, previously nonprofit and independent, was now part of a regional for-profit hospital system. It had also recently formed a close alliance with Health-Sun, one of the state's large managed care organizations. Enrollees of HealthSun now comprised the majority of the hospital's patients. HealthSun was even more aggressive—and successful—than its managed care competitors in keeping its enrollees out of hospitals entirely and shortening their length of stay, when they were admitted. HealthSun was similarly successful in its negotiations with hospitals and other providers. For example, HealthSun got the hospital to agree to its demand that the hospital accept a flat per-diem rate for all of HealthSun's cardiac patients, despite the hospital's misgivings that the rate might not cover its costs.

In response to the more competitive environment and a steadily decreasing inpatient load, the hospital made a number of major adjustments. For example, the hospital adjusted its staffing levels, both by increasing the patient-to-nurse ratio and by transferring some responsibilities from registered nurses to lower-wage and less-skilled employees. As a result, even in the cardiac care units, registered nurses frequently only supervised patient care, while nursing assistants and technicians provided direct patient care. Another adjustment was to transfer patients expeditiously from the hospital's more intensive (and thus more costly) units to less intensive units, for example, from an intensive care unit to a regular floor.

On the day Mr. Nelson was transferred to the special cardiac care unit after his second heart attack, there were thirteen other patients on the unit, three of whom had undergone open heart surgery less than twenty-four hours before and had just been transferred from the cardiac intensive care unit. That evening, the cardiac unit's nurse supervisor had scheduled Ms. Cohen and a recently graduated nurse with no cardiac nurse training to work on the unit. This met the unit's recently established one-to-eight nurse-to-patient ratio (two years ago this ratio had been one-to-five). When Ms. Cohen started her shift, she asked for additional or more experienced staff. She had reviewed the status of her patients and told her supervisor she felt she could not adequately care for them all. Her request for additional help was turned down.

At 10 P.M., while Ms. Cohen was caring for one of the other patients on the unit, Mr. Nelson went into cardiac arrest. The unit's staff responded promptly; however, two of the staff had relatively little experience with cardiac arrests. After a long code, they were able to revive Mr. Nelson's heart. But he never regained consciousness. Several days later, Mr. Nelson was transferred to a nursing home. Yesterday, five months after his heart attack, a neurologist confirmed that Mr. Nelson is in a persistent vegetative state.

Questions for Consideration

➤ What should Ms. Cohen do if she believes the hospital's policies do not enable her to care adequately for her patients?

➤ What obligations does Ms. Cohen have to Mr. Nelson, to the other patients on the unit, and to the hospital? How should she seek to balance these obligations?

➤ Who is responsible for Mr. Nelson's current state of health?

➤ What criteria and processes should institutional providers use to establish patient-to-nurse ratios and other staffing patterns? What role, if any, should bedside nurses have in the process? What role, if any, should health plans have in the process?

➤ What accountability do health plans have to purchase services of sufficient quality?

COMMENTARY

Joanne M. Disch, Ph.D., R.N., F.A.A.N.

While theoretical debates rage as to the pros and cons of managed care, reality plays out at the individual point of service between a patient and caregiver, often a nurse. Within this interaction, the values of the individuals involved, of the institution in which care is provided, and of society as a whole are operationalized. When the values are congruent, the experience can be positive. When they conflict, which seems to occur more and more frequently, problems ensue. Far too often, the nurse is left to "make do."

This commentary addresses the issue of resource allocation, specifically hospital staffing. A basic reality in health care today is that society cannot afford to provide all services to everyone. Resources are limited and decisions need to be made as to how best to use them. When patient care is involved, nurses must be active participants in determining how best to allocate the resources and evaluate the impact of their presence or absence.

Providing Adequate Staffing

A major issue is how to match staffing levels with patient requirements for care in acute care settings. A variety of factors complicate this task: the shortened lengths of stay and increased acuity of hospitalized patients; the fluctuating in-patient census in many health care centers; the growing scarcity of experienced registered nurses; the increased reliance on assistive or paraprofessional personnel, licensed and not; the proliferation of regulatory requirements; and the desirability of working conditions in ambulatory care, which attracts nurses away from acute care settings.

As the Nelson case shows, hospitals are using many strategies to deal with the problem of adequate staffing. These include increasing the patient-to-nurse ratio, transferring some responsibilities from registered nurses to less skilled workers, using temporary help or employing new graduates in critical care areas, instituting staffing incentives or sign-on bonuses, transferring patients to intermediate areas, and discharging patients as soon as possible.

In some instances, these effective strategies are used responsibly to adjust imbalances in staffing. In other situations, health care systems use them to cut costs and thereby jeopardize patient safety. How are nurses able to know the kind of institution in which they are working?

First, Mr. Nelson's hospital should have instituted policies and practices that provide sufficient baseline staffing and options for augmenting staffing levels on a short-term basis when necessary. What is "sufficient" now varies from what was sufficient in previous decades, when the cost of care was not a concern. Sufficient staffing levels depend on (1) involving nurses directly in determining staffing levels, (2) using comparative data to establish norms among organizations caring for comparable patient populations, (3) securing the agreement of a cross section of experienced clinicians in the institution that the levels will ensure safe care, (4) preparing staff through orientation and training, and (5) monitoring outcomes of care and developing plans for what to do when outcomes are not acceptable.

While some nurses or organizations support quotas for ensuring a level of staffing for a given patient volume, quotas do not offer much help: they may even act as a barrier to hiring additional staff when needed, for example, when changes in patient acuity might warrant more staff. A dynamic process that involves nurses with true decision-making authority works best.

The hospital must also be able to augment staffing levels temporarily when the patient census increases or staff numbers decrease. Possible options include float pools, internal agencies or per diem staff, reassignment of staff, use of staff from external agencies, or incentive bonuses for staff to work overtime. In all cases, the nursing staff must be oriented and prepared to care for the particular patient population. New practice models may need to be developed so that the float pool or agency staff serves as a partner with the permanent staff.

Second, the hospital should have clear guidelines and mechanisms in place through which patients and families are informed about their rights and invited to be full partners in decisions about care and care delivery. In addition to a mandated Patient Bill of Rights, the hospital should provide information to the Nelsons in a clear, readable, linguistically appropriate format. Such information should include directions regarding care delivery and options available to them for resolution of issues.

Third, the hospital should have an explicit philosophy and system and also practices to support a healthy work environment and a quality-improvement approach to issues and concerns of patients, providers, and payers. A well-articulated, responsive process in place for dealing with concerns about patient care is the mark of an organization truly concerned about its patient care delivery.

What Should Julie Cohen Do?

At the beginning of the shift, Julie Cohen assessed the situation, asked for more help, and communicated her concern. Her immediate responsibility was to use optimally the resources that she had and provide the best possible level of care. The Nelson case suggests that there is virtually no other assistance available in the organization, even for a few hours. Ms. Cohen might also consider writing up the situation for her supervisor or nurse manager.

After the shift, Ms. Cohen might seek out her nurse manager or her peers to define clearly what the situation was and what could be done about it. They might discuss some of these questions:

1. How often does it happen that an experienced charge nurse believes more help is needed and none is available? If it occurs frequently, what can be done to increase the staffing options in the short- or long-term? Whose assistance or support is needed to obtain the resources? What data are needed?

2. What other changes have been made to help make the workload feasible? Is other staff, such as respiratory therapy or social work, being asked to help when the census rises? When the intensive care units are busy, are patients being maintained in the recovery room or the emergency department until the crunch is over? Is staff working with the nurse manager on possible strategies? Has the nurse manager's supervisor been consulted?

3. What is the plan for orienting new staff or cross-training temporary staff to help out? Are the ancillary personnel appropriately trained? Are they being partnered with professional nursing staff rather than independently assigned to patient care duties?

4. Why is there no experienced code team in the organization? How could one be set up?

In the longer term, the nurse manager could be asked to share information about some of the larger issues, such as the hospital's financial picture, trends in the community, and what is happening at other institutions. Reviewing the experiences of comparable institutions can highlight ways in which Ms. Cohen's hospital does or does not match with similar institutions as well as suggest new ways to address patient care.

The case indicates that the hospital has agreed to accept a flat per-diem rate for all HealthSun cardiac patients. Many hospitals have misgivings as to whether the costs of capitated contracts will be fully covered, since the calculation is very complex. In some instances, hospitals can offset their losses by achieving some margin with other patient populations. In other instances, the hospital may try to reduce its costs. Hospitals will try different strategies because they have different philosophies and are at different points along the continuum of balancing cost and quality. For some, cutting costs is reasonable and defensible; for others, it is not and patient safety could be jeopardized.

The case also raises the question of the accountability of health plans to purchase services of sufficient quality, and of providers to offer it. In reality, health plans are increasingly interested in purchasing quality or "value," that is, the best quality for a given price. This differs from purchasing the best quality at any price. Health care systems that offer good quality at competitive prices will outperform—and be preferred over—systems that offer low quality at either competitive or low prices. The push is toward efficiency—achieving the greatest benefit at the lowest cost. It is in the economic interest of payers to seek value and of providers to offer it.

The Need for a New Values Framework

Situations such as those faced by the Nelsons and Ms. Cohen are not unusual in health care today. They are symptoms of the larger societal shift in the values underpinning the American health care system.

Since World War II six values have driven health care decision making: professional autonomy, patient autonomy, consumer sovereignty, patient advocacy, high quality care, and access to care (Priester 1992). For many reasons, these values have been of limited help in decision making or policy formulation. Some of them are contradictory, for example, maximizing professional autonomy can interfere with enhancing access to care. Second, patient advocacy has traditionally focused on the interests of individual patients, regardless of the cost of care or the impact on the greater community. A community-centered view of health and human welfare must take the place of an individual-centered view (Callahan 1990).

The list of values is also incomplete. For example, society cannot afford to provide all services to everyone. Efficiency must be added to the list of values. Resources are limited and decisions need to be made as to how to use them best. New values and standards must be applicable to both individuals and organizations, reconciling economics and ethics (Whitley and Heeley 1997). They need not be antithetical. The challenge is to balance differing objectives.

The challenge for nurses today is to maintain their role as patient advocates in a changing health care environment that is struggling to balance quality and cost. Nurses have knowledge, skills, and competencies that equip them well for functioning effectively in and shaping the health care environment for their patients, patients' families, and themselves.

What Else Should Nurses Do?

To prevent a situation like the one Ms. Cohen faced or help turn it around, nurses might engage in the following activities:

1. Attend and participate in staff meetings at which these issues are presented. Participate in employee forums; if the institution has a shared governance model of management, become active. Strategize with coworkers and share concerns and observations with the nurse manager or director. If appropriate responses are not forthcoming, speak with the director of nursing or vice-president of patient care.

2. Read and gather information about health care trends in the local health care market. How well is the institution performing financially? How are other organizations dealing with similar contracting and payment pressures?

3. Call peers in other organizations and find out how they have dealt with similar issues. Have they preserved the role of the nurse as the individual primarily accountable for nursing care? How have they minimized the time spent by nurses on nonnursing tasks? Do their paraprofessionals help rather than replace the nurse?

4. Work with the nurse manager or director to pull together available information on the impact of nursing within the organization, for example, how a higher registered nurse skill mix was associated with a shorter length of stay and, thus, lower overall costs; how much nursing time was wasted by stripping beds, running to the blood bank, or drawing up intravenous medications; how nursing care improved wound healing rates and reduced postoperative complications; how the nursing salary budget decreased as a percent of overall hospital costs; how nursing full-time equivalents per patient day have actually gone down, while other full-time equivalents have risen (Aiken and Salmon 1994; Buerhaus 1995). Gath-

ering data on these indicators to be shared with senior management can be part of the organization's quality-improvement effort.

5. Talk with physicians and coworkers about how care could be reconfigured to free up nurses to do nursing and how support systems could provide support to nurses. Perhaps nurses in the cardiac catheterization lab can be cross-trained to assist in radiology when that department is busy.

6. Identify oneself as a nurse through introductions, nametag, and appearance. Part of the challenge in health care today is to make visible nurses' contributions. The public needs to know when nurses are providing the care and what that looks like. Ms. Cohen did this well. In fact, she was able to build on her earlier interactions with the Nelsons. As health care changes, however, this may require her to discuss with the patient and family how what they can expect during this particular hospitalization may differ from other episodes of care.

If Ms. Cohen were meeting them for the first time, she should ask them about their previous experiences with health care: what worked, what didn't, how they coped, what helped. She should then ask them what their expectations are this time, what they hope to achieve, and what role they want to play in Mr. Nelson's care. If she senses that their expectations are not realistic, given the resources available, she should work with them to identify the priorities that could be achieved during this stay in the hospital. Identifying and agreeing upon realistic goals of care is a crucial first step in care planning.

7. Speak directly to the director of nursing, vice-president for patient care, or CEO about concerns for patient care. Institutional leaders committed to delivering value and improving service, and who are aware that the nurse has done all that he or she can do by way of raising the issues through appropriate channels, will welcome the visit.

When Staffing Levels Do Not Improve

In many situations, efforts like those just suggested will produce positive change for nurses and their patients. In some cases, however, a nurse may feel that, despite his or her efforts, staffing levels are still insufficient and that patient safety is routinely being jeopardized. In that instance, the nurse has several options: to report the situation to an external regulatory body, to leave the organization, to reconcile professional values with those of the organization and continue employment, and/or to continue working to effect change. Each situation is unique. A nurse's accountability to the patient occurs on several levels. For the immediate, short-term situation, the nurse needs to do the very best that can be done, given the resources. In this case, Ms. Cohen did all she could under the circumstances. To the extent that the situation was one that could be expected to occur again, Ms. Cohen or any nurse needs to work with other staff and nursing leadership to ensure that systems are in place to provide adequate staffing. Here the nurse manager is chiefly responsible, but nursing staff should also help decide what staffing levels are needed and contribute to the recruitment and retention of staff. The *Standards of Clinical Nursing Practice* (American Nurses Association 1998), under which all nurses must practice, states: "The nurse assists the patient and family in identifying and securing appropriate and available services to address health-related needs"; and "The nurse contributes to a supportive and healthy work environment."

A patient or family member may ask the nurse to whom further complaints or concerns can be addressed. If the relevant issues cannot be addressed by those closest to the patient care area, the nurse could provide the names and phone numbers of other individuals within the administration with whom the patient or family member can talk, or facilitate patients or families contacting individuals directly.

It is *not* appropriate for the nurse to initiate a discussion with the patient or family about the nurse's concerns or issues. If a patient has questions, the nurse should answer them honestly and straightforwardly, while being reassuring—and the nurse should work with the appropriate individuals within the organization to see that needed change is achieved. Complaining about staffing levels, belittling coworkers or management, or sharing personal frustrations are inappropriate and contradictory to the nurse's role as patient advocate. When these occur, the nurse is exceeding the boundaries of a therapeutic relationship. The interaction between patient and nurse should be focused on meeting the patient's needs, not the caregiver's. Ms. Cohen and other concerned nurses can best help their patients and families by working with others to ensure sufficient staffing levels.

Conclusion

Within a managed care environment, the emphasis is on efficiency, effectiveness, and value. Instead of providing the best quality at any price, the challenge is to offer the best quality at a given price or the most benefit for the least cost. This challenge is forcing a clarification of values in health care and a redirection of resource allocation to meet new objectives. Identifying adequate levels of competent nursing staff, and recruiting and retaining them, are major challenges. All nurses in an organization have a responsibility to help in this process.

References

Aiken, L., and Salmon, M. 1994. "Health Care Workforce Priorities: What Nursing Should Do Now." *Inquiry* 31, no. 3:318–29.

American Nurses Association. 1998. *Standards of Clinical Nursing Practice*, 2d ed. Washington, D.C.: American Nurses Publishing, pp. 13, 15–16.

Buerhaus, P. 1995. "Economics and Reform: Forces Affecting Nurse Staffing." *Nursing Policy Forum* 1, no. 2:8–14.

Callahan, D. 1990. *What Kind of Life: The Limits of Medical Progress.* New York: Simon and Schuster, p. 28.

Priester, R. 1992. "A Values Framework For Health System Reform." *Health Affairs* 11, no. 1:84–107.

Whitley, E. M., and Heeley, G. F. 1997. "Forging A Code Of Ethics For Managed Care." *Healthcare Forum Journal* 40, no. 6:40–43.

COMMENTARY

Judith Shindul-Rothschild, Ph.D., R.N.C., N.A.P.

In the Nelson case, Ms. Cohen, a cardiac care nurse with many years of experience, finds herself in an ethical dilemma increasingly faced by nurses across the United States. More and more nurses report to work each day only to find too few registered nurses to provide adequate care. In Mr. Nelson's case, Ms. Cohen believes the staffing is inadequate for two reasons. First, there are not enough registered nurses, given the acute care needs of the patients; and second, the staff assigned does not have the clinical competence to provide safe care to acutely ill cardiac patients.

Faced with such a situation, registered nurses have to weigh whether the risk of harm to the patient is greater if they accept the assignment than if they reject it. Ms. Cohen contacted her supervisor and requested additional nursing staff. Her request was denied. At this point Ms. Cohen places her license and the care of her patients in jeopardy. Many staff nurses are asking for specific direction about what they should do when they are faced with such a professional and ethical conflict.

The American Nurses Association (1995) position statement entitled *The Right to Accept or Reject an Assignment* states: "Neither physicians' orders nor the employing agency's policies relieve the nurse of accountability for actions taken and judgments made," and "Professional nurses are accountable for nursing judgments and actions regardless of the personal consequences."

In the Nelson case, the staff nurses do not take sufficient steps to obtain additional nursing staff, and a patient is harmed. Could that harm have been avoided? Ms. Cohen and the other nurses had several other options available to them, short of flatly refusing the assignment, that could have resulted in a more positive outcome.

Nurses must first respond in a professional manner to protect their licenses and advocate assertively for the patients on their unit. Once a verbal request for additional personnel has been denied, nurses should immediately document their objections in accordance with hospital policies and procedures. Written documentation specifying the number of nurses, their clinical competence, the severity of illness of the patients, the time, and the response of the supervisor to their requests for additional staff should be recorded carefully.

Staff nurses should follow the appropriate chain of authority to expedite a reasonable resolution, at least in the short-term. Often the formality of following hospital procedures and protocols to request additional staff is enough to persuade the immediate supervisor that the situation is indeed untenable and must be addressed immediately. Furthermore, such written documentation is essential in the legal defense of nurses should a patient be harmed and the nurse held individually liable. While hospital management has the authority to make staffing decisions, state practice acts hold registered nurses legally accountable should an untoward event occur as a result of short-staffing.

Nurses' ethical duty to work collaboratively with physician colleagues would include timely notification if there are insufficient nurses to provide competent medical and nursing care. Physician colleagues can be formidable allies in nurses' attempts to ensure that there are enough registered nurses to care for critically ill patients. Physicians have also collaborated with staff nurses to document how the numbers and mix of nursing personnel affect a variety of patient outcomes. Analysis of quality-assurance data is one of the best long-term strategies for demonstrating the impact of staffing cutbacks on both the cost and quality of care.

A registered nurse's primary responsibility is to the patient. The contract between the nursing profession and society is made explicit through the *Code for Nurses* and the *Standards of Clinical Nursing Practice* (American Nurses Association, 1985, 1991). If the ability to provide patients with competent care is threatened in a systematic way, patients and their families need to be informed of the constraints on nursing staff and apprised of the anticipated effect on nurses' ability to provide adequate care. For example, patients and families should be informed that the nurse may not be able to fulfill requests for pain medication in a timely way because the unit is short-staffed. Patients and families who complain to the nurse about the quality of care should be directed to put their concerns in writing to hospital management.

Strategies to Document and Improve Inadequate Nurse Staffing

Until recently, management's prerogative to set nurse staffing levels or assign nursing staff has been considered sacrosanct. In two negotiations in Massachusetts, staff nurses were able to include language in their collective bargaining agreement mandating that staff nurses participate in decisions regarding staffing levels. Most collective bargaining contracts include clauses termed "endorse objection." Such clauses give a nurse the right to submit an "assignment-despite-objection" (ADO) document simultaneously to the bargaining agent and nursing administration. This document puts the health care agency on notice that professional standards of care could not be met.

ADO forms are developed and distributed by the organization or agency representing the nurses for collective bargaining. Most ADO forms consist of checklists and spaces for written documentation about the number of nursing staff and patients. Ample space is available for nurses to delineate why they have specific concerns about the inadequacy of nursing staff. Forms are typically cosigned by a staff nurse and that nurse's direct supervisor and then forwarded to appropriate management and the collective bargaining representatives.

Management's immediate response to an ADO form may be to mandate that nurses from other shifts do overtime. Unionized nurses have been very effective in reducing mandatory overtime by documenting its excessive use and negotiating at the bargaining table for additional staff. ADO forms may be also used in a grievance process if a nurse is disciplined for an error that occurred when the unit was short-staffed. Most important, ADO forms provide clear and sustained written evidence documenting actual or threatened harm to patients from short-staffing. ADO documentation has been used successfully by many state nurses associations in contract negotiations regarding staffing levels and in public relations efforts to educate consumers about the problems of short-staffing in a particular institution.

Unfortunately, nonunionized nurses have little internal leverage to increase registered nurse staffing and may find themselves relying instead on external means such as notifying regulatory agencies of unsafe staffing. Notifying outside licensing and accrediting agencies is useful only to the degree that many nurses within the same institution call the agency and file complaints. Given budgetary constraints, government regulatory agencies are unlikely to pursue an investigation unless they receive numerous complaints from nurses, patients, or patients' families.

A complaint of short-staffing by itself is unlikely to elicit an investigation from a government agency. Complainants—whether nurses, patients, or patients' families—must link the short-staffing to a measurable adverse effect upon a patient. For example, simply saying the unit was short-staffed and several patients went without pain medication is unlikely to result in an investigation. However, saying that a patient is now in a coma because the cardiac care unit was inadequately staffed with inexperienced nurses who made medication errors during a code *is* likely to result in an investigation.

Several states have established hotlines to which nurses can report unsafe staffing anonymously. Based upon these reports, the state Department of Public

Health may conduct unannounced site inspections to ensure that health care facilities meet minimum standards. Some have criticized the state licensing agencies as "paper tigers" beholden to hospital management. State licensing agencies' primary accountability is to the citizens of that state. If the state licensing agency is being less than enthusiastic in investigating allegations of unsafe care, nurses should forward their complaints to the state's Office of the Attorney General, Consumer Complaint Division.

Each state has a peer review organization that handles quality-of-care complaints for Medicare beneficiaries in hospitals, home health agencies, day surgery centers, skilled nursing facilities, and health care management organizations. In most states, the Department of Public Health, Division of Health Care Quality, is the agency responsible for licensing Medicare/Medicaid-certified health care facilities. If nurses find that hospital management is not responsive to internal requests for increased staffing, this is the first place they should go with a complaint about the adverse effects of staffing on quality of care.

The Joint Commission on the Accreditation of Healthcare Organizations (JCAHO) publishes staffing standards that must be adhered to if the agency is to maintain its accreditation. JCAHO standards usually exceed those established by state agencies. Unlike state licensing agencies, JCAHO does not have any legal authority over health care facilities. The fact that federal Medicare reimbursement is tied to JCAHO accreditation is often incentive enough for health care agencies faced with a JCAHO site inspection to increase staffing to registered nurse staffing standards.

Developing and Disseminating Guidelines Regarding Nurse Staffing

Nursing organizations must work aggressively to measure how the numbers and mix of nursing personnel affect outcomes empirically associated with the quality of nursing care. The American Nursing Association's report (1997) entitled *Implementing Nursing's Report Card* found that as the number of registered nurses decreased, the incidence of pressure ulcers, pneumonia, postoperative infections, and urinary tract infections rose. Based on this research, state nursing organizations in Massachusetts, New York, Rhode Island, Oregon, and Washington state have submitted legislation that would require the collection and dissemination of nursing quality indicator data to the public.

The ten nursing quality indicators identified by the American Nursing Association are the nosocomial infection rate, the patient injury rate, patient satisfaction with nursing care, patient satisfaction with pain management, patient satisfaction with educational information, patient satisfaction with care, maintenance of skin integrity, nurse staff satisfaction, the number and mix of nursing personnel, and the total nursing hours provided per patient per day. In a follow-up project, the American Nurses Association convened an expert panel of nurse researchers in March 1998 to develop principles for staffing in acute care hospitals. The project aims to try to answer a complicated question: What is the most cost-effective mix of nursing personnel that will preserve high-quality care?

Recent experience in the Cleveland, Ohio, area, where patient outcome information has been collected and shared among businesses purchasing health insurance, suggests that dissemination of outcome data does cause organizations that are below the community standard to change their practices and improve their performance. The American Nurses Association has introduced a bill into Congress entitled the Patient Safety Act (H.R. 1165) that would require health care institutions to make public information regarding nurse staffing and patient outcomes. With the broad dissemination of such information, consumers may make more informed choices of where they or their families should receive health care services.

Professional Cost of Whistle-Blowing

Whistle-blowing does carry risks. While individual nurses working in unionized hospitals are protected against retaliation for whistle-blowing, nonunionized nurses are not. Barry Adams, a registered nurse, was working in a nonunionized hospital where he felt the staffing was insufficient to provide patients safe care. Mr. Adams systematically documented instances where inadequate staffing had jeopardized or actually harmed patients and provided the information to nursing management, the Massachusetts Board of Registration of Nursing, and the Massachusetts Attorney General's Office.

Although Mr. Adams had previously received exemplary work performance evaluations, he was terminated from his position. Two months later, a patient died from an overdose of morphine. A subsequent investigation by the Massachusetts Department of Public Health found several violations of Massachusetts regulations pertaining to prescriptive authority and administration of medication.

In a hearing before the National Labor Relations Board, a judge ruled that Mr. Adams's termination was "motivated by [the hospital's] desire to silence him and retaliate against him" for complaining about his working conditions. The judge ordered the hospital to reinstate Mr. Adams and pay him for lost wages and benefits. A civil lawsuit (now under advisement by the trial judge) argues that Mr. Adams was fired for fulfilling his legal responsibility to patients under the Massachusetts Nurse Practice Act.

Six state nursing associations (Massachusetts, New Jersey, Alabama, Oregon, New York, and Washington state) have introduced whistle-blower protection legislation. The Patient Safety Act of 1997 also contains whistle-blower protection language. If enacted, these whistle-blower laws would protect nonunionized nurses who report unsafe staffing from retaliation, disciplinary action, or termination from their place of employment. Until such time as whistle-blower protection laws are enacted, the only safeguard for nurses who disclose unsafe health care practices is to be organized under a collective bargaining agreement.

Role of Health Insurance Plans

The purchasers of health insurance in the United States are businesses that offer health insurance as a benefit of employment. As long as health insurance is largely employer-based, the primary obligation of health insurers will be to keep premiums low, not necessarily to uphold quality of care. Clearly, if nurses want to change the economic incentives for health insurers, especially the for-profit insurers, they will have to elicit the assistance of the American public.

Public intolerance to cutbacks in nursing personnel is the most potent weapon against efforts to diminish the quality of care at the bedside. In a nationwide focus group survey commissioned by the American Hospital Association (1996), a key indicator of quality of hospital care was the availability of registered nurses. The American Nurses Association has embarked on a very successful public relations campaign entitled "Every Patient Deserves a Nurse." Because the public trusts registered nurses, public relations campaigns on their behalf have had a strong influence on Americans' views of the health care system.

Corporatization of Health Care—
Profits Before Patients?

The case of the Nelsons and Ms. Cohen ascribes changes in the quality of health care services to the arrival of a for-profit health care insurer, HealthSun. In response to these trends, physicians, nurses, and other health care providers across the United States have joined together in a movement against the corporatization of health care services. Their statement of principles, entitled "Call to Action," was published in the December 1997 issue of the *Journal of the American Medical Association* and was endorsed by over eight thousand prominent nurses and physicians.

Corporatization of health care services, specifically the conversion of nonprofit insurers and providers to for-profit status, is problematic for a variety of reasons. Most relevant to the Nelson case, it drains scarce capital and human resources away from patient care. The largest for-profit hospital chains have a substantially lower percentage of their total budget earmarked for direct care providers than the nonprofits. For-profit health insurers devote far less of every premium dollar to patient care than their nonprofit counterparts. Instead, capital resources are diverted to shareholders and administrative overhead that includes exorbitant salary and benefit packages to CEOs far in excess of those offered to CEOs in other, comparable industries.

Direct care providers are not alone in their efforts to rid the health care system of potent financial incentives that reward undercare. There has been an unprecedented national outcry from the general public for legislative action. By 1996, over eighty bills had been introduced in more than thirty states to either limit or prohibit the conversion of nonprofit health care entities to for-profits. And states introduced over one thousand bills addressing the regulation of managed care companies or consumer protections.

Christine Tanner (1997), editor of the *Journal of Nursing Education*, wrote, "It is unlikely the for-profit managed care train is going to be derailed with anything less than good data, total public outrage, or both." It is reasonable to assume that nurses' protests would have little impact on the selective contracting practices of a for-profit insurer like HealthSun. But nurses, physicians, and the public can use government laws and regulations to prohibit the most egregious activities of for-profit providers, which degrade the quality of health care services.

Conclusion

In a survey conducted of over seventy-three hundred nurses from across the United States, nurses repeatedly described instances in which they were torn between their ethical duty to their patients and unreasonable demands from hospital management to assume greater and greater patient loads (Shindul-Rothschild, Berry and Long-Middleton 1996). Too often nurses are afraid to take a stand against unsafe working conditions. Nurses want someone else to be the risk-taker. They do not want to be labeled as troublemakers; they do not want to risk losing their jobs. Instead, nurses work to the point of exhaustion, triggering a familiar cycle of stress, physical injury, and resignations. Silence is dangerous not only to patients; it is inevitably harmful to nurses and the profession itself.

If nurses find themselves second-guessing what they know to be their ethical duty to their patients, they need reacquaint themselves with the Nursing Code of Ethics, whose third principle states: "The nurse acts to safeguard the client and the public when health care and safety are affected by the incompetent, unethical or illegal practice of any person." Any nurse who has ever filled out an incident report, filed an ADO document, voted to strike, or picketed in front of a hospital has felt fear. It is not easy to take a stand against forces more powerful than yourself and to risk losing your job and your livelihood. Registered nurses must always remember that they are accountable for nursing judgments and actions *regardless* of the personal consequences.

The corporatization of health care and the use of competition to ratchet down health care costs has forced every health care institution to seek ways to improve efficiency. In some institutions, where individual nurses in positions of authority still exert primary influence over the nursing budget, staffing, and work redesign decisions, quality has not been compromised. There are hospitals where nurses report care is excellent, registered nurses have not been cut back, and nursing morale is high (Shindul-Rothschild, Long-Middleton, and Berry 1997). But increasingly, these institutions appear to be in the minority. Despite protestations of hospital management that they can no longer afford registered nurses, as recently as 1997, hospitals' profits continued to soar while the number of registered nurses working full-time was cut back to record low levels.

Staff nurses have the power to influence decisions regarding nurse staffing if they act collectively. Joining their state nurses association and actively participating in collective action either through (1) collective bargaining, (2) political action, or (3) professional activities, particularly research regarding nursing outcomes, are the best long-term strategies to improve nurse staffing and safeguard the public.

References

Ad Hoc Committee to Defend Health Care. 1997. "For Our Patients, Not for Profits: A Call to Action." *Journal of the American Medical Association* 278, no. 21:1733–38.

American Hospital Association. 1996. *Reality Check: Public Perceptions of Health Care and Hospital.* Washington, D.C.: American Hospital Association.

American Nurses Association. 1985. *Code for Nurses with Interpretive Statements.* Washington, D.C.: American Nurses Association.

———. 1991. *Standards of Clinical Nursing Practice.* Washington, D.C.: American Nurses Association.

———. 1995. *The Right to Accept or Reject an Assignment.* Washington, D.C.: American Nurses Association.

———. 1997. *Implementing Nursing's Report Card: A Study of RN Staffing, Length of Stay and Patient Outcomes.* Prepared by NETWORK, Inc. Washington, D.C.: American Nurses Association.

Shindul-Rothschild, J.; Berry, D.; and Long-Middleton, E. 1996. "Where Have All the Nurses Gone? Final Results of Our Patient Care Survey." *American Journal of Nursing* 96, no. 11:25–39.

Shindul-Rothschild, J.; Long-Middleton, E.; and Berry, D. 1997. "10 Keys to Quality Care." *American Journal of Nursing* 97, no. 11:35–43.

Tanner, C. 1997. "A Call to Looms." *Journal of Nursing Education* 36, no. 5:1–2.

PART FOUR

Responsibilities to Patients

12

Purchaser and Plan Responsibility for Benefit Design

CASE STUDY

Commercial insured products are subject to numerous mandated benefits and other state laws that make it virtually impossible to offer potential purchasers an inadequate benefits package. State law may define not only a required minimum comprehensive benefit set but also very specific goods and services that must be covered. For example, a state may require coverage of certain types of transplants, particular supplies for diabetics, substance abuse treatment, or wigs for certain types of baldness. States may further regulate the types of providers whom the plan must include in the network as well as the range of products available to the member. For example, a state may require equal access to chiropractors. Or a state may require that a plan offer a point-of-service product, that is, a product that permits a member to go to providers outside of the network for services in exchange for higher premiums and copayments.

However, most large employers have self-funded health plans, which are exempt from these state mandates. In a self-funded plan, the employer chooses to fund and assume the financial risk of the cost of health care rather than purchase coverage through an insurance company or HMO. Due to the application of the federal Employee Retirement Income Security Act (ERISA), self-funded plans are not subject to mandated benefit laws and many other state regulations such as those described. In self-funded plans, employers retain the discretion to determine the terms of coverage and will often contract with an HMO only to administer the health plan. As a result, an HMO may experience considerable pressure from a self-funded employer to administer a benefits package that may significantly differ from the benefits packages offered to the HMO's other insured enrollees.

Integricare is a large, for-profit southwestern HMO. Integricare offers numerous commercial insured products and administers several self-funded products. The state has a long list of mandated benefits and other regulations governing the insured products offered by Integricare. Approximately 40 percent of Integricare's business is with large self-funded companies, and this is the business Integricare would like to expand in the future.

Mayline Moving, an employer representing over five-thousand employees, recently approached Integricare to administer its self-funded health plan. Mayline wants a benefits package containing no mental health or substance abuse benefits and no coverage for oral contraceptives unless for a medically necessary condition. In addition, Mayline wants to use a very restricted formulary and a restricted network of providers (providers at two clinics on opposite ends of town). Mayline plans to offer only one product to its employees, covering specialty care only with a preauthorization from a primary care provider and only if received within the network. Finally, Mayline insists that it has the right to receive all claims information, including employee names and other identifying information, and that this is consistent with Mayline's role as payer and ultimate decision maker with respect to coverage.

Integricare believes the restrictions on services covered, on plan choice, and on choice of provider mean that enrollees will not have adequate access to basic health care services. This package is certainly more sparse than that included in any of Integricare's insured products and is bare compared even to what other self-funded plans in the community provide. This package would violate a number of the state's mandated benefits and regulations were it not for the plan's exemption under ERISA. In addition, Integricare worries that the claims information requested by Mayline contains highly confidential material that ought not be in an employer's hands. Integricare is also concerned that members of self-funded plans are often unaware that their employer has access to such records and that provision of the information conflicts with Integricare's ethical obligations to preserve member confidentiality. Technically, the law arguably permits the employer access to this information. Nonetheless, many self-funded employers voluntarily choose to restrict or not receive identifying information to eliminate any possibility that they might subsequently use the information in an illegal, discriminatory manner.

Notwithstanding all of these considerations, Mayline is a very attractive potential client, and Integricare risks losing a substantial revenue stream if it does not comply with the employer's specifications. The plan and terms proposed by Mayline are perfectly legal, yet Integricare feels uncomfortable participating in such a plan.

Mayline insists that these are rough economic times and that these are legitimate business decisions. The premiums and copayments associated with this type of bare-bones plan are affordable for both the company and its employees and are thus preferable to layoffs. Moreover, as Mayline reminds Integricare, the company will take its business elsewhere if Integricare attempts to interfere in its business decisions.

Integricare must decide whether or not it should agree to execute the administrative services contract with Mayline.

Questions for Consideration

➤ Should Integricare agree or refuse to administer Mayline's plan? Why?

➤ The legal distinctions under ERISA are, in part, responsible for the problems in this case. Does the plan have an obligation, nonetheless, to promote appropriate benefits packages for members in self-funded plans? An obligation to advocate for changes in the law?

➤ How should an "appropriate benefits package" be defined? Should the same standards apply in both the fully insured and self-funded contexts? Should it be measured against the prevailing standard in the community? Should an employee always have a choice of products? How many providers should be in the network?

➤ How, if at all, should Integricare work with the employer to promote a more appropriate package?

➤ How should Integricare protect the confidentiality of patient information against the employer's demands for this information?

➤ Whose responsibility is it to educate employees about the role of the employer in a self-funded plan? How should such education be accomplished?

COMMENTARY _____

Lisa J. Raiola, M.P.H.

TO: President, Mayline Moving

FROM: CEO, Integricare

RE: Benefit Design Request

We appreciate the opportunity to respond to your request for a sales proposal for Mayline Moving's self-insured business. As you have not asked us to quote one of Integricare's standard products, instead opting for a somewhat unusual benefit design, we felt that we needed to explore a number of questions and issues with you prior to furnishing a formal proposal. In fact, your request prompted an important dialogue within both our sales department and our medical director's committee regarding the nature of the relationship between plan design and care delivery. It reminded us that, as our self-funded business continues to grow, Integricare must stake out a clear and consistent position vis-à-vis our partners in these arrangements.

In order to better frame these issues, we referred your "case" to Integricare's Ethics Advisory Group. Our intent in this letter is to raise several broad issues for consideration by you and your organization, to articulate some specific recommendations that would enable us potentially to align our interests to serve Mayline employees better, and to share frankly some of what we learned from the Ethics Advisory Group discussion.

Commiserating

We begin with the assumption that there is no ideal plan design, that is, coverage that makes all the people happy all the time. A benefits package ultimately represents a cocktail of multiple factors including assumptions about what constitutes comprehensive care, population demographics, and actuarial and economic considerations. As Integricare attempts to keep pace with the cost pressures faced by our purchasers while maintaining or improving quality of care, plan design really becomes a matter of principled trade-offs. These trade-offs take many forms, for example, trading preventive services for richer sick-care benefits or trading an extensive network that is expensive to administer for one that offers less choice at lower cost.

These are not easy decisions, but if one owns the risk—the risk for ensuring that a population is adequately cared for within a finite envelope of resources—one also owns the responsibility for making these decisions. As an increasing percentage of employers opt for self-funded arrangements, they find that *they* are the stewards of this responsibility. We would like to be able to tell you that we have a recipe to ensure success in this role but must admit that we too are scaling a steep learning curve, just a few paces in front of you! In fact, there are probably few more agonizing, less satisfying tasks in American society than determining what health services to pay for with limited dollars. Even the Oregon Basic Health Care Act of 1989, perhaps the best single example of a successful health care resource allocation project in this country, does not offer a model that can be successfully exported out-of-state. The magic of that solution lies not in the outcome but in the process. Meaning that, unfortunately, the result is nearly impossible to generalize as it nests in the value system of Oregonians.

The ERISA Vacuum—Only Fools Rush In

ERISA was originally conceived in 1974 as a package of structural reforms intended to safeguard workers against loss of earned benefits. It contains certain administrative and reporting requirements but is almost entirely silent on the issue of plan content. Some argue that today ERISA potentially imperils workers in two ways. First, ERISA *enables* self-funded employers' access to claims data for the legitimate purpose of administering an insurance risk pool. This, of course, also gives employers access to medical information that violates employees' confidentiality. Second, ERISA *preempts* self-funded employers from state-mandated benefits and other state laws affecting managed care organizations. This is a major legislative void that leaves the self-funded market largely unsupervised. But to depend on this legislative loophole when an employee-member cries foul is a foolish strategy.

Insofar as self-funded plans are exempt from state mandates, employers that construct such plans are working outside the context of prevailing guardrails of what a particular state considers "adequate plan design." However, that a benefit is mandated does not confer an ethical blessing on those self-funded employers that choose to cover it, nor does it cast an unethical curse on those that do not. Some state mandates are simply the result of intense lobbying by special interest groups and have little to do with what is "best" or "fair" for the overall population. An individual employer may be able to craft a benefits package more closely tailored to the needs of its employee population than either a state-mandated plan or a managed care organization's standard plan. Moreover, without the financial drag of regulatory requirements the employer may explore a greater range of trade-offs. For example, Mayline can choose whether to trade a less rich benefits package for increased job security for its workforce. Were it not for exemptions afforded to Mayline under ERISA, this choice would probably not be possible. We recognize, however, that this is the result of a loophole, not an intentional legislative strategy to give self-funded employers a blank check. Within this regulatory vacuum, we—meaning both Integricare and Mayline—must also recognize that abuse can occur.

The question for our organization then becomes, What is our role, the role of the managed care organization, in a self-funded arrangement? We know that we are not ultimately accountable for managing the financial risk. But we do feel responsible to deliver the best possible care to Mayline members within your budget. We know that we are not ultimately accountable for the choices that you make to include or exclude particular services for your employees. But we do feel responsible to ensure that those choices support a standard of care that our providers believe is necessary for meeting their patients' needs. We know that we are not ultimately accountable for the macro trade-offs you make between what Mayline will spend on health benefits and what it will spend, for example, on creating new positions. But we do need to ensure that you spend enough to meet some threshold of health care need that we can both agree is fair to the Mayline employee population.

Holier Than Thou? Hardly!

Let me be clear that we do not claim that Integricare's standard products are carved in two stone tablets and come straight from our holy mount to your cafeteria. We strive to align plan design to the mission and values of *our* organization. But what do the mission and values of our organization have to do with someone else's plan design? In pondering this question, we found the specific examples of those elements in your proposal that were out of sync with our standard coverage and business practices to be useful learning tools. By mining these examples—namely, the exclusions, the restrictions on choice, and confidentiality—our Ethics Advisory Group was able to articulate the reasons that, and in some cases the ways in which, Mayline and Integricare need to come together.

The reason for coming together is not simply that we differ on specific items. It really has less to do with the "what" of the differences than with the "why." And this is where I again invoke the value of process, as I did in the Oregon example. The Ethics Advisory Group's process was to *consider the facts* from Mayline's perspective. The group then *defined the legitimate interests of the various stakeholders* and considered where these interests create organizational conflict of responsibility for Integricare. It then *prioritized competing interests* in accordance with organizational values. Finally, the group *generated options* and *recommended a course of action* reflecting these values. I offer you some snapshots of our Ethics Advisory Group discussion.

Exclusions

In thinking about exclusions, we believe it is essential to anticipate the downstream impact on the doctor-patient relationship. Will the omission of a particular service potentially straitjacket clinical decision making or lower the quality of care provided by the Integricare delivery system? Much of this depends on our sensitivity to the practice culture of the providers within our network. We believe that plan design should facilitate this practice culture in ways that allow for flexibility and the seamless provision of care; it ought to feel transparent to clinician and patient.

Let's use the example of your desire to exclude mental health and substance abuse services. Absent more facts, we speculated that there are several reasons for your request: anticipation of substantial savings on expensive inpatient care, detoxification, drug therapies, and the like; expectation that employees are likely to nonetheless be covered under a spouse's plan through coordination of benefits provisions; and your intention to carve out these services and contract with a specialty vendor for their coverage.

In Integricare's delivery system, mental health and substance abuse services are tightly linked to primary care. We find that excluding or carving out these services is not only likely to fragment care, but our experience suggests that it is more costly in the long run. Allow me to provide you with an example from within our own delivery system. A quality-improvement project sought to reduce hospital readmission rates for high-risk diagnoses. We discovered that certain diagnoses were historically likely to result in a repeat admission within one year. Fifty percent of these were found to be known substance abusers admitted for other reasons including trauma, acute gastrointestinal episodes, and liver problems. Each patient's primary care physician was consulted and, where appropriate, made a referral to a substance abuse treatment program. Fifty percent accepted the referral and did not require a second inpatient admission within one year of follow-up. Exclusion or carve-out of mental health and substance abuse services not only disintegrates the coordination of care that exists within our delivery system and our practice culture but may also put patients at risk for more serious and costly episodes of care.

Mayline's desire to exclude oral contraceptives is also problematic. We guessed that perhaps your census revealed a high proportion of young, single males for whom you wished to trade off this benefit in favor of covering a more widely needed service. If Mayline believes that excluding coverage for oral contraception is a cost-effective decision, we need only point out that the highest proportion of our hospital expenditures is for obstetrics, that is, deliveries. Conspicuous by its absence was an exclusion of abortion services, which might have told us there were underlying religious values motivating the oral contraception decision. The trade-off question can only be answered by profiling your employee population, and we would require this process as a condition of responding to your request for a proposal in any case. On the other hand, the implicit request that our delivery system support the religious beliefs of your organization, when they are known to be inconsistent with our own, would represent a deal-breaker for Integricare. Were the values of our organizations to be seriously misaligned around this issue, we could not ask our providers to carry out your plan design.

Restriction of Choice

One of the fundamental tenets of managed care is "managed choice." The idea is that working with a group of physicians who are aligned with the managed care organization ultimately ensures an appropriate balance of quality and cost. So we cannot say that a highly limited network, such as the one Mayline proposes, is simply a "bad thing." In fact, we have evidence that these types of arrangements can actually provide as high a level of satisfaction, albeit to a self-selected group of members.

Designing a network is not just a matter of consumer satisfaction (although I'll suggest in a moment how this must be counted as a critical factor) but also involves issues of continuity and coordination of care as well as creating options to meet patients' and physicians' needs. So to the extent that one wants to offer a fairly restricted network, one must examine how this affects the existing pattern of doctor-patient relationships among an employee population. This would be the first time Integricare is offered to Mayline employees. You have proposed coverage only for in-network services and only if received at two participating clinics. This means that your employees will need to break existing relationships in transitioning to Integricare coverage.

We do not believe that our doctors are any less well equipped to meet the high standards of quality of care or patient satisfaction than other doctors in the community. However, it surely makes our job more difficult when we must fight to build patient trust when patients' options are limited. Trust and choice have an inverse relationship; when trust is low, as in the case of going to see a new physician, there is a high need for choice. As trust builds, choice may become less important.

We would, therefore, ask that you consider adding three provisions to your current proposal: (1) a point-of-service option allowing patients to seek care outside the network, with a deductible; (2) a continuity-of-care policy that enables patients to receive ongoing care from their existing providers where necessary; and (3) a plan to measure member satisfaction with Integricare providers and share that data with your employees and our physicians, so that we have some assurance that we are doing all that we can to help physicians bond effectively with these patients. These provisions are likely to add cost to the existing plan design at the outset, but they may actually decrease cost within one to two years as more and more patients are comfortable receiving their care within the network. Our aim here is to create the right trust climate, enabling us to pare down choice in the future as appropriate.

Confidentiality

An especially knotty problem of self-funded arrangements involves our desire to balance the employer's legal right to, and legitimate need for, data with the patient's expectation that medical information is private. Consumers are increasingly aware of who has access to their medical records. Yet we recognize that expectations of absolute privacy are unrealistic and may even hamper our own care process; they may also impede your ability to audit claims. But how to explain this to members and how to afford them an acceptable level of confidentiality remain challenges we believe are shared by Mayline and Integricare.

Legalistic notions of informed consent, like those in the subscriber agreement and on the enrollment form, are inadequate to protect member confidentiality. Not only have we found that members do not read these provisions, but member representatives of the Ethics Advisory Group pointed out that even with a detailed explanation members may not understand them. This is particularly true when an employer offers only one choice of health plan rendering meaningful consent illusory. An explanation of this business practice to employees is necessary but not sufficient to protect confidentiality.

We prefer to think of confidentiality as an infrastructure made up of "fair information practice guarantees" that are the result of an explicit understanding between Mayline and Integricare. Can we build a set of guidelines to shape the format, analysis, management, storage, and application of claims data? For example, who in your organization will have access to data and how will the data be secured? Will you accept encryption or scrambling of data? To meet your needs, can we provide you with aggregate rather than patient-specific data? Would you consider outsourcing data analysis to a third party? Most important, do you know what your employees would view as adequate safeguards to protect their confidentiality?

Co-stewarding

The Ethics Advisory Group's attempt to characterize the relationship between Mayline and Integricare, oddly enough, reminded me of a recent argument I had with my husband. He was responsible for purchasing a home computer system, and in an effort to save money decided not to buy a "fully loaded" system configured by an expert systems integrator but to piece together his own hardware and software. Of course there were problems. Each manufacturer blamed the other and diagnosed a "compatibility problem." I told my husband that he should have left the systems design to the experts.

In many ways, Integricare and Mayline must deal with a similar issue. The system will not work if Mayline's software—its plan design—is incompatible with Integricare's hardware—delivery system and operating policies. If we do not address this at the outset, your employees (who are ultimately our patients) may be left holding the bag in the same way I was left between two manufacturers who were more interested in shifting blame than solving the problem.

This is the challenge of "co-stewarding." To co-steward is to recognize the interdependencies that two or more parties have in delivering a product that involves balancing a dynamic tension created by competing values. I suppose one could compare this to old-fashioned teamwork, except that it is much more complicated than that. Decision making against a backdrop of complex trade-offs is hard enough when only one organization is involved. But if two parties must collaborate, they are wise to begin with an examination of their own organizational values and priorities. I suggest that if we are to proceed with this proposal we begin here.

Integricare could easily choose to see our role as an administrative pass-through for claims. We could choose to hire out our delivery system to anyone willing to pay the price. But we choose neither of these options, because of the potential threat to a trusting doctor-patient relationship. Absent a co-stewarded plan design, we could blame any problem on you, the employer that designed this plan. And your human resources office could blame us, the plan that cannot meet employees' needs.

It has taken some courage to write this letter. It reflects the tremendous responsibility I feel to those members who place their trust in Integricare. It would be a great disservice to my organization and our members to turn away business arbitrarily. Yet it serves them no better to accept it arbitrarily. I truly hope we can partner in the future.

COMMENTARY

Raymond G. DeVries, Ph.D.

Should Integricare agree to administer the health plan Mayline Moving desires? The plan Mayline is requesting is so limited and comes with so many strings attached, we are tempted to dismiss the case as absurd. Surely no employer would be so "frugal." But we cannot dismiss this case so easily. The pressures that lead to inadequate product design are real. The high cost of health care is a significant problem for American businesses and the American economy. Mayline notes that "these are rough economic times" and frames its request as a choice between reduced benefits and layoffs. Efforts to make American businesses more competitive will increasingly include reducing the cost of health care. Given the hesitancy of the American political system to impose any sort of control on the price of medical services, companies are forced to act on their own.

Furthermore, many Americans believe that health plans are giving in to employer demands for "bare-bones" products. Public fear about limited coverage, like that proposed by Mayline, is the driving force behind the creation of special referenda to limit cost-cutting measures in managed care. Numerous states have enacted Patient Protection Acts and other consumer protection laws, including limits on certain cost-cutting measures. Perhaps most disconcerting, surveys of physicians suggest that doctors too are pessimistic about the effects of managed care on the quality of medical services (Borowsky et al. 1997).

The conflict between Mayline and Integricare represents the future of medical care in the United States. Companies seeking to remain competitive will choose to avoid requirements by self-insuring, forcing health plans—facing increased competition themselves—to make difficult choices about what they will and will not do to attract and maintain employer business. Providers and users of health care services will find themselves caught in the middle. Can medical ethicists find a way to speak to this increasingly common situation?

Resolution of the disagreement between Mayline and Integricare requires finding a way to balance the conflicting needs (and desires) of business, health plans, health care providers, and those who use health services. This is no easy task; in today's health care market, it is likely that the outcome of this impasse will be determined by bargaining and the "give and take" of business, with little or no ethical input. It would probably be naive to assume that Mayline and Integricare will call for an independent ethical mediator. Perhaps the best we can hope for is "dueling ethicists," where each organization hires an ethicist to negotiate a settlement based on the (ethical) interests of the organizations they represent. In either event, there are some preliminary questions that need to be addressed first.

The first step in resolving the dilemma is obvious: we need to identify the organizational barriers to effective ethical deliberation. There are many places to look when searching for the constraints on effective ethics. We might scrutinize the corporate strategies of Mayline and Integricare or examine the existing relationships between health care providers and Integricare and other health plans. But the first place to look for the barriers to ethical solutions for inadequate product design is the organization of medical ethics itself. Is traditional medical ethics, focusing on the physician-patient relationship in a clinical setting, up to the task of addressing managed care?

A Short Sociological Assessment of Traditional Medical Ethics

It might seem odd to make the ethicists the object of analysis in a case that pits a health plan against an employer, but just as Mayline and Integricare bring their interests and histories to the negotiations, so too ethicists come with a sociological past and a collection of interests that color the approach they take in resolving problems. The ability of medical ethics to mediate the problems of managed care is directly influenced by its historical identity and role in American health care.

In the United States medical ethics grew up in the clinic and the research laboratory: there its reputation was made, and there it developed its way of approaching ethical dilemmas. As a result, American medical ethicists are very good at describing threats to autonomy and at finding ways to balance autonomy and beneficence, but they are ill-prepared to explore the quandaries and questions of social justice presented by managed care (Light and McGee 1998).

Fee-for-service systems and early incarnations of managed care created the illusion that financial arrangements and organizational structures had little influence on the clinical encounter (Rodwin 1993). When fee-for-service reigned, the work of ethics centered around questions about termination of treatment, abortion, experimentation, privacy, and organ donation (Crigger 1998); ethicists rarely, if ever, asked how financial incentives influenced medical decisions. But those days are gone. Recent and dramatic changes in the organization of health care, including the rapid proliferation of managed care and the growth of for-profit medicine, have shattered any illusion that clinical interaction is unaffected by the organization and financing of medical services. It is now plain that nonclinical variables affect what goes on in the clinic and that there is a need to extend the ethical gaze to larger questions about the structure of care delivery.

But habits learned in the clinic are hard to shake. In the face of the sustained public outcry over the deficiencies of managed care, clinically oriented ethicists have had little to say. This conspicuous silence has left ethicists out of discussions of the problems associated with new ways of organizing health care.

Presidential initiatives on managed care by Bill Clinton in 1998 illustrate the perceived irrelevance of bioethics to matters of health care policy and organization. When Clinton needed a response to growing fears about managed care, he did not call on his National Bioethics Advisory Commission (NBAC). He found the NBAC to be a useful source of advice on the propriety of human cloning, but when Clinton wanted a Consumer Bill of Rights and Responsibilities for managed care, he assembled a new group called the Advisory Commission on Consumer Protection and Quality in the Health Care Industry. Its charge was to "recommend such measures as may be necessary to promote and assure health care quality and value and protect consumers and workers in the health care system" (http://www.hcqualitycommission.gov/). No bioethicists were appointed to the thirty-four-member commission.

The issue of inadequate product design requires ethicists to shift their focus, to move ethics out of the clinic and into the realm of the structure and financing of health care delivery. In making this shift, we discover that ideas that helped resolve the microproblems of the clinic have little purchase with problems at an organizational level. For instance, the principle of autonomy (Wolpe 1998) cannot do much work for us in the case of Mayline and Integricare. The dilemma here is extraclinical; to emphasize autonomy would be to encourage the actors in this case—the moving company and the health plan—to find a way to realize their self-interest through negotiation. It is not clear that balancing the rights and "self"-interest of the two organizations will elicit the most just result here.

Ways of Seeing

The participants in any ethical quandary, including the one we face here, have distinctive ways of seeing the problem, views that are rooted in interests and social location. It is no surprise that Mayline and Integricare see the present dilemma as, at least in part, a problem of economics. Mayline's demand for a bare-bones health plan is a matter of economic survival; from its point of view, Integricare is being unreasonable. Integricare, on the other hand, is concerned with its reputation as a health care provider. The health plan believes Mayline is using undue pressure to force it to offer a product that might lead enrollees to associate Integricare with inadequate care. But what about the ethicists? Do they have a peculiar "way of seeing"? While it might be assumed that the ethicist's economic interests are only tenuously tied to the outcome of the case and that they are therefore neutral arbiters, this is a dangerous assumption. Although the interests of the major players in the case are obvious and easily discounted, the interests of ethicists, while less monetary, may be more insidious because they are less visible. The preconceived ethical frame given to a case, a frame influenced by the clinical heritage of ethics, may limit the ethical imagination and introduce arbitrary limits to deliberation.

The case has an adversarial tone common to the traditional ethical analysis of clinical dilemmas: the interests, rights, and obligations of party A conflict with the interests, rights, and obligations of party B. In clinical ethics, where the actors are individuals—patients, care providers, family members—this adversarial frame is easy to apply. But it becomes strained when the principal actors are organizations. First, the conflicts are more complex: in addition to the competing interests of Mayline and Integricare, there are conflicts internal to each of those organizations (for example, Integricare's responsibility to provide "good" plans and its need to generate enough money to stay in business). Second, the dilemma involves more than simply two parties; Integricare and Mayline are not the only participants in this dilemma.

Imagine what the case would look like if framed in terms of the ethical responsibility of Mayline employees. Young, vigorous, and healthy employees might celebrate a low-cost plan. Those with chronic health problems, those who need a drug not on the formulary, and those who have relationships with specialists outside the proposed network would not be so sanguine. What is the nature of the moral duty of employees to each other? If we assume the existence of moral obligations to fellow employees, what is the proper response to a bare-bones health plan? Create and/or join a union? Get involved in political action? Look for work elsewhere?

The case takes on yet another hue if framed in terms of the ethical problems it presents to health care providers. Hearing of Mayline's plans, should providers boycott Integricare? Help organize or educate Mayline's employees? Lobby their state legislators?

It might be argued that these other frames, while legitimate, are red herrings. They are interesting but unnecessary distractions in the consideration of the problems faced by Mayline and Integricare. One dilemma is enough; why add more to the mix?

There are several reasons to expand our ethical frame, to see the question in a context that includes all of the actors and relationships involved. Taken together, these reasons demonstrate that when we see the dilemma in a larger frame, the ethical questions posed by the problem are altered. For example, when we include the ethical perspective of employees of Mayline and care providers affected by the proposed plan, we introduce at least three new social facts into our ethical analysis:

1. The relationship between the American medical profession and the government has changed. After several decades of resisting government involvement in medical care, physicians are now looking to the government to curb the excesses of managed and for-profit medical care. In a startling reversal of their stance in the 1950s, physicians are inviting the government to get involved in medicine, actively lobbying for legislative mandates that limit the ability of health plans to restrict care.

2. The current health care market reflects a growing diffusion of responsibility for medical decisions. In the complicated world of managed care, self-funded plans, and provider incentives, the responsibility for a bad decision—one that harms people—is difficult to locate. In this case it is clear that Integricare will be blamed for poor care, lack of referrals, limited formularies, and failure to protect patient confidentiality. Physicians and patients alike—working with outdated notions of health insurance—will see Integricare, not Mayline, as the culprit in this situation. The research of Borowsky et al. (1997) shows that physicians often incorrectly fault health plans for coverage decisions actually made by self-funded employers (Gervais and DeVries 1997).

3. Ethical dilemmas exist not just in clinical settings or in the conference room shared by Mayline and Integricare but in American society at large, where the marketplace has been allowed to become the primary driver of changes in the relationship between providers and payers. For example, in her commentary about this case, Lisa Raiola suggests that oral contraceptives ought to be included in the plan as a cost-saving measure. Adopting an even wider frame of reference on obsterical care in the marketplace might lead us to also challenge the excesses of

American obstetrics with its overuse of epidural anesthesia, unnecessary electronic fetal monitoring, and inordinately high cesarean section rates.

We might wish for Integricare to work with Mayline to promote a more appropriate package, but is this possible given the current structure of the health care marketplace? Both Mayline and Integricare must advocate for their business interests in a society that has decided to eschew government regulation of health care. In this case, exclusions granted self-funded plans by ERISA remove the minimal limitations the government has attempted to place on the marketplace. The ethical problems we find here do not exist in the regulated market or in countries where the government takes an active role in ensuring adequate health care for all citizens.

When we shift our ethical focus, we discover very important questions about the state of American health care and about the role of ethicists in that system.

Reframing the Task of the Medical Ethicist

In an exchange over the report of the NBAC on the cloning of human beings, Richard Lewontin (1998) accused the commission of concentrating its attention on the technical matters of safety rather than on ethical and religious issues as a way of "finessing the political problems" raised by this new technology. Commission members commented that they heard concerns about the potential of cloning to result in the objectification and exploitation of human beings, but that time constraints made further reflection on these issues impossible. Similarly, the dilemmas presented by the case call attention to the political and social context of ethical decision making. In so doing, managed care raises the stakes for traditional medical ethics. Of course we need ethicists who don white coats and can mediate the clinical problems of medicine; but we also need ethicists to confront the ethical problems that inhere in the structural arrangements of medical care.

Going forward, medical ethicists must ask themselves two related questions. First, is the health care system worth preserving? Second, how do my actions contribute to the preservation or alteration of the system? If an ethicist possessing Solomonic wisdom could find a way to mediate the interests of Mayline and Integricare, whose interests would be served? Solving a problem like this brings with it a certain inherent satisfaction, but a thoroughgoing medical ethics must understand how its expertise affects the delivery of health care. A profession that runs about putting out the ethical fires created by an inherently unjust health care system may, in fact, perpetuate that system.

As ethicists are drawn into the world of managed care, they are realizing the impossibility of separating ethical concerns from the political and social environment. Can we develop mechanisms that will ensure appropriate ethical deliberation in a world of competing corporate interests? Sociology can help to answer this question by pointing to the ways that such mechanisms may be impeded by the predictable consequences of organizational processes and traditional approaches to American medical ethics. This commentary has focused on the latter. The organizational limits on the practice of ethics cannot be confronted until ethicists understand their own biases. Ethicists with expanded frameworks for analysis will be better prepared to solve problems like those posed by Mayline and Integricare. From this expanded perspective, their role in addressing the problems of managed care will not be limited to the interests of individual corporations but will incorporate the interests of all parties involved.

References

Borowsky, S.; Davis, M. K.; Goertz, C.; and Lurie, N. 1997. "Are All Health Plans Created Equal? The Physician's View." *Journal of the American Medical Association* 278 no. 11:917–21.

Crigger, B. 1998. "As Time Goes By: An Intellectual Biography of Bioethics." In *Bioethics and Society: Constructing the Ethical Enterprise*, pp. 192–215. Edited by R. DeVries and J. Subedi. Upper Saddle River, N.J.: Prentice Hall.

Gervais, K., and DeVries, R. 1997. "Doctors 'Report Card' on HMO Care Is Probably a Misdiagnosis." *Minneapolis Star Tribune* November 4:A14.

Lewontin, R. 1998. "The Confusion over Cloning: An Exchange." *The New York Review of Books* March 5:46–47.

Light, D., and McGee, G. 1998. "On the Social Embeddedness of Bioethics." In *Bioethics and Society: Constructing the Ethical Enterprise*, pp. 1–15. Edited by R. DeVries and J. Subedi. Upper Saddle River, N.J.: Prentice Hall.

Rodwin, M. 1993. *Medicine, Money, and Morals.* New York: Oxford University Press.

Wolpe, P. 1998. "The Triumph of Autonomy in American Bioethics: A Sociological View." In *Bioethics and Society: Constructing the Ethical Enterprise*, pp. 38–59. Edited by R. DeVries and J. Subedi. Upper Saddle River, N.J.: Prentice Hall.

13

Advocating for Patients in Managed Care

CASE STUDY _____

Horizon Health Care, a rapidly growing network HMO in a large metropolitan area in the Northeast, is part of a national for-profit managed care organization. To remain competitive, Horizon Health Care has initiated a broad range of cost-containment and quality-improvement strategies. For example, last year Horizon Health Care comprehensively reviewed the use of a variety of high-cost procedures among its enrollees, including the use of neuro-imaging (computerized tomography [CT] and magnetic resonance imaging [MRI]) of the head. It found that the use of these neuro-imaging tests was adding substantially to its expenditures; that since CT and MRI are considered safe, accurate, and valuable in assessing the brain and surrounding structures, they have replaced most other tests in evaluating a patient when an intracranial disorder is suspected; and that only a very small percentage of headaches and other neurological complaints are caused by an underlying pathology (such as brain tumor) detectable by neuro-imaging. To ensure that neuro-imaging tests of the head would contribute more directly to improving health outcomes, Horizon Health Care established a policy of requiring prior authorization for all such tests.

Dr. Ashton, a pediatric neurologist, has worked at Hillside Clinic since completing her residency two years ago. Hillside serves a very diverse population in a multiethnic community in the same metropolitan area where Horizon Health Care is headquartered. More than half the patients seen at Hillside are foreign-born. Dr. Ashton, like many other practitioners at Hillside, is fluent in another language. Still, the clinic often has to scramble to find an interpreter to facilitate communication with its non-English-speaking clientele.

Dr. Ashton works at Hillside three days a week and sees approximately twenty patients a day. Her workload has increased steadily since she began to work there, and she feels mounting pressure to limit the amount of time she spends with each patient. Most of her patients are now in a capitated plan of one form or another, and the clinic has implemented a variety of strategies (including quotas of patients per practitioner per day) to help it remain financially solvent in its increasingly cost-competitive environment.

On a particularly busy day last year, Dr. Ashton saw Sonia, a ten-year-old girl, who had been referred to her by a pediatrician at Hillside. Sonia was the youngest of three daughters of a Ukranian family who had moved to the United States three years ago. The whole family accompanied Sonia to Dr. Ashton's office, and since the parents were not yet fluent in English and no interpreter was available, their seventeen-year-old daughter served as interpreter.

Sonia's parents were concerned that she was acting differently and seemed to be losing cognitive and motor skills. They reported that during the past few months Sonia had begun to shake, especially her right arm and hand. These tremors were bad enough that she would hold her hands together to keep them from shaking. She had lost the ability to tie her shoes, though she could still zip and button her clothes, albeit with difficulty. Sonia moved more slowly and fatigued easily. She had been a cheerleader but two months ago stopped this activity due to her motor problems.

Sonia also had a history of learning problems but had been in an age-appropriate class. Within the past year, her parents felt that her short- and long-term memory were significantly affected, and five months ago she was evaluated by a psychologist who recommended special education placement. Sonia's pediatrician decided to refer her to Dr. Ashton for a consultation.

Her examination revealed marked tremor, significant cognitive deficits, and gait abnormalities. Dr. Ashton suspected that Sonia had a neurodegenerative condition and wanted to order an MRI and screening metabolic studies to establish a diagnosis. Sonia was covered under her father's health insurance plan with Horizon Health Care. Dr. Ashton knew she could not order the studies without receiving prior authorization from the HMO. Accordingly, during Sonia's initial appointment, Dr. Ashton phoned the utilization review program at Horizon Health Care, but even after a lengthy conversation with the nurse reviewer, did not obtain the necessary authorization. She informed Sonia's family that she would pursue this further and then continued with her other scheduled appointments. Some of her patients had now been waiting for over an hour.

Over the next few days, Dr. Ashton spent several hours on the phone and writing letters to Horizon Health Care's utilization review program in her effort to obtain authorization for Sonia's MRI scan. Horizon Health Care's program is staffed by registered nurses, all of whom have had at least several years' patient care experience. The nurse reviewing Dr. Ashton's request, for example, had fifteen years' emergency department experience. If an initial request is denied, the utilization review process provides for several levels of review; final decisions are made by Horizon Health Care's medical director. Dr. Ashton engaged the support of Sonia's pediatrician and through their combined efforts was able to reach the medical director and obtain the necessary authorization. The tests confirmed a neurodegenerative disorder and treatment was promptly initiated.

Sonia's parents thanked Dr. Ashton profusely for her efforts on behalf of their daughter. And, while Dr. Ashton was also pleased that she was able to help Sonia get the diagnostic test, she wondered if spending her time and effort in this way—in her words, "fighting the bureaucracy"—was fair to her other patients, for whom she had proportionately less time as a result.

Questions for Consideration

➤ When treating Sonia, should Dr. Ashton take into account the interests of her other patients? If so, how should Sonia's interests be balanced against the interests of other patients in the waiting room and in the health plan?
➤ What is a physician's responsibility to advocate for an individual patient? What factors, if any, limit a physician's responsibility to "plead the patient's case"?
➤ What obligations do health care institutions and health plans have, if any, to advocate for patients?
➤ How should the health plan balance the interests of a patient like Sonia with the interests of all its enrollees?
➤ What is an appropriate appeals mechanism if requests for authorization are denied?
➤ What mechanisms are most ethically appropriate for encouraging physicians to consider the costs of alternative interventions as they design a patient's treatment plan?

COMMENTARY _____

Susan M. Wolf, J.D.

With the rise of managed care, physicians now routinely face the issues Dr. Ashton confronts in this case: whether to advocate that a patient receive health plan coverage for desired care, how hard to advocate, and when to stop. Similarly, health provider organizations such as Hillside Clinic face questions of whether to support or oppose patient advocacy and when to help directly in that advocacy effort. Finally, managed care organizations such as Horizon Health Care face the issues of what cost-containment measures they may ethically impose, what roadblocks they may erect for doctors and patients, and whether to encourage advocacy for patients.

The problem in this case requires analysis at all three levels. Traditional doctor-patient ethics that ignores organizational context will not suffice. The question of whether physicians have duties of patient advocacy has arisen precisely because physicians practice in the context of organizations that have reasons to say no to patients and physicians. In order to stay afloat financially, Hillside wants to deny patients physician time by imposing quotas of a certain number of patients per practitioner per day. And to save money, Horizon Health Care wants to deny coverage for certain neuro-imaging tests. Such organizations typically put the burden on individual physicians to sacrifice time, see fewer patients, and perhaps suffer negative financial and other consequences if they decide to fight for their patients.

Ignoring the ethical obligations of Hillside and Horizon Health Care would simply dump the full burden on the physician. It would allow these organizations to create terrible conflicts of interest for the physician and constraints bound to cause harm to patients, but it would then leave the doctor to handle the problem alone. In such a framework, an ethical solution would have to be built on the moral heroism of physicians. It would clearly be neither realistic nor fair to expect physicians to solve these problems by themselves.

Thus the old approach to doctor-patient ethics that looked only at that dyad is inadequate here. We have to take a broader view, supplementing physician ethics with organizational ethics. That broader view has great advantages, allowing us to see the doctor as one player within a system. The doctor need not resolve all ethical problems herself, trying to reconcile the need for cost containment with patient welfare within her own aching head. Instead, we can consider a system in which she might advocate for her patient's welfare, knowing that others will sometimes say no. A good analogy is to the defense attorney whose job is to advocate for a client within the criminal justice system. That system does not force the attorney to play advocate and judge; instead, it provides a jury to decide separately whether the prosecution has established guilt. The attorney is thus free, and indeed obligated, to provide zealous advocacy. In a system whose players have differentiated roles we can address the ethics of each and then evaluate the system as a whole. Any other approach is too simplistic, failing to do justice to organizational complexity.

The Physician's Duties

The physician in this case has multiple duties toward her patient, Sonia. Some of these duties are familiar and well accepted. Among them is a duty to render competent care as a pediatric neurologist. Competent care requires performing diagnostic tests to arrive at a diagnosis for this clearly symptomatic patient. Only then will Dr. Ashton know what treatment to recommend to fulfill further well-accepted duties to advance the patient's well-being and avert further neurological harm.

Beyond those duties, Dr. Ashton has obligations to demonstrate loyalty to her patient and act as the patient's fiduciary. The duty of loyalty is a traditional Hippocratic obligation to serve the patient, maintain the patient's confidences, and otherwise pursue that patient's well-being. The fiduciary duty is a related notion, that the physician's commitment to the patient is also grounded in the patient's dependency. The patient arrives with a health problem, bares her body, shares her secrets, and enters into a relationship of dependency on the physician. She depends on the physician's greater knowledge, healing skills, ability to maintain confidences, and commitment to help. This dependency creates obligations on the doctor's part to act as a fiduciary, that is, in the patient's best interests.

These duties alone, which every physician bears in all care settings, drive Dr. Ashton to order a diagnostic MRI and screening metabolic studies. Assuming these tests are medically indicated, which we have no reason to doubt in this case, Dr. Ashton properly takes steps to ensure their administration. The question is how far she should go.

Certainly all physicians ordinarily have an obligation to ensure an ordered test is performed. No physician's obligation ends with a written or verbal order. Physicians in all contexts encounter obstacles such as lack of personnel or available equipment, documentation requirements, and "red tape." They find they must work to overcome these obstacles: pull rank, throw their weight around, jockey for position, call in favors, go to bat. We have phrases for this cluster of maneuvers. These are common techniques that physicians use to ensure that their patients get the tests and care they need and avoid further harm. Physicians using these techniques are facing the reality that health care now is delivered in complex organizations; they have to work the system to get their patients care. In doing so, they are fulfilling traditional duties to render competent care, act beneficently, avoid harm, demonstrate loyalty to the patient, and act as a fiduciary.

However, there must be some limits to this obligation. For example, we ordinarily would not deem the physician obligated to pay for ordered tests directly out of her own pocket or to devote so much time to securing the test that her practice was completely disrupted. Yet we do expect physicians to cope with ordinary obstacles, even if that involves some time and effort.

In this case, the primary obstacle was created by the HMO in requiring prior authorization for neuro-imaging. The HMO has turned to a utilization review program (which may be part of the HMO or a separate entity contracting with the HMO) to respond to authorization requests. As is common in these programs, initial decisions are made by nurse reviewers (Gray 1991).

Dr. Ashton takes the time to phone the utilization review program initially for authorization. When that is denied, she finds she must spend several hours phoning, writing letters, and ultimately enlisting the help of Sonia's pediatrician to obtain approval. She worries about the impact on her other patients of having to spend so much time and effort on Sonia's case.

However, in the face of cost-containment efforts, including utilization review, traditional physician duties of competent care, loyalty, and a fiduciary relationship translate into an ethical duty of patient advocacy (see, for example, American Medical Association, 1995, 1996; Levinsky 1984; Wolf 1994). (For discussion of a legal duty, see, for example, Furrow 1988.) Patients cannot adequately advocate for themselves in these complex organizational frameworks. And the utilization review requirement in this case demands physician justification of the test. Because the physician knows the patient's diagnosis and medical needs best, she is uniquely situated to provide strong advocacy for the patient. Indeed, while others might also perform patient advocacy (Mehlman 1996), ultimately the patient may need the physician's clout and forcefulness.

This case shows how dependent patients are on their physicians to act as advocates. It suggests that when patients initially choose a physician, especially their primary care physician, they should inquire carefully about that physician's commitment to patient advocacy. Physicians may range from those who rarely advocate for their patients to those who often advocate; where a physician falls on that spectrum may greatly influence the patient's care (Sulmasy 1992).

The literature does not yet offer adequate guidance on where a physician should fall on that spectrum (Macklin 1993). Haavi Morreim (1995) argues for a duty of advocacy, but with a limitation: "Each time the physician contemplates pressing for extra resources, he should consider what would happen if all other physicians did the same under similar circumstances." I have suggested elsewhere that the extent of a physician's duties of advocacy is a function of the patient's need for treatment; those duties are highest when the patient needs treatment to avoid great medical harm or to realize great medical benefit (Wolf 1994). The American Medical Association's Council on Ethical and Judicial Affairs (1995) has urged that physicians advocate for all "materially beneficial care," though the report unfortunately never defines the term. The prevailing notion is that physicians should advocate for care likely to offer the patient benefit. Certainly that would include competent diagnosis in Sonia's case.

One might argue that the HMO and the utilization review program are not deciding whether Sonia receives the MRI, merely whether her MRI is covered by the HMO. Under this theory, the question is what obligations physicians have to advocate for coverage, not care. Realistically, however, patients are often dependent on their health plan or insurer, so that a denial of coverage amounts to a denial of care. Sonia's family, having moved to the United States only three years ago, may well be in that position. Even a family of means, though, is entitled to rely on their health plan and health care providers for basic care. And competent diagnosis in response to Sonia's symptoms would certainly be basic care.

The fact that Dr. Ashton fulfills her duties of advocacy in this case does nothing to allay her sense that she may be inadvertently penalizing other patients. In truth, many of her patients will probably require time-consuming advocacy at some point; then it may well be Sonia who has to wait an extra day to see the doctor or has to bear some other burden. No patient should be forced to suffer serious harm in this process, and Dr. Ashton may have to arrange assistance from other physicians to avoid that. The question remains, though, of whether the systems at the clinic and within the HMO are set up in ways that unfairly burden patients and physicians. That forces us to take the ethical analysis to the organizational level.

The Clinic's Duties

Hillside Clinic is an organization providing health care. The clinic thus shoulders obligations to the patients receiving that care. In addition, the clinic has obligations to support the physicians who practice there as they discharge their own duties to patients.

There is no indication in this case that the clinic is doing anything to help ensure that its patients in capitated plans are getting the coverage and care they need. Nor is there any indication that the clinic is helping its physicians discharge their advocacy obligations to those patients. Hillside could have designated a patient advisor or other individual to help patients understand and deal with their health plans. Because most of Hillside's patients are in capitated plans and the clinic often needs an interpreter to assist its foreign-born and non–English-speaking patients, such an advisor would undoubtedly be invaluable. Indeed, without that kind of help, many or most of the clinic's patients probably have little understanding of the health care delivery systems with which they are dealing and the cost-containment mechanisms influencing their care. When patients remain in the dark on these matters, it raises a host of ethical problems. Such patients have not knowledgeably subscribed to their health plan, have not knowingly consented to the plan's restrictions and cost-containment techniques, and cannot advocate for their health interests within the plan.

In such circumstances, an extraordinarily heavy burden falls on the treating physician. It is she who must explain the health plan's restrictions when they interfere with desired care and she who must bear the full burden of advocating for the patient. Hillside Clinic seems to have done nothing to alleviate this burden, even though the clinic is in a far better position than the individual physician to address the systemic problems that this patient population faces in capitated plans.

Indeed, the clinic seems to have exacerbated the problem by imposing on physicians quotas of patients they must see per day. While the clinic feels an understandable need to respond to financial pressures, this particular strategy takes no account of the fact that at different points in time some patients will require more time-consuming care, including patient advocacy as in Sonia's case. By imposing daily quotas on each individual physician, the clinic fails to support the physicians' discharge of their obligations to patients such as Sonia. Such quotas (which may be backed up by financial and other penalties) are akin to a type of financial incentive condemned by the American Medical Association's Council on Ethics and Judicial Affairs (1995). The council found incentives that simply penalize physicians for devoting too many resources to a patient (such as hospitalizations, tests, or referrals) to be unethical, because such incentives consider only the quantity of resources, not whether they are needed or cost-effective. Hillside Clinic's quotas (controlling the resource of physician time) are similar to the blunt, quantitative incentives the council condemned. Indeed, if Hillside actually calculates quotas on a daily basis and for each individual physician, then the clinic has adopted a system with those features the council found most problematic. The council's report urged that physician resource utilization be calculated over substantial periods of time and by physician group, not by individual. That way, the system gives physicians more latitude to care properly for those patients whose needs require more resources.

Hillside Clinic thus seems to have dropped the ball in meeting its own obligations to render and support good patient care. Indeed, the clinic has created a conflict of interest for physicians through the quota system. Yet in Sonia's case the most serious problems in organizational ethics seem to lurk at the HMO level.

The HMO's Duties

Horizon Health Care is a for-profit HMO that has instituted a range of cost-containment strategies, including required prior authorization for neuro-imaging tests. Authorization requires application to the HMO's utilization review program. There, nurse reviewers who may have no expertise in neurology may deny authorization, as in Sonia's case. Several levels of review are then available, with final decisions made by the HMO's director. However, the case suggests that a physician must expend considerable time and effort to obtain that highest level of review. And it was only at that highest level that Sonia's physician succeeded in getting authorization.

The HMO has instituted an extremely problematic program, raising questions about whether it is shirking its own obligations to support good patient care and physician advocacy as part of a good patient-doctor relationship. Required prior authorization for neuro-imaging may help save money and serve shareholders, but it may also undermine competent care and disserve patients. The HMO has an obligation to evaluate its requirement to see whether it is supporting or undermining such care. There is no indication in the case that the HMO has performed any such evaluation.

Further problems arise in the structure of the HMO's utilization review system. Utilization reviewers (and thus the HMO for which they work) can have a direct impact on the content and quality of a patient's care. They thus have obligations to act with due care and medical competence (Gray 1991). It is not at all clear that health professionals with no training in neurology can competently evaluate the need for neuro-imaging. Moreover, some utilization review systems will permit a nonphysician to authorize coverage but not deny it, insisting that denials automatically be reviewed by a physician. In any case, appeals must be readily available so that the treating physician who is persuaded that denial is wrongful can obtain review and a reversal if appropriate. Yet appeals in this case seem time-consuming and cumbersome.

If HMOs were entities whose only obligation was to serve shareholders, one might try to defend this system. But even under the rules of business ethics, the HMO in the business of supplying patient health care coverage and exercising a strong effect on actual care has an obligation to do so in a way that does not unreasonably harm its patient-customers (Velasquez 1997). Indeed, under stakeholder theory, both patients and physicians are stakeholders in the organization whose interests must be taken into account (Freeman 1997). Yet because HMOs exert control over both coverage and care, they bear not only business ethics obligations but also medical ethics obligations. Various writers have suggested what medical ethics would require at the organizational level (see, for example, Wolf 1994). Few would fail to critique the utilization review system in this case.

Conclusion

Rejecting the familiar dyadic ethical analysis for this more complex analysis of both individual physicians and organizations permits the development of a robust ethics of patient advocacy. Even a more ethical system of utilization review and cost containment will sometimes deny health care coverage. And even a better system for balancing the clinic's obligations to individual patients against its interests in maintaining financial viability and serving all of its patients will result in some pressure to cut back in serving certain patients. But precisely because the system will sometimes refuse desired care, either through outright denial or more subtle pressure, the patient needs someone to act as her champion. It is the physician who knows her medical needs and can advocate that they be met. If we rob patients of this natural advocate and dismantle the tradition of physician loyalty to the patient, there will be no one left to see that patients receive good care. They will be at the mercy of large impersonal organizations committed to cost containment. Patient advocacy is critical to maintaining ethical and competent patient care, and health care organizations themselves have a duty to support it.

References

American Medical Association, Council on Ethical and Judicial Affairs. 1995. "Ethical Issues in Managed Care." *Journal of the American Medical Association* 273, no. 4:330–35.

———. 1996. *Code of Medical Ethics: Current Opinions with Annotations, 1996-1997 Edition.* Chicago, Ill.: American Medical Association, pp. 6, 126–28.

Freeman, R. E. 1997. "A Stakeholder Theory of the Modern Corporation." In *Ethical Theory and Business*, 5th ed., pp. 66–76. Edited by T. L. Beauchamp and N. E. Bowie. Upper Saddle River, N.J.: Prentice Hall.

Furrow, B. R. 1988. "The Ethics of Cost-Containment: Bureaucratic Medicine and the Doctor as Patient-Advocate." *Notre Dame Journal of Law, Ethics & Public Policy 1987–88* 3, no. 2:187–225.

Gray, B. H. 1991. *The Profit Motive and Patient Care: The Changing Accountability of Doctors and Hospitals.* Cambridge, Mass.: Harvard University Press, pp. 312–20.

Levinsky, N. G. 1984. "The Doctor's Master." *New England Journal of Medicine* 311, no. 24:1573–75.

Macklin, R. 1993. *Enemies of Patients: How Doctors Are Losing Their Power and Patients Are Losing Their Rights.* New York: Oxford University Press, pp. 158–60.

Mehlman, M. J. 1996. "Medical Advocates: A Call for a New Profession." *Widener Law Symposium Journal* 1:299–323.

Morreim, E. H. 1995. *Balancing Act: The New Medical Ethics of Medicine's New Economics.* Washington, D.C.: Georgetown University Press, pp. 89, 91–92.

Sulmasy, D. P. 1992. "Physicians, Cost Control, and Ethics." *Annals of Internal Medicine* 116, no. 11:920–26.

Velasquez, M. G. 1997. "The Ethics of Consumer Production." In *Ethical Theory and Business*, 5th ed., pp. 201–09. Edited by T. L. Beauchamp and N. E. Bowie. Upper Saddle River, N.J.: Prentice Hall.

Wolf, S. M. 1994. "Health Care Reform and the Future of Physician Ethics." *Hastings Center Report* 24, no. 2:28–41.

COMMENTARY

Genevieve Noone Parsons, M.D.
Peter A. Ubel, M.D.

The need to contain health care costs creates conflicts among health care organizations, health care providers, and their patients. Physicians and other practitioners must grapple with the reality that the drive to control costs may interfere with patient advocacy, as in the case at hand. Dr. Ashton is a pediatric neurologist whose patients subscribe to Horizon Health Care, an HMO that attempts to save money in a variety of ways, including requiring preauthorization for expensive tests. Horizon Health Care initially denies Dr. Ashton's request for an MRI to evaluate a child with worsening neurologic symptoms, forcing Dr. Ashton to spend significant time appealing the decision. Horizon Health Care eventually authorizes the MRI, which reveals that the child has a neurodegenerative disorder. The time Dr. Ashton spends advocating for this test, and for this child, limits the amount of time she can spend with her other patients.

Clearly, this child's neurologic signs warranted diagnostic imaging. And clearly, Dr. Ashton did a morally laudable job of advocating for her patient. But readers should not conclude from this case that clinicians should do everything they can to fight HMOs. Instead, this case should remind health care providers that, in an era of cost-containment, when their traditional duty to advocate for their patient's best interests has been weakened, they must decide when to accede to cost-containment efforts and when to fight the battle for their patients.

Should Clinicians Ever Ration at the Bedside?

Traditional professional norms hold that physicians should do what is best for their patients (American Medical Association 1997). They should promote their patients' best interests and should never ration beneficial interventions at the bedside. If there is any need for health care rationing, this need should be fulfilled at a "higher level." Formulary committees, managed care organizations, or the federal government may make rationing decisions, but not physicians at the bedside taking care of specific patients (Sulmasy 1992).

How do we interpret these norms in the context of a health care system driven to contain health care costs and in the face of managed care organizations doing the best they can to restrain physicians from pursuing patients' best interests without attention to costs? In recent years, clinicians have increasingly faced "higher-level" efforts to change their practice patterns. In many cases these efforts are directed at improving physicians' quality of care by decreasing their use of unnecessary procedures or by urging them to follow practice guidelines or clinical pathways that have been shown to improve patient outcomes. But in other cases these efforts are meant to encourage physicians to use less expensive therapies despite the fact that more expensive therapies offer greater benefits.

Clinicians and ethicists continue to debate the morality of bedside rationing. This debate continues in large part because many cost-containment efforts rely on bedside rationing to succeed. The case at hand provides a good example. The case illustrates a common method of containing health care costs—utilization review. With utilization review, third-party payers supervise clinicians' judgments to decide whether or not they are appropriate or reimbursable. In the present case, utilization review took the form of preauthorization, whereby physicians must obtain approval from the HMO prior to providing therapies to their patients. Preauthorization schemes can be used to control the use of expensive medications, diagnostic tests (like the MRI in this case), or even hospital admissions.

Most cost-control methods do not tie physicians' hands but leave them with discretion about whether or not to pursue patients' best interests. To the extent that utilization review ties physicians' hands, the knots are often quite loose. As this case illustrates, physicians can appeal utilization review decisions. Sometimes these appeals require only a brief phone call; other times, perhaps with increasing frequency, appeals require a significant time commitment, and the physician must battle an increasingly bureaucratic health care system before getting authorization. Physicians are also free to ignore utilization review by ordering diagnostic tests or continued hospitalization without worrying about whether the care will be reimbursed. Managed care organizations, in fact, are adamant that they do not make clinical decisions but only make reimbursement decisions, stating that clinicians can choose to offer free care if they think it is medically necessary.

Suppose physicians agree that they have a duty to promote patients' best interests, regardless of cost. What should they do when the pursuit of patients' best interests requires them to spend one minute filling out paperwork? Or five minutes making a phone call? Or twenty-five minutes arguing with the utilization reviewer? And what if patients' interests require that they go without pay? How should physicians balance their duties to individual patients with duties to their other patients? To spend time promoting one patient's best interests might leave them with less time to pursue other patients' best interests. Or in closed health care systems like county hospitals, with limited budgets, how do physicians balance the interests of specific patients with the knowledge that ordering a marginally beneficial and expensive test may leave fewer resources for other patients within the health care system?

Bedside Rationing:
A Debate About Ethics or Language?

The debate about the morality of bedside rationing often gets bogged down in confusion about what it means to ration at the bedside. There is no general agreement about what it means to ration health care (Ubel and Goold 1998a) or about what specifically constitutes bedside rationing (Ubel and Goold 1997). Ubel and Goold have defined bedside rationing as the withholding by a physician of a medically beneficial service because of that service's cost to someone other than the patient. Not everyone may agree with this definition, and this definition leads to many gray areas: what constitutes "beneficial" health care, for example, and when can we say that clinicians have "control" over the use of health care resources?

Confusion about the language of rationing was demonstrated in a survey of general internists in the United States, in which over 70 percent of respondents thought it was appropriate to choose a $100 colon cancer screening test for a patient even though a $400 test was available that is slightly better at detecting cancer (Ubel and Asch 1997). Despite general agreement that physicians should withhold the more effective screening test, there was no agreement among general internists about whether this constitutes "rationing." Several other studies show that physicians are occasionally willing to do less than the best for their patients in order to save money (Ayres 1996; Brody et al. 1991; Jecker and Berg 1992; Lessler and Avins 1992). This willingness on the part of some physicians to do less than the best for patients, while they also express ambivalence about rationing, suggests that some physicians who oppose rationing may make peace with withholding beneficial services from patients by using terms other than rationing to characterize their actions. Sometimes clinicians appeal to the "standard of care," which is often based on higher-level rationing judgments. Cancer screening is a classic example. Some national cancer societies recommend Pap smears every three years for low-risk women even though studies show that yearly Pap smears identify slightly more cancers. (In these low-risk women, it takes approximately $1 million worth of yearly pap smear testing to find one additional cancer [Eddy 1990]). To some physicians, endorsement of Pap smear testing at three-year intervals by these respected cancer societies shows that this type of testing is not an example of rationing but is simply the professional standard of care. This ignores the possibility that the standard of care itself often encourages rationing.

Confusion or disagreement about what constitutes rationing should not divert us from the more important question of when it is morally appropriate for clinicians to allow their patients to go without the best possible health care. There are times when physicians ought to fight managed care efforts to deny important health care services for a patient. The case presented here is a good example. But at other times it may be appropriate for physicians to accede to managed care cost-control efforts, even when specific patients' best interests are not pursued. For example, if a managed care formulary restricts the use of proton pump inhibitors (an expensive medicine that treats stomach ulcers, among other things) until H_2 blockers can be used (a less expensive class of medicines that are almost as effective as proton pump inhibitors at curing most ulcers), many physicians would comply. Whether or not this cooperation would entail bedside rationing, clinicians need to decide whether the cooperation is morally acceptable.

When Is Less Than the Best Care Acceptable?

Unless physicians relax their advocacy duties and occasionally allow their patients to make do with less than the best possible health care, it will be nearly impossible to control health care costs. Physicians are notoriously talented at "gaming" the system (Morreim 1991). If an insurance company tries to limit the use of prostate cancer blood tests or prostate biopsies, physicians can always say they felt a prostate nodule on a patient's examination. If a formulary committee allows the use of proton pump inhibitors for severe reflux disease but not for ulcer treatment, then every ulcer patient will suddenly be diagnosed with reflux disease. If a physician wants to get a CT scan or an MRI to evaluate a patient with a headache, then that patient will have "blurred optical disks," an often fuzzy diagnostic finding that nevertheless is an immediate indication for diagnostic imaging.

In the face of controversies about whether health care should ever be rationed, and whether physicians, in particular, should ever do the rationing, as well as controversies about what it means to "ration health care," it should be no surprise that there has been very little effort to help clinicians decide when it is morally justifiable to do less than the best for their patients (Ubel and Arnold 1995). Indeed, many clinicians and ethicists do not accept the view that bedside rationing, or allowing patients to do without the best possible health care, is necessary to control health care costs and can sometimes be morally appropriate (Ubel and Goold 1998b). Thus, there has been little effort to develop guidelines to help clinicians decide when it is morally acceptable to withhold beneficial health care services from their patients.

But even if there were general agreement that physicians should occasionally do less than the best for their patients, the nature of clinical medicine would make it very difficult to come up with clear rationing guidelines. In deciding when it is appropriate to ration health care, clinicians need to consider the medical benefits being withheld from patients (compared to the benefits they are receiving), the medical risks of the service being withheld (compared to that being offered), the financial savings of withholding the beneficial service (including the patients' out-of-pocket costs and societal costs, more generally), the amount of time it would take to obtain the best possible service (including how much time it will take to fight with utilization reviewers), and the likelihood that any money saved by withholding this beneficial service will bring health care benefits to other people.

Medical benefits, risks, costs, and time all come on a continuum, and often they are unpredictable. What might begin as a quick call to a utilization reviewer could turn into a thirty-minute argument. What seems like a potential medical benefit could turn into an adverse event. With all this uncertainty, clinicians must make difficult judgments about the importance of offering the best possible care to patients when the next best is almost as good. At one extreme are decisions where the best possible health care is significantly more expensive than the next best and offers only tiny benefits. These are instances where doing less than the best is most justifiable. At the other extreme are instances where the next best alternative is a pale shadow of the best possible care, and where the best possible care is only slightly more expensive.

While these judgments are very difficult, clinicians have a great deal of experience making similar judgments. Often clinicians and patients must balance risks and benefits of multiple alternatives, where no one alternative dominates the rest. One alternative might be slightly more effective but carry a risk of a more severe side effect. These are difficult judgment calls, and there is no simple rule to help clinicians make them. Nevertheless, clinicians make these judgments all the time.

Conclusion

Many clinicians and ethicists think that physicians, when treating individual patients, should play no role in helping contain health care costs. For those who think physicians should pursue patients' best interests regardless of financial costs, the moral decisions will still be plentiful. These physicians will still have to decide when their obligations to pursue patients' best interests have been fulfilled. Is a ten-minute fight with a utilization reviewer enough to fulfill their advocacy duties? How about an hour-long fight? Must they fight utilization reviewers each time they deny a marginally beneficial health care service? Or only when the benefits are important enough? For those physicians who think that their duty to pursue patients' best interests is not absolute, their moral task comes down to deciding how to balance patients' interests with society's.

In caring for their patients, practitioners face difficult decisions every day. To these difficulties has now been added the challenge of acting both as patient advocate and controller of rising health care expenditures. Much more needs to be done to help clinicians decide when it is appropriate to provide less than the best for their patients and when they ought to fight any efforts by third-party payers or others to keep their patients from receiving the best possible care. We can only hope that clinicians do as good a job in making these decisions as Dr. Ashton did in the case described.

References

American Medical Association, Council on Ethical and Judicial Affairs. 1997. *Code of Medical Ethics: Current Opinions with Annotations*, 1996–97 ed. Chicago, Ill.: American Medical Association.

Ayres, P. J. 1996. "Rationing Health Care: Views from General Practice." *Social Science and Medicine* 42, no. 7:1021–25.

Brody, B.; Wray, N.; Bame, S.; Ashton, C.; Petersen, N.; and Harward, M. 1991. "The Impact of Economic Considerations on Clinical Decisionmaking: The Case of Thrombolytic Therapy." *Medical Care* 29, no. 9:899–910.

Eddy, D. M. 1990. "Screening for Cervical Cancer." *Annals of Internal Medicine* 113, no. 3:214–26.

Jecker, N. S., and Berg, A. O. 1992. "Allocating Medical Resources in Rural America: Alternative Perceptions of Justice." *Social Science and Medicine* 34, no. 5:467–74.

Lessler, D. S., and Avins, A. L. 1992. "Cost, Uncertainty, and Doctors' Decisions: The Case of Thrombolytic Therapy." *Archives of Internal Medicine* 152, no. 8:1665–72.

Morreim, E. H. 1991. "Gaming the System: Dodging the Rules, Ruling the Dodgers." *Archives of Internal Medicine* 151, no. 3:443–47.

Sulmasy, D. D. 1992. "Physicians, Cost Control, and Ethics." *Annals of Internal Medicine* 116, no. 11:920–26.

Ubel, P. A., and Arnold, R. M. 1995. "The Unbearable Rightness of Bedside Rationing: Physician Duties in a Climate of Cost-containment." *Archives of Internal Medicine* 155, no. 17:1837–42.

Ubel, P. A., and Asch, A. 1997. "The Appropriateness of Cost-Quality Trade-Offs in Cancer Screening: A National Survey." *Journal of General Internal Medicine* 12, supplement 1:105.

Ubel, P. A., and Goold, S. D. 1997. "Recognizing Bedside Rationing: Clear Cases and Tough Calls." *Annals of Internal Medicine* 126, no. 1:74–80.

———. 1998a. "Rationing Health Care: Not All Definitions Are Created Equal." *Archives of Internal Medicine* 158, no. 3:209–14.

———. 1998b. "Does Bedside Rationing Violate Patients' Best Interests? An Exploration of 'Moral Hazard'." *American Journal of Medicine* 104, no. 1: 64–8.

14

Similarly-Situated Patients with Different Benefits Packages

CASE STUDY _____

Sara Anderson is a physical therapist at a skilled nursing facility in a small South Dakota town. She has been on the job for less than a year and, as her responsibilities have grown, now struggles to keep up with a full caseload. Her fellow therapists in the small (three-person) department are similarly stretched.

About four weeks ago, Ms. Anderson began providing physical therapy to both Mrs. Jones and Mrs. Smith. Dr. Davis, a leading orthopedic surgeon in the region, had performed a total knee replacement on each of the women. Both surgeries went smoothly and Dr. Davis recommended similar follow-up care for both.

Mrs. Jones is a sixty-two-year-old retired salesclerk who moved to South Dakota with her husband shortly before he died, five years ago. Originally from southern Georgia, Mrs. Jones has never felt at home in the Midwest. She had moved at her husband's suggestion but made few friends in their new location, and she now finds herself alone most of the time. Her only relative in the area is her frail older sister-in-law. Mrs. Jones complains that the long South Dakota winters keep her indoors too much and restrict her physical activity.

Since the surgery, Mrs. Jones, who is overweight and has cardiopulmonary problems, including shortness of breath when she walks, has had difficulty follow-ing through with the walking schedule the physical therapy department has recommended for her. The facility's nursing staff has responsibility for walking with patients. Unfortunately, the nursing department appears to be as understaffed as the physical therapy department—to the point of not being able to carry out this portion of its duties. Though her sister-in-law visits once a week, she is not able to walk with Mrs. Jones herself. Accordingly, Mrs. Jones is not meeting her physical therapy goals and is becoming increasingly frustrated.

Mrs. Smith is a very healthy sixty-four-year-old retired school teacher. She is also a widow but, unlike Mrs. Jones, is a lifelong resident of South Dakota and receives a great deal of support from her large family, most of whom live in the area. With her family's help, Mrs. Smith easily manages the walking schedule Ms. Anderson has set out and is rapidly achieving her other physical therapy goals. Mrs. Smith has asked Ms. Anderson to help her meet more ambitious goals. She is willing to pay out-of-pocket for any extra services.

Ms. Anderson is troubled by the differences in the amount of care and attention she is able to provide to her two knee replacement patients. Mrs. Smith has excellent health care coverage with a managed care plan through the school system. Benefits for a total knee replacement include twice daily physical therapy treatments of one hour per treatment. Mrs. Smith has received this level of care since her surgery.

Mrs. Jones, on the other hand, is enrolled in a large HMO that provides for only thirty minutes (two units of fifteen minutes each) of physical therapy each day. She, too, has received her allotted care since the surgery. Mrs. Jones is financially unable to pay for any extra physical therapy services herself.

The skilled nursing facility's own written policies require physical therapists to comply strictly with the patients' insurance coverage and to charge only for the treatments for which the facility will be paid. The facility's management has reprimanded therapists who have treated and charged for services in excess of a patient's insurance coverage, as well as those who have provided additional services but charged only to the limit of the patient's coverage.

Ms. Anderson believes that despite her best efforts, the amount of care she is able to give to Mrs. Jones, as dictated by the HMO's and the nursing facility's policies, is simply inadequate. And, while Ms. Anderson is pleased with Mrs. Smith's progress, she is concerned that honoring Mrs. Smith's requests for additional care would interfere with the care she gives her other clients. She is also reminded of the American Physical Therapy Association's Guide for Professional Conduct, which states that "providing services more frequently than necessary for maximum therapeutic effect is unethical."

Questions for Consideration

➤ How should Ms. Anderson distribute her services among her clients? On what basis should she decide?
➤ Should Ms. Anderson honor Mrs. Smith's request for additional services? Why or why not?
➤ What should a practitioner do if a patient's insurance plan does not cover what

the practitioner believes is an adequate level of services? What should a practitioner do if, as a result of a plan's limits and expectations, patient care is being compromised?

➤ Who should ensure that Mrs. Jones receives adequate and appropriate care—the physical therapist, the skilled nursing facility, the HMO, her physician?

➤ Does a health plan have an ethical obligation to provide a minimally adequate benefits set? Does the consumer have an obligation to purchase a minimally adequate benefits set?

➤ When, if ever, should a facility refuse to accept managed care contracts that offer patients less than a minimally adequate benefits set?

COMMENTARY

Larry R. Churchill, Ph.D.

Sara Anderson faces a cluster of interrelated ethical issues. How should she allocate her scarce time and skills among clients who have different needs for her services, especially when those in greater need have less insurance coverage and fewer financial and personal resources? This problem is compounded by an employer intolerant of uncompensated services. At least one response to the deteriorating condition of Mrs. Jones—whose managed care plan has inadequate coverage for rehabilitation following total knee replacement—would be simply to provide the needed services without compensation. Yet here this option is at best difficult, given the record of the facility for reprimanding therapists who provide uncompensated services. Moreover, Ms. Anderson is already working at full capacity, so it is unclear where she would find time for Mrs. Jones, even if her insurance plan were adequate.

Professional Ethics

None of this would necessarily occasion a direct ethical conflict were not Ms. Anderson a professional, with an obligation to make financial and other considerations secondary to the needs of clients. While anyone might find it difficult to work in an environment that attends so closely to the bottom line, for professionals this presents special ethical difficulties.

Historically, a profession was a vow or oath made upon entrance into a religious order. Even in the modern, secular environment of late twentieth-century America, professionals are thought to have a higher calling than mechanics, technicians, and laborers, no matter how skilled. Professionals are given more discretion in the use of their skills and a greater range of authority in making judgments, primarily because their goodwill toward those they serve is taken as a given. Most professionals are to some extent fiduciaries, whose relationships with their clients are grounded not solely in contracts but also in trust. Relationships based in trust differ from purely contractual ones in that the obligations engendered by trust are more open-ended. In contemporary American society professional work is not necessarily religious in its motivation or sanctions, but it is still thought to be set apart by concerns for service that exceed the desire for money. It is this motivation that presumably makes professionals trustworthy. When compensation or self-interest comes into direct conflict with clients' well-being, professionals are directed by their fiduciary obligations to choose in favor of their clients' good rather than their own. At least this is the common understanding for how health professionals will function.

The *Code of Ethics and Guide for Professional Responsibility* of the American Physical Therapy Association (1991) is very explicit in setting forth a professional standard. It says: "Physical therapists are to be guided at all times by concern for the physical, psychological, and socioeconomic welfare of those individuals entrusted to their care." The extent to which Ms. Anderson takes this guideline seriously is the extent to which she is faced with ethical problems. The term "problem" rather than "dilemma" is used deliberately. Dilemmas are typically situations in which persons must choose between two courses of action, those actions embodying competing values, both of which the agent wants to honor. Dilemmas require discernment about which of these competing values has priority or, sometimes, which of two unsavory alternatives would be least burdensome or harmful. Ms. Anderson is not here faced with a dilemma, at least not in the usual sense. Rather she has the apparent problem of being unable to do what presumably she knows is the right thing to do, that is, to provide the needed physical therapy to Mrs. Jones. The problem arises because Mrs. Jones's managed care plan does not provide adequate coverage, and the facility in which Ms. Anderson works is unwilling to allow uncompensated services. That the better insured and physically more robust Mrs. Smith desires an even more ambitious course of rehabilitation, requiring more of Ms. Anderson's time, complicates the situation. How should she approach these problems?

Perhaps it is important to say at the start that Ms. Anderson may be unable to resolve this problem to her satisfaction, simply because it will not be within her power to do so. The aspirational definition of professional obligations outlined by the American Physical Therapy Association presupposes sufficient power and control over one's work, and one's work environment, to be able not only to make choices but to alter circumstances. This may be unrealistic for physical therapists, especially if they are seen by the managers of the facilities in which they work as employees rather than as professionals. If managed care continues to be guided by market forces rather than professional norms and client needs, the expectation that one can change the circumstances for delivering care may be increasingly unrealistic for any health professional. At best, interventions to rectify systemic problems are partial, and success must often be measured over long periods, and with many clients, not just one. Yet Mrs. Jones's situation requires action now, and judging how Ms. Anderson might act effectively requires an accurate understanding of current managed care practices and how these practices affect professional ethics and client welfare.

Managed Care

"Managed care" loosely identifies a variety of ways of organizing and financing the delivery of health services. Traditional staff-model health maintenance organizations (HMOs), discounted fee-for-service preferred provider organizations (PPOs), and even closely scrutinized indemnity insurance plans are sometimes called "managed care." The common elements are active participation and oversight by the financing agency in monitoring costs and quality and incentives for holding down costs for both providers and patients (Madison 1997).

Yet the success of managed care in achieving its chief objective of controlling costs is still unclear. To date only the nonprofit, prepaid group practice form of managed care has been in existence long enough to have established a clear record of cost reduction with quality comparable to traditional fee-for-service, indemnity insurance plans. For other forms of managed care, and especially for the aggressively managed for-profit organizations, the evidence is still out, and there is room for skepticism. For example, managed care plans that seek efficiency through detailed utilization review require legions of new managers and create hassles for practitioners. Beyond the ill will engendered by approval requirements and second-guessing of professional opinions, there are substantial inefficiencies entailed by seeking approvals and providing extensive and detailed justifications for decisions about diagnosis, treatment, and hospitalization. Another cost-cutting measure used by managed care plans is simply to offer fewer covered services. Coinsurance requirements, deductibles, limitations, and exclusions on coverage are obvious ways of limiting the managed care plan's liability. Yet these measures may also result in lowering the quality of services and the health status of persons covered, as is the case for Mrs. Jones.

Some of the efficiencies and cost reductions claimed by managed care organizations are more accurately described as cost-shifting. While the purchasers of services have experienced reductions, or at least a lessening of the escalation of costs, clients have seen their out-of-pocket costs rise, while the income of professional providers has been flat or declined. Moreover, many health insurers have learned from their fire, accident, and life insurance experiences that the easiest way to control costs is simply through a very careful selection of risks. Some insurers would refuse Mrs. Jones coverage altogether. Her current insurer simply provides inadequate benefits.

It is also sobering to note that in the recent past the established nonprofit HMOs have had to adopt the more aggressive cost-cutting strategies of their market-oriented, for-profit competitors in order to survive. This parallels the adjustment that Blue Cross and Blue Shield organizations were required to make several years ago, dropping their practice of community rating for health insurance premiums, in which everyone is charged basically the same, and adopting the risk-rating practices of its competitors, in which those who are ill and likely to use more care are charged much more than the young and healthy. Such practices exacerbate even further the problems of those like Mrs. Jones, who are categorized as "high users" of the system.

In the aggressive market environment for health services, clients such as Mrs. Smith and Mrs. Jones are being treated increasingly as if they were simply consumers in the health care marketplace, expected to make savvy choices as comparison shoppers for their coverage and then to live within the terms of the contract they have chosen. This system might work if they were truly able to be comparison shoppers, choosing freely and knowledgeably among competing plans with adequate information about price, quality, and extent of coverage readily available. These conditions do not now prevail, since much important information about services is usually only sketched, rather than spelled out in detail, and often the efficiency measures that managed care organizations use are treated as trade secrets, or confidential, proprietary strategies that give these organizations a competitive edge. Moreover, the majority of Americans with employer-sponsored health benefits are given no choice about who will provide their health services or the extent of their coverage. This is clearly the case for Mrs. Jones. Finally, she has the added burden of being overweight and suffering with cardiopulmonary problems. As long as risk-rating dominates health insurance practices, Mrs. Jones will be considered an "undesirable" and avoidable risk for most insurers. Whatever her choices might be in theory, her actual choices about price and quality in health care are nonexistent.

Market-oriented managed care practices affect the shape of this case in yet another way. While insurers seek to reduce the services for which they will pay, facilities are also caught in the cycle of cost reductions. They must use their personnel with greater efficiency in order to compete with other facilities offering the same or similar services. So the skilled nursing facility in which Mrs. Jones and

Mrs. Smith reside must be sure it uses all its resources, including the services of Ms. Anderson, to maximal efficiency. Moreover, it cannot afford to have very many patients whose needs are as great and whose private resources are as few as Mrs. Jones. Time spent caring for the extra burdens of Mrs. Jones is time taken from other residents and other tasks. The ideal situation, from the standpoint of the financial health of this skilled nursing facility, would be a population of clients like Mrs. Smith—clients who have few health needs, extensive coverage for the needs they do have, and private means to satisfy their demands for a higher level of health services.

To assess the situation in this way is not to imply that the managers and owners of the skilled nursing facility do not care for their clients. Rather this assessment points to the ways in which a market-oriented managed care system, driven by cost containment and ultimately by profitability, will be motivated to act. The owners and managers of this nursing facility might well wish that they could provide a better level of service for their clients, and they may well wish they had the means to provide discretionary time for physical therapists like Ms. Anderson to give attention to clients like Mrs. Jones. Yet in the world in which they work efficiency is the means of survival. There is little or no room for largesse. And as an organization the facility has its own obligations to others besides Mrs. Jones, or any of the current residents. If this skilled nursing facility is owned by a for-profit corporation that is publicly traded, that corporation has fiduciary obligations of a legal nature to its shareholders. This is yet another way in which the obligations to clients so simply expressed in the professional codes of health practitioners become entangled in webs of larger obligations and priorities, and finally are subordinated to forces that have little to do with their clients' needs, or their own consciences. Aggressively market-oriented managed care places the very notion of professionalism in jeopardy.

Given this context, what actions is Ms. Anderson obligated to undertake? What can she realistically hope to achieve?

Client Advocacy, Equity, and Justice

The first course of action should be a call to Mrs. Jones's HMO, perhaps most effectively channeled through her primary care provider. Efficiency and cost-containment measures should never mean substandard or inadequate coverage for needed services, especially when those services are a routine part of care. Different patients will require different amounts of rehabilitation, and the HMO's services should be flexible enough to accommodate such differences.

Ms. Anderson may or may not succeed in this effort, but she has several powerful arguments in her favor. She herself is being asked to provide inadequate services for Mrs. Jones, and this is a violation of her professional duties. Moreover, this inadequate care adds an additional burden to the skilled nursing facility, since the care of Mrs. Jones when immobile is more time-consuming than if she were ambulatory. If the facility itself is already understaffed, the failure of Mrs. Jones to achieve her rehabilitation goals will only make the understaffing problem more acute. The facility should be an ally for Ms. Anderson in her conversations with the HMO.

Beyond the economic rationale, any health care facility—no matter how financed or organized—must be committed to providing a standard of care adequate to the needs of its clients. Not just individual professionals but facilities and institutions as well have fiduciary obligations to their clients. As noted previously, these are not the only obligations health facilities have, but without this obligation to clients, they are no more than landlords renting housing units.

The skilled nursing facility's policy of discouraging private contracting by its physical therapists can be interpreted as a recognition of this obligation and, moreover, an effort to achieve some justice in discharging this obligation. Private contracting for additional services erects a barrier to achieving equitable attention to the needs of *all* clients by favoring those with greater purchasing power. Yet the facility must go beyond this passive advocacy of discouraging or restricting private arrangements to active advocacy for their clients in receiving an adequate level of care. This will not be easy to achieve. For-profit managed care facilities have dual obligations—to their shareholders for a profit margin and to their patients for high-quality services. These dual obligations can and do conflict, since resources spent on physical therapy for Mrs. Jones will reduce profits. Yet a health care facility that routinely sacrifices patient well-being for profits will not sustain a reputation adequate for referrals, so that a short-term profit-maximization strategy would be ultimately self-defeating. Still, there will be temptations to cut and trim services, for not every case like Mrs. Jones will be noticed by a concerned professional or a family member. Given the current competitive environment, and the subsequent temptation to squeeze services and enhance profit margins, patient welfare must finally be guaranteed through patient rights legislation and other means of regulating facilities for both the individual and the public good. No set of regulations will eliminate all the possible conflicts of interest between the profitability of institutions and the well-being of patients. Yet regulations will reduce the number of occasions in which conflicts arise by providing a floor for quality beneath which institutions cannot fall and remain accredited.

The same sense of justice that should govern the policies of the facility should function within the thinking of Ms. Anderson herself. This will lead her to decline the additional, privately contracted services desired by Mrs. Smith, so long as Mrs.

Smith is receiving adequate care and Mrs. Jones is not. Mrs. Smith is not harmed by such a norm, and Mrs. Jones could certainly be helped. It is also important for Ms. Anderson to be candid and explicit in relating to Mrs. Smith why she is declining to provide the additional services. Encouraging and promoting an environment in the facility in which fairness is acknowledged and embraced by the residents, as well as the professional staff, is important. To this end, the nursing facility should not accept managed care contracts that call for substandard care, and it should encourage such a criterion for the industry. Only if all nursing facilities play by the same rules in developing standards of care can those facilities that insist on quality survive. This is another argument for uniform standards and practices for facilities, enforced through regulation.

If professional and institutional responsibilities are to have any weight at all, they must do so in situations where differences in power, authority, and social and financial resources threaten to affect the quality of health care and the subsequent health status of individuals. Professional advocacy must mean advocacy for the least well-off, for persons unable to speak adequately on their own behalf, and for persons whose injuries and illnesses threaten to disenfranchise them even further. Managed care, in its current market-driven form, is only the latest test for how substantial and lasting the advocacy for clients needs to be. Unless they provide this advocacy, health providers cannot remain professionals and health institutions cannot be trusted. Markets are designed to shake out those who cannot compete, to reward efficiency and effectiveness, and to create winners and losers. Yet an unregulated market for health services, a market in which no professional values modulate economic measures of success, will make losers of us all.

References

American Physical Therapy Association House of Delegates. 1991. *Code of Ethics and Guide for Professional Responsibility.* Alexandria, Va.: American Physical Therapy Association.
Madison, D. L. 1997. "Paying for Medical Care in America." In *The Social Medicine Reader,* p. 439. Edited by G. E. Henderson, R. P. Strauss, S. E. Estroff, and L. R. Churchill. Durham, N.C.: Duke University Press.

COMMENTARY

Michael Felder, D.O., M.A.

Patients' and health care providers' experience of the health care system has changed dramatically over the last few years. It is not at all clear which changes can be attributed to managed care and which ones might have occurred as a result of the evolution of traditional indemnity insurance. This commentary will attend to some of the organizational structures within the facility and the health plan relevant to Sara Anderson's problem with her two patients; assumptions about clinical care, policies, and guidelines; professional caregivers' (clinical and ethical) obligations to their patients and other "customers"; and patients' responsibilities.

Medical, ethical, and lay publications have described many of the ethical tensions that are commonly experienced and perceived as inherent in managed care. When patients' outcomes or even predicaments seem "unfair," one seeks a locus of responsibility. Increasingly, that locus is not an individual but an institution or a complex organizational structure, where the responsibility for clinical decisions is often diffused.

In the spirit of "preventive ethics," it may make sense to raise some questions about this case that would or should have predated the current "dilemmas." That is to say, by careful deliberation and anticipatory guidance, one often has an opportunity to *prevent* ethical dilemmas. Asking and answering key questions, even at this point, may help identify those with some responsibility for having created the current situation and perhaps those willing and able to resolve it.

Preoperative Review and Quality Planning

While our two patients, Mrs. Jones and Mrs. Smith, have surgery, widowhood, and age in common, there are some clinically important differences between them. From the psychosocial standpoint, Mrs. Jones is retired and has limited economic means, few friends, and apparently limited health insurance coverage for services she may need. Her medical conditions include obesity and cardiovascular disease. Mrs. Smith, on the other hand, has considerable social and family support, liberal health insurance coverage, and sufficient resources to pay for the additional services she desires. Her underlying health is quite good.

A careful initial review before any health care intervention, with regard to the indications, value (for the patient), likely benefits and harms, and short- and long-term goals, is always valuable. Patients and physicians alike are accustomed to balancing harms and benefits when making decisions about medications as well as therapeutic and investigative procedures. In the current clinical scenario, an initial review would have been instructive, not only to our patients but also to Dr. Davis, the surgeon, and Ms. Anderson, the physical therapist. In the common chaos of the current health care system, a comprehensive and holistic preintervention review rarely occurs. It is neither encouraged nor subsidized.

Reimbursement issues aside (but hardly with the intent of minimizing them), the best interests of the patient suggest that the "health care team" perform a comprehensive review of a patient's entire situation, prior to making a decision about surgery. Surgeons commonly request "medical clearance" by a patient's primary care physician in order to identify significant surgical risks and ensure that the patient is likely to survive surgery. There are many other psychosocial and medical dimensions of the case (including the patients' insurance coverage) that powerfully influence patients' postoperative courses. While physicians do not usually make a point of knowing this information, its relevance to clinical outcomes in this case is obvious. For Mrs. Jones, nonclinical factors have placed her at additional risk for a suboptimal outcome. A conversation with the patient that includes all of these issues should become a routine step in the informed-consent process.

The preoperative review should incorporate the relevant clinical information, probable clinical outcomes, and the most likely (financial and insurance-related) complications. The review should also be tailored to the specific patient and not a "population" of patients. Many areas of clinical medicine are simply not amenable to "population-based medicine," despite the growing use of this term in the lexicon of managed care.

The preoperative "conversation" should include the patient (who must be empowered to accept some level of responsibility), members of the rehabilitation facility and physical therapy departments, the HMO's discharge planners, the primary care physician, and the surgeon, all of whom ought to have an interest in designing a high-quality care plan. Approvals, denials, and appeals related to predictable complications should be handled when they are anticipated, and therefore prior to their actual occurrence.

The postoperative dialogue should include the same participants and continue to orient planning around "quality." The ability of caregivers to fulfill their obligation to patients postoperatively can be limited by what they understand their obligations to be. In addition, caregivers' perspectives on the patients' outcomes will be influenced by their relationships to patients and their positions in the health care team. For Mrs. Jones and Mrs. Smith, Dr. Davis may describe each of the operations as "successful" simply on the basis of their postoperative survival. Dr. Davis, however, may be alone in his sanguine assessment of Mrs. Jones's clinical situation. Once she is in the rehabilitation facility, he may not apprehend any further obligations on his part.

Inadequate provision for postoperative complications, which should or could have been anticipated and communicated to the patient, is morally unacceptable because it unwittingly exposes patients to medical risk. Based on a thorough preoperative review, Mrs. Jones's caregivers might have advised her to delay or cancel surgery. Or, perhaps her HMO should have anticipated a higher "intensity" of postoperative needs and approved a more liberal physical therapy benefits package prior to surgery. Perhaps Mrs. Smith's extensive support system and resources should have prompted her HMO to modify her postoperative benefits to suit her needs. Since it is uncommon for HMOs to tailor benefits packages to an individual patient's needs, Mrs. Jones should have been told that, while her health plan would underwrite the cost of the surgery itself, the standard benefits package probably would not provide adequately for her expected postoperative needs. For a caregiver to initiate treatment without assurance that a patient's insurance coverage will allow the patient to complete treatment reveals a narrow view of the caregiver's obligation to the patient.

Trends in health policy and managed care decision making include growing emphases on (1) evidence-based medicine, (2) caregiver accountability for patients' clinical outcomes, and (3) quality. As the patients' physicians, Dr. Davis and the patients' primary care physicians should have considered relevant medical and socioeconomic factors prior to surgery. If they had assumed this responsibility for "quality" planning, to the extent that quality can be defined—the medical/surgical planning and outcomes may have been very different.

The fact that we cannot predict long-term outcomes accurately mitigates the effectiveness of the preoperative review. The process, however, is valuable, since clinical decisions are often made in light of uncertainty. In the case of Mrs. Jones, for whom there will not be enough accurate data, her caregivers could not have predicted exactly how well or poorly her postoperative needs would be met by her covered benefits. Nonetheless, such a review would most likely have predicted Mrs. Jones's difficult postoperative course and poor outcome. For Mrs. Smith, a similarly informed preoperative review would probably have predicted the excellent outcome she actually experienced.

With accountability issues in mind, Dr. Davis's ethical obligations to the patient and contractual obligations to the managed care organization expand beyond performing the operation excellently. His obligations include some responsibility for taking the longer view on both patients and ensuring an optimal final outcome.

The comprehensive quality planning described here can successfully marry patients' needs with caregivers' professional and moral obligations and managed care's growing emphasis on cost-effectiveness, quality care, demonstrable outcomes, and evidence-based medicine. "Quality," when used in this way, can help to incorporate the process of patient care along with service and outcome.

Sara Anderson's Obligations

Absent a preventive ethics or quality planning approach, Ms. Anderson has unfortunately inherited a number of value dilemmas and ethical challenges, practical as well as theoretical. She must decide how she will distribute her time and services among her patients. In addition, she must examine carefully her ethical obligations to her patients and her employer, and attempt to identify the ethical obligations of others, since she may rely on their support later on. Ultimately, she must develop a plan of action. Based on a history of reprimands from facility management, and guidance by the American Physical Therapy Association (1991), she is aware of important constraints. She is expected to provide only care covered by the patient's plan. And she is not to provide care beyond what is "necessary for maximum therapeutic effect." In other words, "No skimping, but no extras, either."

Ms. Anderson must clarify the medical facts. She believes that Mrs. Jones needs more care than either the HMO or the facility will allow. If Mrs. Jones is limited, however, by her medical conditions, it may be that no amount of physical therapy can help her overcome them. Perhaps she needs a nutritionist and/or a cardiologist more than she needs a physical therapist. Perhaps Ms. Anderson should advise against any physical therapy at all if Mrs. Jones is likely to have only limited and painful use of her leg despite ongoing but limited physical therapy. Conversely, Ms. Anderson may believe that Mrs. Smith does not need all the services to which she is entitled. After all, she has a supportive family that is voluntarily providing valuable care.

It is important that Ms. Anderson review the basis of her beliefs. Caregivers' patterns of care are often based on the traditions of their associates or the intensity of care for which insurance companies have historically reimbursed. They are less often founded upon evidence-based studies or outcome measures. Given the trends in managed care clinical decision making, whenever Ms. Anderson believes that her patient will benefit by deviating from established policy, the burden of proof will most assuredly fall on her to demonstrate the likelihood of benefit. Alternatively, she may have to convince the plan that her patient is an "outlier." Though HMOs and purchasers agree that approval for additional services should be conditional upon some evidence that those services will improve patients' outcomes, there has not been universal agreement on what outcomes are important and valuable to patients.

Advocacy

As with all caregivers, Ms. Anderson's primary obligation is to the best interests of her patients. Of course she must balance and advocate for the needs of Mrs. Jones and Mrs. Smith. The clinical scenario suggests that while Mrs. Jones has considerable yet unfulfilled rehabilitation needs, Mrs. Smith is unlikely to benefit from additional services. Mrs. Smith does not need an advocate at this point. Mrs. Jones, however, might benefit from any advocacy Ms. Anderson could offer, since there is reason to think the limitations on her care may be truly harmful. Even if it were useful to Mrs. Smith, it is highly unlikely that Ms. Anderson could justify providing her with additional care if it would hamper Ms. Anderson's care of Mrs. Jones or any other patient.

If Ms. Anderson believes that Ms. Smith is receiving too much care—presumably, more than that from which she can benefit—one might argue that Ms. Anderson has an obligation to advise the facility and/or the HMO to decrease the intensity of Mrs. Smith's coverage to the "right" amount. If Mrs. Smith received less care from Ms. Anderson, perhaps Ms. Anderson would have more time to devote to Mrs. Jones. While it seems extremely unlikely that Ms. Anderson would ever pursue this course of action, this is precisely the kind of action that may be mandated by a population-based approach, where the caregiver is asked to consider the needs of an entire population of patients instead of the individual patient.

Advocating for her patients will most likely require Ms. Anderson to support Mrs. Jones's appeals to the HMO, either verbally or in writing. While most HMOs have well-developed and well-intended appeals processes, it is also unlikely that Mrs. Jones will have the energy and resourcefulness to initiate an appeal. Realistically, Ms. Anderson will probably have to adopt an assertive posture on behalf of Mrs. Jones if she is to have any hope of securing additional services for her.

Ms. Anderson must also acknowledge some risks if she were to meet resistance from the facility, physicians, or HMO. Although advocating for her patients may jeopardize her position, Ms. Anderson may be ethically obligated to do so if the potential harm to patients is sufficiently great and immediate. Prior to accepting her position, Ms. Anderson should have carefully read her contract to be sure she was not accepting contractual obligations that conflicted with her moral, legal, or professional ones. Caregivers are often confronted with divided loyalties, especially as more become employees of larger organizations. Obligations to her employer, the HMOs, the American Physical Therapy Association, and any other party must be secondary for Ms. Anderson. The pressure on caregivers to conform to the expectations of their employers, patients, peers, and parent professional organizations is typically quite subtle. Incentives (financial and otherwise) often exist to overtreat as well as to undertreat. There might be harms in both, though the harms will differ in kind and degree.

If Ms. Anderson treats her two patients differently, it should be because she believes that the different care plans are appropriate to their different conditions. If she believes her two patients deserve the same treatment, the expectations and obligations she faces will be difficult to fulfill.

Physician Obligations

In addition to the obligations outlined, Ms. Anderson should also consider turning to Mrs. Jones's primary care physician or Dr. Davis for support. It is not only appropriate but also obligatory for either one or both of the physicians to embrace the goal of providing the highest quality patient care and achieving the best outcome. Whether any of the physicians (including the facility's medical director) actually acknowledges and accepts an advocacy role for these two patients postoperatively is quite a different story. It can be a time-consuming and frustrating process.

Obligations of the Rehabilitation Facility

Although the rehabilitation facility is unlikely to be in a position to provide a unilateral and favorable response to Ms. Anderson's appeal, its support may increase the chances that she will succeed. In the current environment, in which the facility is unlikely to apprehend any ethical obligations of its own, it is also unlikely to make a serious effort on behalf of a single patient. While many institutions have patient-centered mission statements, translating abstract commitments into concrete initiatives creates special challenges. A health care facility that takes seriously its mission to provide the "highest quality care that is affordable in the marketplace" (or some similar theme) must consider the profound implications this commitment will have for its relationship with insurance plans. This commitment may require facilities to examine the policies of the insurers with which they contract before they accept any of the insurers' patients. If this commitment is taken seriously, facilities may refuse to contract with any HMO or other insurance plan that would interfere with the provision of high-quality care based on the most current clinical guidelines. This is one mechanism, but only one, through which to enforce accountability in health care. Patients and caregivers are seeking reassurance that health care organizations and insurers are committed to patients' best interests and that when these conflict with business interests, the patients' best interests will prevail.

Joint Responsibility

Broad agreement on the definitions of health care terms such as "right," "appropriate," "medically necessary," "futile," and so forth has been elusive. All who provide and receive health care—including patients and purchasers—share responsibility in shaping health care goals. But who are the purchasers? If patients have joined managed care plans through the plan's Medicare products, for example, are the "purchasers" the patients, the government, or the HMOs themselves? Because it is difficult to identify and assign the responsibilities of each of the players, the attempt to do so is often half-hearted—or forgone altogether. Consequently, little effort is made to define the substance or determine the direction of accountability, either.

Given our joint responsibility for addressing the scope and content of health care, it is important not to blame those who have failed to fulfill their responsibilities. Patients often contribute, at least in part, to their ill health. Yet the causal relationship between failed responsibilities and undesirable results is hardly clear or direct. Examining the role responsibilities of the purchaser creates other challenges, not the least of which is clarifying the boundaries between business ethics and medical ethics.

This commentary began by focusing on the importance and content of a preventive ethics and quality planning approach to avoid some ethical dilemmas, an approach that requires all members of the health care team to participate and to focus on the desired ultimate outcome. It also assumes that there are obligations incumbent on the physical therapist, physicians, and the rehabilitation facility. If the HMO is truly committed to the best interests of the patient, then it also has an obligation to ensure that the clinical policies are evidence-based and guided by the patients' medical condition and desired outcomes. Differences in personal and family resources, willingness to pay extra for additional care, more liberal insurance benefits, and so forth offer no moral purchase for different medical treatment.

References

American Physical Therapy Association House of Delegates. 1991. *Code of Ethics and Guide for Professional Responsibility*. Alexandria, Va.: American Physical Therapy Association.

15

Respecting Patients' Cultural and Religious Beliefs

CASE STUDY _____

Request for Exception for Cultural Reasons

Mai Vue is a twenty-one-year-old Hmong woman whose husband brought her to the emergency department of a hospital in a West Coast city. She had a fever and was complaining of stomach pain. The emergency room physician quickly diagnosed acute appendicitis and admitted her to the hospital for surgery.

Despite a long discussion aided by an interpreter regarding the risks of delay and the medical necessity of a prompt operation, her husband explained that the decision would need to involve other family members, including her parents and brothers, who live in Wisconsin and Thailand, and could therefore not be made that evening. The physicians caring for Mrs. Vue determined that her life was not in imminent danger but that it was important that she remain hospitalized. They stressed the urgency of reaching a decision and avoiding a ruptured appendix, which can be very serious, prolong hospitalization and recovery, and may lead to complications such as infertility. Two days later, the patient's husband and brothers authorized the surgery.

The surgery was performed and the hospital billed four inpatient days to Mrs. Vue's HMO, West Coast Care. Although the surgery and two inpatient days were authorized and covered by the West Coast Care policy, as is usual for an appendectomy, the plan denied as medically unnecessary charges for the two days that it took to obtain consent.

The medical director of the benefits committee at West Coast Care has been asked to consider whether to make an exception in this case. Hmong families often take more time to make decisions concerning surgery than is typical for Western patients and families, because a poor decision can have serious adverse consequences for their family relationships as well as for the family's well-being for generations to come. Absent extenuating medical circumstances, however, the plan's policies are supposed to be equitably applied to all members.

Request for Exception for Religious Reasons

John Harris, a Jehovah's Witness, had experienced two severe gastrointestinal bleeds due to deep duodenal ulcers. The bleeds were brought under control with great difficulty because consistent with his religious beliefs, Mr. Harris refused transfusion of blood products.

Mr. Harris received his health care coverage through a preferred provider organization, Preferential Treatment. His primary care physician, as well as all other physicians he accessed through Preferential Treatment's network, is paid on a discounted fee-for-service basis. Preferential Treatment also contracts with several area hospitals for discounted rates for its members.

Mr. Harris's physician informed him that he was at serious risk for another bleed and that the many doctors who had assisted in his care during his two recent health episodes concurred that he could die if he had a similar medical emergency again. The physician recommended that a surgical procedure called a vagotomy and pyloroplasty be performed to heal the ulcers. Mr. Harris consented to the surgery, but only on the condition that under no circumstances would he receive transfusions of blood products.

Mr. Harris's physician sought a surgeon in the Preferential Treatment network to perform the surgery. Although there were a number of well-qualified surgeons, none of them was willing to perform the procedure on the patient's terms. An out-of-network surgeon was finally located in another part of the country, himself a Jehovah's Witness, who agreed to perform the surgery.

Like most preferred provider organizations, Preferential Treatment offered complete coverage for health care services Mr. Harris received in-network and coverage for a percentage of the cost of any health care service he received out-of-network. He was required to pay 20 percent of any medically necessary health care services he received from out-of-network providers. He also had to pay for travel and other expenses for himself and his wife to get to the surgeon whom Preferential Treatment had located for him. For Mr. Harris and his wife these additional expenses were prohibitive. Mr. Harris therefore requested that an exception to his coverage policy be made and that Preferential Treatment pay all costs associated with the procedure, as well as the travel and living expenses.

Preferential Treatment's review of the request noted that the plan had responsibility for 80 percent of the costs of Mr. Harris's out-of-network treatment and no obligation for any other costs he would incur. However, Preferential Treatment indicated that it would be willing to pay Mr. Harris's health care costs up to the amount it would have paid for the surgery if it were performed by a network surgeon at a network hospital.

Even under these circumstances, Mr. Harris could not afford to have the surgery. He initiated an appeal for complete coverage of his surgery and related expenses. While his case was being appealed, Mr. Harris suffered a massive bleed and despite all efforts to save him consistent with his beliefs, he died.

Questions for Consideration

➤ Should the additional time necessary to make a treatment decision by Mrs. Vue's family be considered an "extenuating medical circumstance"?

➤ Who should pay for the two extra days in the hospital that the family required to reach a decision?

➤ If the delay had resulted in a ruptured appendix, or if consent to surgery had been refused and the treatment costs were far more costly over the long run, how should responsibility for the health care costs be assigned?

➤ Was Mr. Harris's preferred approach to surgery medically necessary?

➤ Was Preferred Treatment's compromise with Mr. Harris appropriate? Why?

➤ Does a health plan have extracontractual responsibilities to plan enrollees who have religious beliefs that conflict with dominant Western health care assumptions and practices?

➤ What obligation does the health plan have to find a physician willing to respect the patient/family's request for treatment that deviates from the standard of care?

➤ What obligation does a health plan have to respect a health care professional's personal conscientious objection or professional integrity-based objection to honoring a patient/family's treatment wishes?

➤ When is it permissible for a health plan responsible for the fair distribution of shared resources to give preferential treatment to a class of enrollees? When does the detriment to the plan's population outweigh the advantage to the individual enrollee or class of enrollees?

COMMENTARY _____

James Lindemann Nelson, Ph.D.

Mrs. Vue's case presents a problem to West Coast Care. What is typically seen as a virtually cost-free procedure—obtaining informed consent for a routine intervention—is far from cost-free in her case; it doubles the time she has to stay in the hospital. Who should pick up the bill for the two days West Coast Care considers "extra"?

Of course, obtaining informed consent is never really cost-free. One of the most interesting features about Mrs. Vue's situation is that it highlights questions generally hidden: How much does informed consent cost? How much should managed care plans and their subscribers be willing to pay to obtain valid consents? These questions in turn raise deeper ones: How should we think about the informed consent requirement in the age of managed care? Is informed consent an intrinsic part of the delivery of acceptable quality health services, basic to any defensible standard of care? Or is it rather an alien imposition on health care, a constraint that hails not from medicine's own constitutive values but from foreign ethical theories and cumbersome legal practice, a ritual of little value to consumers? Should the construction of informed consent be differently shaped under the current dispensation than in the heyday of fee-for-service?

John Harris's case—or rather, his legacy—leaves Preferential Treatment with a problem, too. What are a plan's responsibilities when a patient's integrity conflicts with the professional integrity of every provider in its network? If extra costs are generated due to this conflict, whose duty is it to pay the bill?

Mr. Harris's need to go out-of-network for surgery is as much a function of the moral commitments of the surgeons in Preferential Treatment's panel who refused him care as it is of his own commitment to what he takes to be Jehovah's will. As in Mrs. Vue's case, a responsible reaction to Mr. Harris's death will involve thinking through rather broad issues: What latitude should physicians be given to risk the health of their patients as a result of their moral or professional scruples? What kind of scruples *should* physicians have in cases such as Mr. Harris's? What is the role of a health care financing system in supporting or undermining various understandings of medicine's values that may be in place within its system?

And both these cases present a problem. They are presented as instances of culturally or religiously based dissent from what otherwise is a "mainstream," "Western" consensus about the right way to handle appendicitis and duodenal ulcers. How much should managed health care plans be willing to spend to accommodate "diversity"? How much would be too much—an unfair burden on the plan, its providers, and the plan's membership?

Yet focusing on the cultural and religious dimensions of these cases can be misleading in important ways. The threat lies in an all-too-inviting habit of thought: the way that "we" (in the present context, we mainstream Western types) commonly order things, our shared understandings about how the world is arranged and what matters in it, constitute something like the "natural attitude" to have toward reality and how to get around in it. Against this backdrop, "reasonable accommodation of difference" suggests itself as the best analytic framework. If getting a patient to agree to a relatively straightforward treatment typically takes two minutes, allowing two hours in unusual cases might be reasonable, but two days looks pretty outrageous. If patients demand certain forms of medical interventions on religious grounds, our commitment to freedom of religious practice must be tempered; expecting a plan to pick up plane fares and hotel bills when it has already gone beyond the explicit policy limitations seems unreasonable.

Because of their built-in commitment to cost control, the various forms of managed health care make determining the appropriate degree of deference to difference seem a more compelling question than do traditional systems. Properly seen, however, these cases are not so much invitations to refine our grasp of what constitutes reasonable accommodation but a challenge to the assumptions that support the accommodation perspective. Is West Coast Care's problem Mrs. Vue's reluctance to consent without familywide consultation or its misunderstanding of what role informed consent plays in the provision of morally acceptable health care? Is Preferential Treatment's problem Mr. Harris's values or the values of the surgeons on its panel?

What Mrs. Vue Might Help Western Medicine See About Informed Consent

Consider the following thought experiment: Imagine that health law and bioethics had proceeded more slowly and managed care more quickly than actually happened in American medicine. Imagine, then, a world very much like ours, but with a few striking exceptions. For example, a ten-patient-per-hour rate for primary care providers is an industry standard, an efficiency achieved in part because nobody's ever heard of "informed consent." When you visit your physician, nothing much is explained or discussed; they just run you through, tell you what to do, send you on, or send you home. Now imagine further that some brilliant bioethicist in this alternative world discovers seemingly irresistible arguments for implementing an informed consent requirement, arguments quite as good as any we have in our world, resonating equally with common cultural, moral, and legal understandings. The impact is as though the scales had dropped from the eyes of health care providers and ethicists in this alternative world.

However, managed care organizations quickly commission studies of the economic impact of this new proposal, and they find that incorporating an informed consent requirement would add about two minutes to the average primary care office visit. Primary care physician productivity would thus drop from ten patients per hour to about seven. The aggregate expense of instituting an informed consent requirement would add tens of millions of dollars to the health care budget, increasing the cost of insurance and ultimately the number of the uninsured. Positive therapeutic impacts for individual patients are hard to demonstrate.

Under these conditions, should informed consent be excluded as too costly? Should it be offered as an extrapremium service to those whose personal circumstances or moral traditions make it particularly attractive? Or should informed consent be regarded as an instance of genuine progress in the alternative world's understanding of what constitutes good health care, an expression of respect for patients as persons that, once appreciated, is not a moral option?

The choice among these alternatives would, presumably, reflect the character of the brilliant bioethicist's arguments. But they are much like those available to us, drawing heavily on convictions that people are not objects to be manipulated, not even with benevolent motivations, not even when they are patients. Such convictions, when brought to bear on health care, suggest that informed consent ought not to be bartered away for extra efficiencies in the alternative world; the fact that they stumbled onto informed consent's importance only after strong cost-containment mechanisms were in place in their medical system should not be allowed to coarsen their sense of the importance of respecting patients as persons.

Nor should the imposition of strong cost-control measures in our system be allowed to coarsen ours. If informed consent is not as important as bioethicists have commonly alleged, it will take something other than simply discovering that consent costs money to show this. It is interesting to note that, despite the divides between Hmong culture and the West, apparently Mrs. Vue and her family do not think of informed consent as a dispensable amenity. If Mrs. Vue requires extra support in her effort to make a health care decision that meets the purpose of the informed consent requirement—avoiding subjugating patients to a schedule of values they do not endorse—why should that be regarded as different in kind from other forms of extra support she might need if it were her physiology that were at unusual risk from "standard" interventions?

Indeed, the smartest thing to do as a response to Mrs. Vue's case might be to ask whether our informed consent procedures *in general* are doing a good job of achieving their ends. If her situation is not thought of as a problem whose solution is subject to whatever we decide constitutes a "reasonable accommodation" of difference, but as a serious challenge to our standard practices, we might come to see the medical establishment in a decisively new way—not as something mainstream Westerners find cozily familiar but as itself a powerful culture, generally well disposed but decidedly alien to the "laypeople" who enter it as patients or visitors. The health care culture has its own prevalent and distinctive understandings and practices, many of which are undergoing rapid change in the wake of managed care, and it is not only Hmong people who find it disconcerting. If we see medicine in this fashion, informed consent is more clearly visible as a way of trying to create some effective space in the medical world for the values that people live by in their quotidian worlds. It may then occur to us that the support of our own family and friends is something that we could use more of than medicine typically allows us in our forays into its realm. Perhaps the structure of medicine as a whole allows only (contestably) "reasonable accommodations" to "divergent cultures"—the divergent cultures that even people who have lived all their lives in, say, East Lansing, or Knoxville, or Lake Wobegon, bring to it. Managed care's vaunted interest in "evidence-based medicine" is relevant here; what we may need is outcomes research into the effectiveness of techniques of obtaining informed consent, leading to better practice guidelines for this important feature of medical care.

Conversely, if good arguments do come along to show that informed consent is not best seen as something uniformly required as an acknowledgment of people's moral status—and therefore if Mrs. Vue's special needs are seen as chargeable to her own idiosyncracies—then perhaps we ought to do cost-benefit studies of the sort performed in that imagined alternative world. Perhaps we should "unbundle" informed consent, cost it out, and let consumers use the savvy they have gained in their other marketplace transactions to decide whether or not they want to pay the tab for it.

If we assume, though, that further reflection will confirm that sacrificing informed consent to efficiency is not a moral option, Mrs. Vue's case ought not be seen as a problem of how much to accommodate difference. The issue should rather be how she can make what she would accept as a sound and authoritative decision in the most efficient way. It is means, not ends, that should be in question here.

Jehovah's Witnesses Versus Asclepius's Witnesses

But cultural and religious differences will sometimes cut more deeply, as is illustrated in John Harris's case. Let's raise the question bluntly: Who killed Mr. Harris? An equally blunt answer: Mr. Harris did. He was informed of the risks and chose to negotiate to save hotel and travel costs. Perhaps we're only talking a few thousand dollars, but we do not know just what that amount represented to this patient. In any event, he did his best as a canny self-interest maximizer to drive a hard bargain, and he did win some concessions. Unfortunately for him, the negotiations were ultimately unsuccessful.

There are, of course, other ways of answering the question. Perhaps it was the surgeons on Preferential Treatment's list who killed Mr. Harris. Why did they all refuse to operate? Did they consider the intervention without transfusion futile, or at least futile under their hands? Were the odds of success too low for them to be "comfortable"? Did they feel manipulated by a patient whose religious convictions would force them to practice what they considered bad medicine?

Reasons for refusing treatment of this sort might well be collected under the heading "physician integrity," a notion worthy of respect. But it is not a moral trump card. The more specific worries that underlie the appeal to integrity are complex and contestable. "Futility" is a notoriously tricky idea, and "feasibility" is about as obscure. It is at least unclear why or how much "comfort" matters, and one is certainly tempted to ask whether the surgeons would have rejected equally low odds of success if the complicating factor had been biological rather than spiritual. Was Mr. Harris abandoned by his own physicians? Did their scruples justify their washing their hands of his case?

And this brings us to the question of Preferential Treatment's culpability. Apparently, the plan allowed its surgeons to play the "integrity card" as a trump and to do so with complete impunity. The problem was identified as "how do we deal with Mr. Harris's values," not "how do we deal with the clash between Mr. Harris's values and the surgeon's values." We hear of no attempts by Preferential Treatment to persuade any of its surgeons that performing the surgery might be what Martin Benjamin (1990) has called an "integrity preserving compromise," not a sellout of their own values, or of "medicine's values." We hear nothing of returning to any of the plan surgeons after it has been determined that Mr. Harris regards the out-of-network doctor, even with Preferential Treatment's compromise, as prohibitively expensive. Nor do we ever hear that a surgeon's decision to opt out on conscientious grounds places him or her at any kind of risk. It surely might be argued that if Mr. Harris was enrolled in a plan in which those surgeons participated, they already had a responsibility to provide him care. If they could not provide him with care for which he had already paid, did they not have some obligation to make it possible for him to receive the care they were unwilling to provide? Perhaps the extra costs generated by the surgeon's scruples should be picked up by Preferential Treatment but later reflected in the plan's fee negotiations with its providers.

Of course, clinician values are not the only plausible culprits in this case. Mr. Harris may well have had an obligation to himself that he did not take seriously enough. While his financial circumstances might have been very strained, his reluctance to meet the extra costs might have stemmed from the attitude that, as someone with health insurance, he simply had no further responsibility for the costs of his care. Further, perhaps he was blameworthy for his credulity, for not having challenged a deadly dogma. The case as presented does not provide sufficient information to sort out the first issue, and discussing a person's moral responsibility for the content of their religious beliefs would take this commentary rather far afield. But both of these questions are relevant to an issue not often enough examined in discussions of managed care: Do managed care consumers assume moral obligations different from those accompanying traditional indemnity arrangements?

And perhaps the Jehovah's Witness community is implicated in Mr. Harris's death. The Witnesses, after all, helped land him in this fix to start with. It is the Witness community that makes adherence to their distinctive views about blood transfusions so important a feature of spiritual well-being. If there are forms of medical intervention that reduce the risk of foregoing transfusions, shouldn't the Witnesses help their members obtain such help if they are unable to do so on their own?

The difficult questions about the moral responsibilities of Mr. Harris or his religious community should not, however, be allowed to distract attention from the moral liability of this preferred provider organization and its panel of surgeons. For even if both Mr. Harris as an individual and the Witnesses as a body were to blame for his death, it does not follow that all other agents are thereby exculpated. The surgeons may be blameworthy for misunderstanding their own values; Preferential Treatment, for its apparent assumption that Mr. Harris's convictions alone generated this problem and that its providers' convictions are "natural" and "right," needing no scrutiny.

There is, of course, a good deal more that could be said about both these cases, some of which does squarely involve the particular cultural and religious differences they present. There are, for example, particular historical circumstances that have led to the recent presence in the United States of Hmong people. Do these circumstances give rise to any special duty on the part of this country to respond to their needs, and if so, on whom is this duty properly enjoined? And it is hard not to wonder why the need for vagotomy and pyloroplasty was discussed with Mr. Harris only after his second severe bleed. Did it really just not strike anyone that a bleeding problem raises special difficulties for a Jehovah's Witness? But there are other general morals to be derived from these cases as well. Here is one: West Coast Care, Preferential Treatment, and their kin need not only to manage problems like these but to learn from them as well. What is informed consent, why is it important, and how can it be efficiently and effectively obtained from patients with many different presenting circumstances? What is the value and what are the limits of providers' conscientious refusals to provide treatment, and with what kinds of educational or fiscal responses should such refusals be met? And how can the best answers to these questions be incorporated into the structures of daily life in the many varieties of managed health care?

As Martha Minow (1990) has taken pains to remind us, even attempts to attend carefully and respectfully to difference can be perilous, particularly if we allow ourselves to think of those differences as "possessed" by The Other, in distinction to the inevitable naturalness of our own norms. Difference, rather, is an inherently relational idea; differences emerge out of human interchanges. Managed care's encounter with the Hmong or with the Jehovah's Witnesses is not a challenge to its largesse. It is, rather, an opportunity to reflect on the character of the cultural assumptions of mainstream Western medicine, and to acknowledge that to which it witnesses.

References

Benjamin, M. 1990. *Splitting the Difference*. Lawrence, Kans.: University of Kansas Press.
Minow, M. 1990. *Making All the Difference*. Ithaca, N.Y.: Cornell University Press.

COMMENTARY

Kathleen A. Culhane-Pera, M.D., M.A.

Due to traditional kinship medical decision-making patterns, a Hmong woman's appendectomy is delayed for two days. Due to religious beliefs about blood products, a Jehovah's Witness man's gastrointestinal hemorrhage is impossible to control and he dies. Due to belief in the primal healing powers of prayer, a Christian Scientist's treatment for pertussis is delayed. Due to historical distrust in the medical system, an African American man's uncontrolled hypertension causes a cerebral hemorrhage. Due to fears about insulin therapy, a Mexican American woman's uncontrolled diabetes mellitus leads to end-stage renal failure. Due to tobacco addiction and a belief that "you've got to die of something someday," a European American man continues to smoke cigarettes, which contributes to atherosclerosis, with multiple admissions for angina, myocardial infarctions, angiograms, and a coronary artery bypass graft operation.

Cultural beliefs, values, and practices influence health, disease, and treatment of all patients. Sometimes patients' beliefs conflict with biomedicine's standards of care and managed care's cost-containment goals. Four questions arise from the conflicts between Mai Vue and John Harris and their managed care plans:

1. Should Mrs. Vue's and Mr. Harris's health plans make exceptions and pay for services not usually required, on account of "extenuating medical circumstances"?

2. What effects do Mrs. Vue's and Mr. Harris's cultural and religious perspectives have on the costs to their managed care plans?

3. Does it constitute unfair preferential treatment for Mrs. Vue's and Mr. Harris's health plans to cover their health care bills?

4. How should managed care plans and individual providers respond to patients' cultural and religious beliefs so that they optimize health and minimize disability?

Payment

Should Mrs. Vue's and Mr. Harris's health plans make exceptions and pay for services not usually required on account of "extenuating medical circumstances"?

The health plans should pay for both patients' costs, but not because these uncustomary costs are due to extenuating medical circumstances. Managed care organizations are in the business of providing efficient and effective health care services as well as fiscally sound services. Paying the costs of addressing patients' needs related to treating their diseases and improving their health is within the realm of a managed care organization's fiscal responsibilities.

Managed care organizations should not consider the additional, uncustomary costs due to Mrs. Vue's or Mr. Harris's cultural and religious beliefs as extenuating medical circumstances because neither the Hmong family's decision-making practice nor Mr. Harris's spiritual needs constitute extenuating *medical* circumstances. Rather, managed care organizations need to track the real causes of extended length of stays (The Oak Group 1997), extraneous costs, and poor medical care outcomes. Once the factors that contribute to increased costs and poor health outcomes are accurately identified, managed care organizations can develop systems that contain costs as well as improve health care delivery and improve health outcomes.

What effects do Mrs. Vue's and Mr. Harris's cultural and religious perspectives have on the costs to their managed care plans?

These two clinical encounters do not provide enough data to evaluate the influence of cultural beliefs on health care costs, for Mrs. Vue, for Mr. Harris, or for the American population in general. Any additional cost due to cultural and religious beliefs in these two cases (two additional hospital days and travel expenses) is small and inconsequential. Compared to the substantial costs of the effects of tobacco, alcohol, illegal drugs, domestic and community violence, high-fat and high-calorie diets, and lack of exercise, which managed care organizations deal with everyday, the costs are minuscule. And calculated in terms of the financial benefits of patient satisfaction, it may be cost-saving. It may be that *not* dealing with health beliefs increases cost, and that dealing with health beliefs decreases the overall costs of health care.

What could be the financial impact of not dealing with Mrs. Vue's and Mr. Harris's health beliefs? Let us suppose that instead of taking appropriate cultural steps to make a family decision, Mrs. Vue agrees to the operation without her family's consent and a life-threatening complication occurs. Having made the decision alone, she must bear the responsibility of her actions and may be ostracized for her independence. Outcast, she becomes depressed and suicidal, which results in extensive and expensive mental health treatment. Or perhaps after a complication, members of the Hmong community blame the hospital for forcing Mrs. Vue to undergo the operation, for performing an unauthorized tubal ligation (as has happened in Thailand and as the Hmong community believes has happened in the United States), or for acting in the doctors' and the hospital's own financial and educational interests. The resulting loss of trust in the hospital results in increased medical costs as Hmong people postpone medical care and attempt to avoid early medical treatments.

Similarly, if Mr. Harris receives a blood transfusion, he could lose the support of his community, resulting in depression with a significant mental health bill. Or the Jehovah's Witness community could become angry and express their disapproval of the hospital system by taking its business elsewhere. When cultural beliefs and needs are not respected, the damage to patient-physician trust and to community-hospital relations, while difficult to measure, is real (Culhane-Pera 1989). When patients' cultural beliefs and concerns are ignored, moreover, their satisfaction with medical care is reduced. This can result in increased doctor shopping, noncompliance with medications, and tests to investigate potentially missed diagnoses (Kleinman, Eisenberg, and Good 1978).

Paying attention to cultural and religious beliefs can decrease costs over the long run as well as improve health outcomes. In Mrs. Vue's case, perhaps the Hmong interpreter was not trained, or perhaps the physicians were not skilled at working with interpreters. Misunderstandings may have occurred, and the family may have needed to deal with suspicions and concerns before agreeing to the operation. While hiring trained interpreters and teaching providers to work with interpreters require a substantial financial outlay, the rewards of the investment in decreased hospital time and fewer office visits, unnecessary laboratory and radiological tests, misdiagnoses, mistreatments, and potential fatal outcomes with expensive lawsuits are well worth the costs.

What could be the financial benefit of dealing with cultural beliefs? Understanding patients' knowledge, attitudes, beliefs, and practices about health, disease, and optimal therapies, and then targeting preventive therapies and healthy lifestyle changes to patients' beliefs, could result in a significant decrease in medical costs. Responding to consumer demands has already resulted in improved health care delivery and in changed standards of biomedical care, some of which have decreased costs as well as improved health. For example, Jehovah's Witness demands for bloodless operations spurred technological advances that have decreased the dangers of blood products to all patients. Patients' desires to be home rather than in hospitals have resulted in home-based intravenous therapies. Women's desires for vaginal deliveries after cesarean sections with earlier pregnancies resulted in acceptable "trials of labor" and vaginal births after C-sections. Women's demands for alternatives to radical mastectomies immediately after frozen sections resulted in alternative diagnostic and therapeutic approaches for breast cancers.

There are no good actuarial tables demonstrating that attention to patients' cultural or religious beliefs increases costs significantly, but there are good arguments to suggest that dealing with cultural issues can decrease costs. To imply, as these two cases do, that people who are "in step" with the Western biomedical perspective (that is, people from mainstream ethnic and religious backgrounds) have lower health care costs, and those who are "out of step" with Western biomedical ideas (people from nonmainstream ethnic and religious backgrounds) have higher costs is empirically unfounded, ethnocentric, and probably racist. Justice requires that we treat people equitably.

Justice

Does it constitute unfair preferential treatment for Mrs. Vue's and Mr. Harris's health plans to cover their health care bills?

The short answer is no. As they exist now, medical care institutions—hospitals, clinics, insurance companies, managed care plans, universities—preferentially treat certain groups of patients, diagnoses, and therapies over others. The health care system gives preference to English-speaking people with high literacy skills from middle and high socioeconomic classes; focuses on acute, curable patho-physiological disease processes; and values invasive procedures and high-technology approaches performed by specialists. It is not self-evident that addressing the health care needs of people with different cultural and religious beliefs from those of mainstream American society, and/or non-English-speaking, nonliterate, socioeconomically disadvantaged people, should be considered unfairly "preferential." Should plans refuse, for example, to cover the two "extended days" that result from the mainstream value of leisure weekends, the observance of which means that some tests, procedures, and consultants are not available to hospitalized patients on Saturdays and Sundays? Should plans refuse to pay for appendectomies performed on normal appendices, when waiting might have differentiated true surgical candidates? Should plans refuse to pay for complications from blood transfusions when surgeons could have used bloodless techniques? Managed care systems are facing diverse professional, folk, and lay beliefs, values, and practices that sometimes increase the cost of medical care; the challenge will be deciding which beliefs, values, and practices we (plans, health care providers, government, and society) are willing to change and which we are not, irrespective of cost.

Is the health plan obligated to find physicians willing to respect Mrs. Vue's and Mr. Harris's requests for treatments that deviate from the standard of care? Yes.

Both of these patients have a right to receive care from physicians who respect their beliefs and values. Mrs. Vue's physicians agreed to deviate from the standard of care of an immediate appendectomy and provided her with services, while Mr. Harris was unable to obtain the potentially lifesaving operation in a timely manner because his plan's surgeons were not willing or not able to perform an operation using bloodless surgical approaches. While the financial compromise offered by the managed care plan was not unreasonable, it was unreasonable that the plan had not ensured that surgeons within their network both knew how and were willing to perform bloodless procedures.

When the insurance company refused to pay Mrs. Vue's full hospital bill, she and her family—if they understood their rights to an appeal—could have asked for a review through the plan's appeal process. Once they explained how seriously their culture values making a family-based decision, the family may well have won an appeal, especially in view of the biomedical values of autonomy and informed consent and their relevance in this case. In future situations, physicians will probably consider administering intravenous antibiotics at home under the supervision of a public health nurse, an expense the insurance company would likely pay. In the case of Mr. Harris—despite the fact that he won his appeal—it is surprising and ultimately tragic that the two parties could not agree on a final solution.

To what extent might bias against cultural and religious beliefs be a factor in clinicians' and managed care organizations' refusals to perform care and provide coverage? Patients with different world views who refuse biomedical recommendations or request deviations from biomedical standards of care often challenge providers. If such challenges violate providers' value systems, they may refuse to provide care, but providers should not do so lightly or based on prejudices. In challenging situations, clinicians are likely to explore their beliefs about disease and treatment, their legal liability, and their standing in their professional community as they decide how to proceed. As part of their self-examination, providers also should explore to what extent their egos are threatened; their own cultural biases regarding health, disease, and optimal treatment are challenged; and their stereotypes about people are negatively influencing their clinical judgments. Respect for diverse cultural and religious perspectives is necessary for providers as they develop trusting therapeutic relationships with a wide range of patients. Without elemental respect toward patients as human beings with varied belief systems, the trust between doctor and patient is eroded. Without respect and without trust, there is no basis for a therapeutic relationship, which is the key to healing (Brody 1987). Managed care organizations must support the diversity of human experience of health and disease by providing medical care to all members without bias (Emmanuel and Dubler 1995).

Justice requires that we not refuse coverage to patients because of their cultural and religious beliefs, even those that increase the cost of care.

Recommendations

How should managed care plans and individual providers respond to patients' cultural and religious beliefs so that they optimize health and minimize disability?

Managed care organizations should evaluate how cultural, social, and spiritual beliefs, values, and practices influence how people maintain health and manage disease and then use this information in their design of effective delivery systems.

In Mrs. Vue's situation, perhaps the physicians, health care workers, or hospital system contributed to the two-day delay by not being proficient in culturally sensitive or culturally competent health care delivery. Communicating clearly and respectfully with Hmong families, inquiring about concerns and traditional therapies, and being willing to negotiate alternatives can build trust between the health care providers and the Hmong community, which may decrease delays, decrease costs, and improve patient satisfaction. Managed care organizations can increase their capacity to provide culturally competent health care by hiring trained interpreters, employing bilingual and bicultural staff, teaching providers to work effectively with interpreters, requiring providers to become proficient in patient-centered communication techniques, and promoting negotiated approaches between patient desires and biomedical standards of care (Berlin and Fowkes 1983).

Some surgeons within all networks should be familiar with bloodless surgical techniques and should be willing to use them for patients who wish to avoid the adverse effects of blood products. Health plans need to support a diverse provider population that can form therapeutic relationships and meet the diverse care needs of the plan's population. As managed care organizations continue to ask to control expenditures, plans, providers, and patients must work together to create cost-effective approaches that respect human values and improve medical care outcomes.

Managing cost is not the only aim of managed care. In competitive health care environments, plan administrators understand that satisfied customers and improved health care outcomes are important corporate values as well. Addressing cultural issues is a key to the future provision of cost-effective medical care. In the end, addressing cultural needs is the right thing to do, both ethically and financially.

References

Berlin, E. A., and Fowkes, W. C. 1983. "A Teaching Framework for Cross Cultural Health Care." *Western Journal of Medicine* 139, no. 6:934–38.

Brody, H. 1987. *Stories of Sickness*. New Haven: Yale University Press.

Culhane-Pera, K. A. 1989. *Analysis of Cultural Beliefs and Power Dynamics in Disagreements about Health Care of Hmong Children.* Master's thesis, University of Minnesota.

Emmanuel, E. J, and Dubler, N. N. 1995. "Preserving the Physician-Patient Relationship in the Era of Managed Care." *Journal of the American Medical Association* 273, no. 4:323–29.

Kleinman, A.; Eisenberg, L.; and Good, B. 1978. "Culture, Illness, and Care: Clinical Lessons from Anthropological and Cross-cultural Research." *Annals of Internal Medicine* 88, no. 2:251–58.

The Oak Group. 1997. *Managed Care Appropriateness Protocol (MCAP).* United States of America: Utilization Management Associates.

PART FIVE

Managed Care for Vulnerable Populations

16

Managing Care for the Seriously Mentally Ill

CASE STUDY

Mr. Smith, a twenty-five-year-old patient with schizophrenia, recently suffered an acute episode that led to a brief hospitalization, his second. Mr. Smith is soon to be discharged back to his home. Even though he lived at home successfully for several years following his first hospitalization and diagnosis four years ago, his parents, who have always been strongly committed to providing their son with the security of family and home, now feel unable to cope with the demands his return to their home will make on them.

The county in which Mr. Smith lives addresses the needs of clients like him through an array of services and activities provided by a team that includes a psychiatrist, case manager, nurses, persons trained in occupational skill development, social activity coordinators, and volunteers. After a difficult adjustment period, Mr. Smith's case had been managed very smoothly before his second hospitalization through weekly nursing visits and other interventions to support and monitor his progress. Like many patients whose disease is managed with the help of psychotropic medications, Mr. Smith did not think he was sick; he did not think he needed to continue taking his medication and he had difficulty remembering to take it. Weekly nurse visits and frequent meetings with his psychiatrist were therefore essential. His psychiatrist was available to him at the same location as the other support services the county provided, including weekly drop-in opportunities for planned activities and coffees. As Mr. Smith adjusted to this support system, the frequency of nursing visits was reduced, but his condition and needs continued to be monitored, and his psychiatrist coordinated his medical care on an ongoing basis.

Many of Mr. Smith's needs were nonmedical social services, without which his medical needs would likely have resurfaced. For example, when he was discharged from the hospital, the county provided case management services in the form of one nursing visit per week, in his home or elsewhere, if he preferred. With support from Mr. Smith's parents, the case manager pursued the issues central to his stabilization and reintegration into the community. Mr. Smith needed to apply for disability benefits, an overwhelming task for him on his own. The case manager arranged for others to work with him on skill development and on finding a suitable volunteer job. His parents attended a monthly support group for families and had a help line available to them. Community support workers provided a range of nonbillable services that neither insurance nor Medicaid would cover.

Four months ago, the service and coverage arrangements for medical, social, and rehabilitative services were changed. The state where Mr. Smith lived entered into a prepaid public assistance managed care contract with the for-profit Whole-Body Health Plan. WholeBody Health Plan subcontracts with a for-profit behavioral health managed care company, BrainCare. Since Mr. Smith was receiving Medicaid due to his disability, management of his mental health services shifted from his county's Assertive Community Team to BrainCare.

When BrainCare assumed the management of Mr. Smith's care, the state had no overall plan for the delivery of complex mental health care services. The state's contract with WholeBody Health Plan included behavioral health care coverage, which it subcontracted to BrainCare. But the state had no explicit contract with BrainCare. BrainCare's responsibility to cover the range of services needed so that Mr. Smith could continue to access medically necessary mental health services was not addressed. Nor was there a clear delineation of responsibility between Brain-Care and the county.

Because BrainCare had no provider in Mr. Smith's town, his care shifted to a provider in a clinic twenty miles away. He did not drive a car, and public transportation did not conveniently serve his area, so his link to a provider was imperiled from the start, as was the ability of his team of providers to collaborate effectively.

Three months after his transfer to BrainCare, Mr. Smith's condition began deteriorating. He had forgotten to take his medication on several occasions. He did not understand that he needed to see his new psychiatrist for authorization of any ancillary services, nor had he been informed of the ancillary services he could access. With Mr. Smith's behavior becoming increasingly uncontrolled and threatening, and their accustomed support system unraveling, his parents arranged for him to see his new psychiatrist for the first time.

Mr. Smith's new psychiatrist noted that the medication he had been taking was not included in BrainCare's formulary. Resentful of BrainCare's cumbersome process for physician requests for exceptions to the formulary, not to mention the uncompensated time this required of him, the psychiatrist explained that Mr. Smith would either have to pay for the more expensive drug himself or be switched to the drug BrainCare's formulary did include. In no position to pay or object, Mr. Smith went home with a new prescription and an authorization for four days of home visits by a nurse over a four-week period to monitor his compliance with his new medication regimen. The nursing visits helped him get back on track with his new medication, but the drug made him nauseous and unable to sleep at night. The nurse conveyed this information to the psychiatrist, who adjusted the dosage but was unwilling to change the drug order.

The nursing visits stopped after the four-week period, and Mr. Smith stopped taking the medication. He was unable to take the initiative to request authorization for more nursing visits. He wanted to see his psychiatrist because he remembered feeling better when he had been taking the other medication; but he could not manage the process of seeing the psychiatrist or communicating his wish to go back on the old medication.

Mr. Smith became withdrawn. When his parents tried to intervene, he became physically threatening to them. Unable to cope with their son's behavior, his parents contacted his psychiatrist again. The psychiatrist labeled Mr. Smith "non-compliant," and a case manager at BrainCare warned them that this could alter the terms of his coverage. Concerned that Mr. Smith had become a danger to his parents and possibly to himself, however, the case manager authorized an inpatient evaluation. BrainCare's criterion for authorizing inpatient care, dangerousness to self or others, is also the standard for commitment to the state hospital. Thus, on the same grounds that BrainCare has allowed hospitalization for Mr. Smith, it may, if it sees fit, pursue commitment proceedings for Mr. Smith and thus shift the costs of his care from the health plan to another part of the state system.

Questions for Consideration

➤ What are the respective obligations of the state, the health plan, and the mental health managed care organization in transitioning patients like Mr. Smith to a managed care arrangement?

➤ Should the notion of medical necessity be expanded, or should the range of services managed care organizations are obligated to cover be explicitly expanded to include social and rehabilitation services? Why?

➤ Should managed care's approaches to cost containment be reserved for populations that are predominantly healthy rather than chronically ill? Why or why not?

➤ What approach to monitoring managed care ensures that the needs of the most vulnerable groups in society are being fairly and adequately met?

COMMENTARY

James E. Sabin, M.D.

If a local newspaper wrote an exposé about Mr. Smith's clinical decompensation under BrainCare, the headline would almost certainly say something like: "Twenty-five-year-old deteriorates rapidly after state introduces for-profit managed care." Such a headline would be deeply misleading. Mr. Smith's story gives us pointers about how to manage care well and poorly, but it says nothing about managed care as such. Understood properly, all of Mr. Smith's care has been "managed."

All health care systems are struggling to come to grips with the unsolved problem of meeting patient needs fairly under reasonable resource constraints. Any enterprise that operates within resource constraints (a budget) must be managed. The United Kingdom manages care through a National Health Service. Canada manages care through a provincially administered "single payer" insurance program. Only the United States has chosen competitive market forces as its framework for managing care. Although all three countries must manage care, only the United States uses competing "managed care" insurance programs to do the job, and only the United States conducts its national policy without articulating a clear vision of values and objectives that might educate the public about the fundamental task (Sabin 1995).

The county program under which Mr. Smith received highly efficient and effective treatment for schizophrenia during the past four years represents managed care at its best. Like all community mental health programs, it provided treatment to members of a defined population (the county's) under a budget (funded by local taxpayers). Mr. Smith's excellent regimen included careful discharge planning after his first hospital admission, assertive community treatment tailored to fit the kinds of limitations associated with schizophrenia, attentive medication management, and family support and education. All of the components of comprehensive care appear to have been provided, and nothing that was included sounds wasteful or excessive.

Since the colonial era, the state has taken responsibility for providing mental health care to citizens with severe mental illness. Until the community mental health movement in the 1960s, public sector care consisted largely of the state hospital system. Under this system, Mr. Smith's state and county paid for and provided the excellent care that he received.

The key ethical failure in Mr. Smith's situation under BrainCare is a grossly flawed contracting process. Like many other states, Mr. Smith's state has chosen to purchase private delivery of the Medicaid insurance services that it had formerly provided directly. Typically, public purchasers hope to achieve a combination of improved services and decreased costs by "buying" rather than "making" the service in question (Stroup and Dorwart 1997). The contract is the vehicle through which purchasers and providers make the terms of their agreement explicit. The case lets us infer that the state, WholeBody Health Plan, and BrainCare entered into a contract that failed to spell out purchasing specifications, performance standards, and the relative responsibilities of the three parties.

Although a court would almost certainly not hold WholeBody Health Plan or BrainCare responsible for providing services that the state did not specify in the contract, all three parties should be held ethically accountable for Mr. Smith's clinical deterioration. The state clearly failed to exercise due diligence as a purchaser. This is especially egregious, given the fact that prior to contracting with the private vendor, the state was delivering high-quality services, so it clearly understood and appreciated high-quality care.

However, even though the state did not specify its contractual expectations with any clarity, since WholeBody Health Plan and BrainCare are providing a public good (health insurance), they have an ethical obligation to inform the state if the services they intend to provide under the contract deviate substantially from the current standard or from widely accepted standards of good care. Although *caveat emptor* (buyer beware) may reflect the legal standard for the contracting process, it is not the correct standard for the present situation for two reasons. First, since the time of Hippocrates health care ethics has required *fidelity* to the interests of the patient as the primary value. Although WholeBody Health Plan and BrainCare are contracting with the state, their insurance services will determine what kinds of services patients receive, and their conduct must be guided by the ethics of clinical practice as well as the ethics of contracting. Caretakers—a category that includes purchasers, insurers, and clinical program managers as well as clinicians—have a covenantal relationship with patients that requires more than honest conduct within the limits of the law (Berwick, Hiatt, and Janeway 1997). Second, patients like Mr. Smith, for whom the state is purchasing insurance services, often have no choice among insurers and cannot therefore exert the fundamental market power of taking their business elsewhere. Even if *caveat emptor* were an acceptable standard for health care services, it could not legitimately be applied to service recipients who have no realistic choice of service provider (Daniels and Sabin 1997).

The fact that WholeBody Health Plan and BrainCare are both for-profit organizations introduces the passionately debated issue of the ethics of for-profit versus nonprofit health care. Zealots on both sides of the debate have—alas—distracted the public from the real issues. Believers in the market attack government ineptitude and assert that the discipline of the market and for-profit organizational structure produce superior outcomes. Their opponents attack corporate greed and assert that for-profit health systems produce inferior outcomes. The real issue, however, is performance, not corporate structure. Mr. Smith, and presumably other patients like him, are receiving substandard treatment under the new arrangements. That, and not the hypothetical explanation for why poor care is being provided, is the ethically relevant fact (Sabin 1996). Good care is preferable to bad care irrespective of the corporate structure within which the care is provided. Evidence does not yet allow generalizations about the relative merits of for-profit and nonprofit systems (Clark, Dorwart, and Epstein 1994).

Mr. Smith's case invites reflection about how many resources a managed care organization should devote to patients with serious and persisting mental illness. From Mr. Smith's perspective, the question concerns the kinds of services he is entitled to expect from his care system. Since most insurance programs in the United States are contractually required to cover "medically necessary" treatment, the question of what Mr. Smith can reasonably expect is ultimately a matter of how "medical necessity" is defined.

According to the "normal function" model for determining "medical necessity" in mental health practice, the central purpose of health care is to maintain, restore, or compensate for the restricted opportunity and loss of function caused by disease or disability (Sabin and Daniels 1994). Under this model, Mr. Smith can reasonably expect his state, through WholeBody Health Plan and BrainCare, to provide services aimed at restoring the range of capabilities he would have had without the intrusion of schizophrenia or, insofar as restoration is not currently possible, preventing further deterioration. In terms of the current state of the art, this means the kinds of services he previously received from the county program.

It is much easier to define "medical necessity" for acute conditions that impinge on relatively healthy baseline functioning than for conditions like schizophrenia that may have profound chronic impacts on cognition, emotion, and behavior as well as cause acute episodes of illness. For example, with previously healthy patients suffering from severe depression, treatment that restores them to their prior level of function is both medically necessary and sufficient. For patients like Mr. Smith, treatment of the acute symptoms of schizophrenia is medically necessary but not sufficient. While we do not wish to treat Mr. Smith as a helpless child unable to take any responsibility for himself, his difficulty applying for disability benefits or planning for remediation of basic skill deficits, and his belief that no illness was present and no medication was required, are almost certainly products of the brain dysfunction associated with schizophrenia. As such they are legitimately the target of insurance-supported intervention.

If a person colloquially described as "of sound mind" makes an informed decision not to take medication or participate in other forms of treatment, the responsibility of the health care system is to ensure that the person has adequate knowledge of the consequences and to remain available if the person changes his or her mind. However, when these "decisions" occur in the context of brain function that has been altered by schizophrenia, as in Mr. Smith's case, clinically and ethically sound care requires assertive outreach, not passive waiting for the patient to present himself for care. This is the rationale for covering these services under health insurance.

The case tells us that under the county program, a nurse would come to Mr. Smith's home if he preferred to meet there, a case manager would help him with the bureaucratic demands of applying for disability, and others would work with him on augmenting his skills. Suppose someone with the ordinary range of neurotic quirks, but luckily without a serious illness like schizophrenia, were to request similar services from his or her own health care system, arguing that if Mr. Smith can have these desirable services, so should they have access to them.

A proper answer to this request would rest on a distinction between treatment of an illness as opposed to enhancement of well-being or, put differently, on the distinction between "needs" and "wants." While well-being might be enhanced by services like those Mr. Smith received, health insurance is designed to address the impacts of illness. Mr. Smith does not simply find bureaucracy tiresome—as a result of his illness, he is not able (at least at present) to meet the bureaucratic requirements. The assistance of the case manager is not a luxury—it compensates for an illness-imposed deficit. Having his clinician come to his home is not merely the kind of convenience we might all appreciate but a necessity, if treatment is going to occur and if he is to stay in the community as opposed to the hospital. And receiving some level of skill training is not to make up for previous laziness about school or to give him a competitive advantage in the marketplace, but rather it is directed to the unfortunate fact that schizophrenia may interfere significantly with skill development and retention. For Mr. Smith, skill training is more like speech therapy for someone who has had a stroke or gait training for someone who has had a knee replacement than like computer training for someone who wants a better job. However desirable and beneficial the computer training may be, the health system is not responsible for helping us improve our employment opportunities unless our employment problems are the direct result of a disorder. The request for services like those provided to Mr. Smith should be denied.

When tax revenues pay for health insurance and provision of the supportive services important for rehabilitation and recovery from the impacts of an illness like schizophrenia, deciding how these services will be financed, organized, and delivered is primarily a matter of logistical convenience. Whether the health budget includes housing and vocational training funds or whether these are paid for by other budgets is a question of practicality, not ethics. Since services for people with schizophrenia require special configuration to allow for cognitive, behavioral, and emotional symptoms, states may choose to locate these in the health sector.

The fact that supported housing or skill training are not conventional "health" interventions is not, however, a reason for the state not to include these services under health insurance. They are well documented as important components of comprehensive treatment for schizophrenia. The ultimate aim of health insurance is to remove or prevent the loss of capability produced by illness and injury. For acute illnesses like infections, appendicitis, and injuries, the key interventions are typically delivered by health professionals. For chronic illnesses like schizophrenia, many of the most effective interventions may be delivered in community settings in which health professionals play a much smaller role. To neglect these services because they are not "health care," and to preferentially use available funds for services (like psychotherapy) delivered by professionals without considering patient preferences and relative contribution to clinical outcomes, can be criticized as a form of elitism or profession-centrism.

The fact that assertive outreach and a range of rehabilitative services should be *eligible* for coverage under Mr. Smith's health insurance does not dictate that they *must* be covered. As ample as our health care resources are, they are limited, and it is ethically appropriate for a purchaser of health insurance to set priorities within its overall budget. However, although it has been common insurance practice to constrain mental health services in ways that are not applied to other health services, there is no ethical justification for such a policy, which must be regarded as discriminatory. As the National Alliance for the Mentally Ill and other advocates have argued so powerfully, psychiatric disorders are health conditions and cannot ethically be excluded from consideration for coverage on the same footing as other health services.

The point is not that the mental health services must be included, but that they must be allowed to compete for coverage on a level playing field with other kinds of disorders. Interestingly, in Oregon, which has conducted the major experiment in public priority setting, mental health services were allowed to compete with other health services in just this way. Mental health ranked very well on the priority listing, with schizophrenia ranking just behind asthma and respiratory failure, well above the cutoff point set by the legislature's allocation (Sabin and Daniels 1997).

If Mr. Smith's state had intended to stop paying for the kinds of services it had previously been providing, it would have been obligated to publicize the scaled-back plan and subject it to the usual form of public debate and legislative oversight. If the state was not intending to scale back its services, its contract with WholeBody Health Care (which subsequently "carved out" mental health services through its contract with BrainCare) should have specified its expectation that these services would be provided.

Historically, private insurance has discriminated against mental health conditions, often altogether excluding them from coverage. Even insurance that included equal coverage for mental health care has relied on the public sector to provide the kinds of outreach services Mr. Smith received from his county program. As a result, many private insurers and managed care organizations do not have experience providing the kind of care the best public programs have provided to patients like Mr. Smith.

There is no intrinsic reason why managed care organizations could not provide the same kinds of services, but a responsible public purchaser would need to assess the organization's competence at providing these services, clearly specify its expectations in the contract, and monitor performance to ensure that its purchasing expectations were met. While some managed care programs appear to be delivering high-quality services of the kind patients like Mr. Smith need (Sabin 1998), a recent review of managed care programs that serve Medicaid recipients gives the "industry" a failing grade and provides a warning signal about quality of care (National Alliance for the Mentally Ill 1997).

Understood properly, managed care is not a distinctive philosophy of care but an approach to aligning means with ends. To a large extent, employers have asked managed care to control the escalating cost of mental health insurance. Managed care has achieved substantial success in meeting this requirement. If public purchasers like Mr. Smith's state ask managed care organizations to reduce costs without adequately spelling out what kinds of services they want patients like Mr. Smith to receive, and if organizations like WholeBody Health Plan and BrainCare fail to warn naive purchasers about the clinical implications of the purchasing plans they are proposing, Mr. Smith's unfortunate and avoidable story will occur again and again.

A poor country can justify not providing services of the sort Mr. Smith received from his county program if it chooses to invest in immunization, clean water, and malaria control instead. A country as wealthy as the United States, however, cannot justify providing services of the kind his state is providing through WholeBody Health Plan and BrainCare. Although the United States is in an early phase of a steep learning curve regarding the effort to deliver publicly funded mental health services to vulnerable patients like Mr. Smith through contracts with private managed care organizations, a substantial body of knowledge on how to conduct the process well is beginning to emerge (Bazelon Center for Mental Health Law 1997; Rosenbaum, Silver, and Wehr 1997). Managed care has proven that good-quality mental health services can be provided within an acceptable budget. No one in the United States needs to or should receive the kind of mismanaged care delivered to Mr. Smith.

References

Bazelon Center for Mental Health Law. 1997. *Protecting Consumer Rights in Public Systems: Managed Mental Health Care Policy.* Washington, D.C.: Bazelon Center for Mental Health Law.

Berwick, D.; Hiatt, H.; and Janeway, P. 1997. "An Ethical Code for Everybody in Health Care: A Code That Covered All Rather Than Single Groups Might Be Useful." *British Medical Journal* 315, no. 7123:1633–34.

Clark, R. E.; Dorwart, R. A.; and Epstein, S. S. 1994. "Managing Competition in Public and Private Mental Health Agencies: Implications for Services and Policies." *The Milbank Quarterly* 72, no. 4:653–78.

Daniels, N., and Sabin, J. E. 1997. "Limits to Health Care: Fair Procedures, Democratic Deliberation, and the Legitimacy Problem for Insurers." *Philosophy and Public Affairs* 26, no. 4:303–50.

National Alliance for the Mentally Ill. 1997. *Stand and Deliver: Action Call to a Failing Industry.* Arlington, Va.: National Alliance for the Mentally Ill.

Rosenbaum, S.; Silver, K.; and Wehr, E. 1997. *An Evaluation of Contracts Between State Medicaid Agencies and Managed Care Organizations for the Prevention and Treatment of Mental Illness and Substance Abuse.* Washington, D.C.: Center for Health Policy Research, George Washington University.

Sabin, J. E. 1995. "Lessons for U.S. Managed Care from the British National Health Service I: 'The Vision Thing'." *Psychiatric Services* 46, no. 10:993–94.

———. 1996. "What Should We Advocate for in For-Profit Mental Health Care, and How Should We Do It?" *Psychiatric Services* 47, no. 10:1061–62ff.

———. 1998. "Public Sector Managed Behavioral Healthcare I: Developing an Effective Case Management Program." *Psychiatric Services* 49, no. 1:31–33.

Sabin, J. E., and Daniels, N. 1994. "Determining 'Medical Necessity' in Mental Health Practice." *Hastings Center Report* 24, no. 6:5-13.

———. 1997. "Setting Behavioral Health Priorities: Good News and Crucial Lessons from the Oregon Health Plan. *Psychiatric Services* 48, no. 7:883–84ff.

Stroup, T. S., and Dorwart, R. A. 1997. "Overview of Public Sector Managed Mental Health Care." In *Managed Mental Health Care in the Public Sector*, pp. 1–12. Edited by K. Minkoff and D. Pollack. Amsterdam, The Netherlands: Harwood Academic Publishers.

COMMENTARY

Mary L. Durham, Ph.D.

The clinical quality and access problems Mr. Smith is experiencing are the result of poor managed care practices. Instead of melding care coordination and incentives for health enhancement with capitated financing, BrainCare appears to have done little more than contract for services to be delivered to a defined population of severely mentally ill clients, with little accountability to anyone for the clinical results.

Incentives for care management can be imbedded into a managed care model, providing important clinical care benefits to patients and financial benefits to payers in truly "managed care" systems. In managing only the finances and ignoring the importance of keeping patients functioning at their optimal levels, WholeBody Health Plan and its contractor, BrainCare, may experience short-run gains (profits). Ultimately, however, they will lose their credibility as health caring organizations, as well as their ability to finance services for this vulnerable population. Mr. Smith is at present a hapless victim of this arrangement.

A managed care model—properly constructed—can serve the needs of Mr. Smith and other people with complex needs. However, to establish and maintain a successful managed care model requires clarifying responsibilities among the partners (WholeBody Health Plan, BrainCare, and the state) and establishing and aggressively monitoring contractual performance objectives regarding patient outcomes.

In and of itself, managed care is a neutral concept. The definition of the term does not signify removing clinical decision making from providers, denying needed services, or tolerating shortcuts that undermine high-quality patient care. In fact, plummeting patient functioning and the need for hospitalization signal failure of the patient care objectives as well as the financial objectives of a managed care system.

Managed care, combined with capitated financing, alters provider incentives and encourages high-quality, cost-effective care in three ways: (1) it removes the motivation to provide ineffective treatments, (2) it focuses on prevention and keeping patients functioning at their optimal level, and (3) it reduces the use of expensive treatments of little clinical value.

Capitation

In capitated systems, providers (or their organization) receive a fixed income or reimbursement per patient, regardless of the amount of service rendered. As a result, they have no incentive to provide treatment that is not effective or medically necessary. This disincentive to provide ineffective or unnecessary care stands in sharp contrast to fee-for-service coverage, where treatment that has no proven value (and/or may pose unacceptable risks to patients) may be reimbursed and encouraged.

In a managed care system where payment is capitated, it is extremely important to use treatment methods that work and to avoid using resources on treatments that are ineffective or provide no additional benefit. Reliable evidence of treatment effectiveness is especially crucial, since investing in ineffective therapies takes precious resources away from all patients.

Thus, treatment effectiveness should be the central focus of a capitated delivery system. Unfortunately, far too little is known about which mental health treatments work and which do not (Weisz et al. 1995). This lack of information on a clear array of cost-effective treatments is a disadvantage for mental health services, regardless of payment method. Within managed care arrangements, the lack of clear evidence about what works and what does not makes financing trickier and performance targets more crucial.

Funding of mental health services suffers as a result of the assumption by many that people with psychiatric symptoms can pull themselves together if they choose and that the health care system can do little to treat their condition. The presumed open-endedness of treatment and the chronic nature of psychiatric conditions have made payers at all levels reluctant to put resources into mental health services. Because of the severe limits placed on funding for mental health care by state governments, employers, and Medicare, evidence of treatment effectiveness is especially crucial.

For example, state governments that fund services for severely mentally ill people require rigorous scientific data evaluating the effectiveness of extremely expensive psychoactive drugs. They need to know whether investments of limited public dollars in sheltered workshops or back-to-work programs achieve important goals for people with chronic mental illnesses. Providing expensive care that is clinically ineffective does not serve the purposes of payers, patients, or families.

Capitated payment rates must be properly risk-adjusted to reflect the severity level of patients in the population. Reimbursement rates can be set too low to cover the costs of essential, effective services. This can result from inadequate risk models, vendors that undercut the market to gain entry and drive out competitors, or contractors that choose to provide too little for too many clients instead of adequate resources for fewer patients. Inadequate reimbursement will guarantee the failure of managed care systems for vulnerable populations. Proper risk-adjustment removes the financial disadvantages of assuming responsibility for treating a sicker population. If very unhealthy populations are to benefit from managed care systems, sound approaches to risk-adjustment are essential.

Preventing Declines in Function

Whereas fee-for-service reimburses providers for treating illness, capitated providers profit most when enrollees are at their maximal level of functioning and require only routine health services. A general population will include a mix of healthy along with sicker people. This mix is a financially sustainable one. In a Medicaid contract like the one BrainCare is now servicing, the organization is challenged to identify treatments that improve patient function, stabilize chronically ill individuals like Mr. Smith, and prevent future episodes of costly care. Only through risk-adjustment is this a financially sustainable arrangement.

Therefore, capitated financial incentives ought to reward providers for preventing episodes of illness, encouraging early diagnosis, and promoting the active pursuit of proven treatments. Preventing declines in function for Mr. Smith should be an urgent priority for capitated providers. Even fragile individuals with chronic conditions have periods of stability and variations in their need for resources. Pooling resources can work effectively, even when periods of high resource demand are certain—as long as risk-adjustment for the population reflects the higher overall level of need for the total population.

Carve-out Programs

Mr. Smith is enrolled in a so-called carve-out program. Treatment of his mental illness has been contracted to BrainCare, apart from all other medical or other social services. Virtually all of BrainCare's patient population have serious mental illnesses. In theory, carve-out programs have the advantage of developing more easily accessible, specialized, intensive interventions than are available to people like Mr. Smith in comprehensive health care plans. Carve-out programs can negotiate capitation rates that reflect higher risk and use those dollars to develop broad-based service packages that go beyond traditional mental health services. The range of service and coverage—including a broad definition of "medical necessity"—can be negotiated for this unique population. If employment support programs or aggressive outreach to people living at home or in foster care help patients like Mr. Smith maintain their ability to function in the community, then such programs can and should be developed. Fee-for-service is likely to reimburse specific, approved services and disapprove others not on the list. Managed care with capitation should make it possible for companies to use funds more flexibly to support the complex needs of such patients.

Incentives to Maintain Mr. Smith's Function

The *financial* and *care management* goals for BrainCare should be identical: to maintain Mr. Smith at his optimal level of functioning and prevent a crisis or exacerbation of his illness. If Mr. Smith returns to the hospital because he can no longer live at home, BrainCare, the managed care company that is fully "at risk," will incur the cost of that hospital stay. In fact, it appears that the state has negotiated a contract with WholeBody Health Plan that does not put BrainCare at risk for the cost of hospitalization and allows BrainCare to transfer Mr. Smith to the civil commitment system, where his care will be covered at someone else's expense. This is a poorly structured contractual arrangement that the state, as the responsible party, must remedy.

Expensive Treatments with Little Clinical Value Are Avoided

Early intervention, outpatient treatment, and social support in the community are always favored over an expensive and restrictive inpatient admission—especially in the eyes of most patients. Outpatient treatment, including aggressive medication monitoring, is as effective as, and less expensive than, hospitalization. Since managed care contracts must cover expenses, regardless of the actual health care costs for an individual during a given period, incentives should point toward less expensive treatment alternatives when they are available (Durham 1994; Stuart and Stockton 1973). But despite these facts, Mr. Smith's condition deteriorated without BrainCare's intervention. In fact, it was the total collapse of a previously successful care program that led to his hospitalization. What went wrong?

Because of his distance from a BrainCare provider, Mr. Smith was not seen by a provider until his condition had begun to deteriorate. The new psychiatrist had to prescribe from a formulary and cope with a difficult and frustrating approval process for nonformulary drugs. Even when the psychiatrist was advised of significant problems with the new medication, he failed to take steps that would increase the likelihood of making the medication work (or changing back to the old prescription).

Formularies are intended to list drugs that yield clinical results equal or superior to their competitors. If a new drug is more expensive than others currently in use, it should be substituted only if it is associated with better patient outcomes—not just because it is being marketed aggressively by a drug company. However, it is foolish to slavishly adhere to a formulary when a specific formulary drug has a detrimental effect on an individual patient. The exception process must be flexible enough to encourage cost-effective prescribing, while allowing psychiatrists to exercise clinical judgment. Rigorous evaluation of the impact of formulary-based prescribing on patient health and functional status is the final test of how well the closed formulary works.

In an exemplary model of managed care, it is not the length or the intensity per se of the treatment that determines one treatment choice over another; rather, it is the cost relative to the effectiveness of the intervention that should count. The formulary drug prescribed to Mr. Smith, group therapy, and the use of a social worker instead of a psychiatrist cost less only if they keep Mr. Smith functioning at his maximal capacity. They are bad clinical and financial choices if they allow him to deteriorate to a condition that requires more intensive (and expensive) treatment.

Managed care systems must be designed to optimize each of the three provider incentives mentioned earlier. Taken together, systems of care can "incent" evidence-based and preventively oriented care in the least restrictive setting. Because Mr. Smith's original treatment program worked so well, the new program should achieve at least that level of success. But as it now stands, Mr. Smith's case is an example of a poorly structured, profit-oriented system that has failed to yield the potential benefits of managed care. Indeed, his case appears to have harvested short-run profits by denying needed care in the absence of longer-term prevention or care management. His providers allowed his condition to deteriorate, causing him personal harm as well as requiring more expensive hospital-based care. Clearly, the managed care model with which the state contracted failed Mr. Smith.

In the short run, BrainCare and WholeBody Health Plan may achieve this year's profit margins and give their shareholders an adequate return on investment; in the long run, however, their programs will fail to serve the patients they have contracted to cover. They will find an ever more disabled group of clients for whom they are still responsible. It appears BrainCare managed the finances without managing the care.

The State's Responsibility

The state, as the responsible party, contracts with WholeBody Health Plan for Mr. Smith's care. Can the state structure a managed care contract with WholeBody Health Plan (and BrainCare) that takes advantage of the health-enhancing incentives of managed care with capitation and minimizes care motivated by financial incentives alone? What kinds of mechanisms might be put in place to ensure a different outcome for Mr. Smith within a managed care environment, given his diagnosis, his geographic location, and his need for extensive nonmedical supports?

Contracts with managed care organizations should go far beyond negotiation of the capitation rate or payment schedules. The state should be responsible for ensuring that the quality of care—not just the payment schedule—is negotiated with WholeBody Health Plan and its agents. Assurances of quality, financial performance, and patient satisfaction with the experience of care are now commonly reported for physical health care contracts. An expanded list of performance requirements, including measures of function and satisfaction by key constituents (for example, measures of satisfaction with BrainCare by patients and families compared to those of users of competing services), should be a part of service contracts for patients with chronic, severe mental illnesses. The contracts can specify targeted levels of quality, satisfaction, and financial performance.

Further, the state and WholeBody Health Plan should require BrainCare to disclose the contents of the formulary as well as how it was created and updated; doctors should be well versed in how to seek approval to use off-list products; and there should be evidence that exceptions are granted promptly when medically appropriate. These contracts should be executed between the state and WholeBody Health Plan as well as between WholeBody Health Plan and BrainCare. States can turn to their colleagues in other state mental health departments or the National Institute for Mental Health (NIMH) for assistance in establishing successful contracts.

The state can mandate a basic benefits package for each beneficiary, and it can empower contractors to go outside traditional medically oriented services to meet the psychosocial needs of this unique client group. The state can also insist that its contractors develop provider networks in rural communities or establish more aggressive outreach to clients like Mr. Smith who live in more remote areas. In the general medical care market, health care organizations that lack provider networks in certain geographic areas simply do not get the contract.

Focus on Function

Many managed care companies—especially for-profit organizations—have inserted utilization review managers and case managers to review certain clinical treatment decisions. For example, these administrative staff may be required to scrutinize off-formulary drug use, outpatient visits, and hospitalizations. These practices tend to remove decisions from clinicians and place them in the hands of someone outside the health care team. This is deplorable in primary care, internal medicine, or specialty care; it is disastrous for people with chronic, severe mental illnesses. It is even more difficult for reviewers to second-guess the many complicated factors associated with mental health treatment, compared to medical conditions, since few clear-cut diagnostic or laboratory tests exist as markers for clinical decision making in mental health. These aspects of current managed care practices should be discouraged and eliminated.

Coverage decisions and individual care plans should be made by the health care team with clear clinical—not financial—objectives in mind. Here managed care can provide distinct advantages over fee-for-service incentives. If Mr. Smith's care team were put at financial risk for Mr. Smith's functional status rather than for the services he receives, they would be motivated to develop a treatment plan that provided the maximum likelihood of success. For example, clinicians at BrainCare could be rewarded on the basis of Mr. Smith's symptom remission or stable management of symptoms. When and if Mr. Smith needed to be hospitalized, the team would be accountable for timely follow-up after discharge and for review and implementation of the care plan. Paying providers on the basis of reduced hospital days or reductions in the number of outpatient visits is a recipe for disaster because clinicians will have to choose between denying care or reaching those perverse performance targets. Rewarding providers on the basis of improved functional status (Mr. Smith's ability to carry on usual activities of daily living) or enhanced quality of life is more difficult—but more clinically and fiscally responsible in the long run.

This type of accountability—for improved or stable function—will motivate providers to develop outreach programs that deter loss of function. Mr. Smith's physician will not choose a less expensive drug if he believes it will derail Mr. Smith's functional status. Companies will seek out and develop (and clinicians will insist on) tested methods of community support (such as subcontracts with the county's Assertive Community Team) and abandon alternatives that cost money but do not produce desired results.

Paying for Care of the Seriously Mentally Ill

All of this costs money. At present, managed care companies like BrainCare are engaged in a race to the bottom. They may have contracted "on the cheap" with the state—accepting payment that was too low to provide adequate services for severely ill people. Given their for-profit status, they have diverted some portion of that revenue into profit, thus reducing the dollars available to build proper incentives to providers for high-quality care. It is likely that both factors are at work.

Mental health services have always been the poor stepchild of medical care. Competitive cost pressures throughout the health care world have shortened the length of time clinicians spend with their patients, tightened the rules for prescribing drugs off-formulary, and broken long-standing contractual relationships with community providers (as in the case of the Assertive Community Team in Mr. Smith's county). These changes come not from provider interest in modifying their practice but from the lack of resources to give patients more attention. It is time to debate how high capitation rates must be for health care companies to provide efficient care under the most streamlined and carefully monitored systems. The appropriateness of for-profit health care must also be reconsidered, especially for serving the needs of the most vulnerable of individuals.

What does the future hold for companies like BrainCare? In the long run, BrainCare probably will not survive the growing scrutiny of payers: state governments, major employers, and the federal government. These payers are insisting on ever more sophisticated performance standards for quality, satisfaction, and cost control. But will states, employers, and the federal government be willing to place enough priority on the care of vulnerable populations like the severely mentally ill to allow health care organizations to design successful managed care programs? Adequate resources must be paired with incentives to balance the financial temptations of blunt capitation with the care-enhancing features of managed care.

References

Durham, M. L. 1994. "Healthcare's Greatest Challenge: Providing Services for People with Severe Mental Illness in Managed Care." *Behavioral Sciences and the Law* 12:331–49.

Stuart, B., and Stockton, R. 1973. "Control Over the Utilization of Medical Services." *Milbank Memorial Fund Quarterly/Health and Society* 51, no. 3:341–94.

Weisz, J. R.; Donenberg, G. R.; Weiss, B.; and Han, S. S. 1995. "Bridging the Gap Between Laboratory and Clinic in Child and Adolescent Psychotherapy." *Journal of Consulting and Clinical Psychology* 63, no. 5:688–701.

17

Quality Care for Elderly Nursing Home Patients

CASE STUDY

The Tamarack Health System owns a large delivery network that includes physician practices, clinics, hospitals, nursing homes, and a hospice and home care company. Over the years, it has intentionally created a values-driven organizational culture. All managers and employees are schooled in the meaning and application of the system values of caring, quality, dignity, and stewardship. Their performance evaluations are focused on the extent to which they implement these system values in their actions and decisions.

Tamarack has a contractual arrangement with the OptiHealth Health Plan that enables physicians of OptiHealth to practice in Tamarack's health care facilities. OptiHealth is a staff model HMO (that is, an HMO whose physicians are salaried employees) that has a large Medicare contract. Dr. Wilson, a geriatrician employed by OptiHealth, has several Medicare-covered patients in one of Tamarack's nursing homes. Recently, OptiHealth initiated cost-containment measures to lower physician use of laboratory services. According to plan data, laboratory use rates among its physicians, particularly for its Medicare enrollees, are significantly higher than the rates of other physician groups. To incline physicians toward greater restraint, the health plan has implemented new practice guidelines designed to discourage laboratory tests that are not medically necessary for Medicare enrollees.

Mrs. Erickson, a ninety-year-old woman, is one of Dr. Wilson's patients. She was admitted to Tamarack's nursing home from another long-term care facility over a year ago. Her admitting medical problems included stage-four decubitus sores, arthritis, scoliosis, paralysis following a stroke, and dementia. Upon admission, she was poorly nourished.

Over a fifteen-month period, her oral intake improved, and she gained thirty pounds. Numerous treatments for her decubitus were unsuccessful in healing the wounds. Medications were given for pain management, and physical therapy made recommendations for positioning techniques to alleviate Mrs. Erickson's discomfort and to promote healing.

A disagreement between Mrs. Erickson's nurses and Dr. Wilson has developed because her nurses believe a special bed would be of great help to Mrs. Erickson, not only to promote healing but also to ameliorate some of her discomfort from her arthritis and scoliosis. Accustomed to seeing non-HMO Medicare enrollees with similar problems receive Medicare coverage for the special bed if laboratory tests demonstrate appropriate albumin levels, the nurses expressed to Dr. Wilson their concerns about Mrs. Erickson and their feeling that the bed might benefit their patient. Dr. Wilson was unwilling to order the routine laboratory test to determine Mrs. Erickson's albumin level because, in his view, the bed would, at best, have only marginal benefit for her.

Convinced that the bed would be of great help to Mrs. Erickson, the nurses believe that Mrs. Erickson is entitled to this intervention and that a failure to provide it is a failure to provide medically necessary, quality, and compassionate care. As employees of Tamarack, they feel Mrs. Erickson is being treated unfairly by her physician. Non-HMO Medicare enrolled residents in similar circumstances receive the laboratory tests necessary to justify Medicare coverage for the special bed. Mrs. Erickson's nurses feel that Dr. Wilson's decision requires them to continue providing her more painful and less successful interventions. They also worry about their involvement in activities that they think violate the Nursing Code of Ethics and compromise Tamarack's values.

Tamarack trusts its employees' ability to recognize when patient care is inconsistent with its values and has a strict policy of employee protection for disclosures of serious departures from these values. Mrs. Erickson's nurses and physician differ on the benefit the bed would have for Mrs. Erickson. Essentially, Dr. Wilson has stated that the benefit of the bed is not worth the cost of the lab test, while her nurses consider the bed sufficiently beneficial to be worth it. Further, the nurses believe Tamarack commits them to a philosophy of patient care different from OptiHealth's and Dr. Wilson's.

Questions for Consideration

➤ What features of this case are unique to managed care?
➤ What should Mrs. Erickson's nurses do in response to their perception of inequitable and qualitatively inappropriate treatment?

➤ Should Tamarack's values apply to physicians attached to Tamarack facilities through contractual arrangements between Tamarack and the health plan that employs the physician? Why?

➤ When system issues (for example, contracts, practice guidelines, and incentive arrangements) may be affecting patient care adversely, who is responsible for calling for an ethics consultation? At what level in the system should such issues be addressed? What kind of ethics mechanism is needed for consideration of such situations? To whom should an advisory opinion be transmitted? The delivery system? The health plan? The nursing home's administrator? Dr. Wilson?

➤ What trade-offs do the elderly face when choosing between fee-for-service and managed care Medicare contracts?

➤ What special considerations should guide the design of managed care contracts for the elderly?

COMMENTARY

Rosalie A. Kane, D.S.W

This case seems to be a setup. Tamarack Health System, on the side of the angels, has created a "values-driven organizational culture" and its employees are steeped in ideals of "caring, quality, dignity, and stewardship." It wants only the best for its residents, which, for Mrs. Erickson, means a high-tech bed to promote healing her stage-four decubitus ulcers and perhaps relieving her discomfort from arthritis and scoliosis. The bedsores as well as her malnutrition were the fault of her previous nursing home. Tamarack's nursing care has brought about marked improvements. Without the bed, the work is stymied.

Standing between the bed and the patient, a woman with dementia who cannot advocate for herself, is OptiHealth's Dr. Wilson, a geriatrician who attends Mrs. Erickson under a Medicare managed risk contract. He and his colleagues have been warned by OptiHealth's administration to cut back on laboratory tests, since Opti-Health physicians have exceeded industry standards in those expenses. As a member of a staff model HMO, Dr. Wilson has an incentive to withhold even this inexpensive test from a needy, suffering patient. Nurses are pitted against more powerful doctors, men against woman, and a values-based organization against a bottom-line-oriented managed care corporation. What to do? Should Tamarack call for an ethics consultation or form its own ethics committee to address such dilemmas on-site? To whom should the advisory opinion of the ethics consultant be transmitted? Should Tamarack sever its connection with OptiHealth and refuse to take its patients?

The Managed Care Context

Mrs. Erickson is enrolled in a Medicare risk contract as enabled by the 1982 Tax Equity and Fiscal Responsibility Act (TEFRA). In theory, she enrolled voluntarily and, under current Medicare policy, may disenroll at any time. Each month, OptiHealth receives 95 percent of the adjusted average per capita costs (AAPCC) for Mrs. Erickson's care. This means that OptiHealth gets 95 percent of the average costs of all fee-for-service Medicare beneficiaries in Mrs. Erickson's home county, adjusted to consider her advanced age, gender, residence in a nursing home, and Medicaid status. For this sum, OptiHealth must provide her with all the care she would receive under Medicare Parts A and B. If Mrs. Erickson resides in a low-ACPCC county, OptiHealth receives much less per month than if she resides in a high-AAPCC county. The enormous variation in AAPCC both within and across states directly reflects the variation in fee-for-service Medicare costs from area to area. Thus, Medicare capitation schemes are inequitable to begin with, complicating the different equity question put by the case: Is Mrs. Erickson, an HMO member, being treated unfairly compared to fee-for-service patients?

The hardest test of managed care comes when enrollees have serious and chronic illness. (For well people, health care hardly matters, and obtaining the lowest price is reasonable.) But, why would Mrs. Erickson or her agent exchange customary Medicare benefits for what may be the more restricted allocations of OptiHealth? Why would someone in dire need or at imminent risk of expensive health care expose themselves to the do-less, spend-less incentives that go with the territory of Medicare managed care? Why would it be prudent for them to choose a Medicare risk contract?

The answer lies in the flaws of the Medicare fee-for-service program. Despite Medicare protection, older people still have substantial out-of-pocket medical expenditures. Drains on the wallet include the deductibles, premiums, and co-payments built into Medicare; the supplemental Medi-gap insurance policies many seniors carry; and prescription drugs, dental care, eye care, hearing care, and long-term care (LTC). Depending on the details of the risk plan, a Medicare managed care organization may eliminate many front-end expenses and add many benefits not ordinarily covered by Medicare (such as outpatient drugs, dental care, and preventive care). The higher the AAPCC, the more likely are extra benefits. Also, the beneficiary is spared the anxiety of dealing with health care bills, paying in advance and collecting Medicare payments when providers refuse consignment, and paying for uncovered and denied expenses when providers accept consignment. Furthermore, despite the hand-wringing about the high costs of health care for older people, the typical hospital and physician know little about the nuances of high-quality diagnosis and treatment for very old people. Under business as usual, high costs do not equate to high quality.

Moreover, managed care could be an attractive vehicle to bring the best of geriatric medicine to older people with serious health problems. Its incentives encourage investment in health. Such an investment might include enhanced emphasis on primary care; comprehensive geriatric-assessment programs; preventive activities, such as flu shots; Alzheimer's disease workups; case management for high-risk enrollees; medication reviews; assistance with medical compliance and transportation to outpatient settings; and rehabilitation to enhance functioning beyond what Medicare usually allows. Whenever activities such as these lower the risk of subsequent expensive events like hospitalizations, they are advantageous to both the managed care organization and the patient. Mrs. Erickson, for example, apparently received primary care services from a geriatrician, which is quite unusual for most Medicare beneficiaries and most nursing home residents. Obviously, however, the downside for Mrs. Erickson relates to OptiHealth's incentive to reduce services, which might curtail her access to specialist care and other ancillary services, including lab tests and special beds.

With some effort, OptiHealth can provide other structural advantages for its Medicare beneficiaries. The HMO can structure itself around episodes of care and organize systematic medical follow-up after hospitalizations. Unlike most medical practices, it can afford management information systems that track patients over time, a common record system to help coordinate care across outpatient and inpatient units, and educational programs offering state-of-the-art information to its primary care practitioners based on the best guidelines for practice. When the science warrants, it can treat and monitor high-risk patients aggressively. It can invest in patient education, too. Of course, not all TEFRA HMOs follow these exemplary practices, but the potential is there.

An HMO can also be more flexible than fee-for-service Medicaid in its use of funds. For example, it need not insist on "home-boundedness" to send a home care nurse out to visit. It may act creatively to maximize health. The main way that a Medicare HMO saves money is by keeping Mrs. Erickson and others out of the hospital. Thus, it may behoove the HMO to invest in improving the nursing home's capability to treat her there. Of course, the HMO will also be alert to costs in other areas, including prescription drugs and durable medical equipment. The laboratory test as a gateway to Mrs. Erickson's bed is a red herring. The HMO is free to order the bed without the hoops that Medicare statutes and fiscal intermediaries impose in fee-for-service cases in their own efforts to erect barriers to utilization. The issue in this case is the bed, not the test.

Incentives of OptiHealth and Tamarack

Medicare managed care organizations come in many species and subspecies. One cannot assume one knows the incentives of the various participants without additional information. Dr. Wilson belongs to a staff HMO, which means he is salaried. Perhaps his income is unrelated to what he authorizes for Mrs. Erickson. Perhaps, however, Dr. Wilson is part of a group practice arrangement where physician salaries are augmented or reduced depending on how well they control the total expenses of the Medicare group. In that case, he indeed has a monetary incentive to avoid expensive treatments for Mrs. Erickson, but only to a point. It would be economically foolhardy to knowingly court a costly hospital admission. Sometimes physicians in Medicare risk contracts are paid on a fee-for-service basis, in which case the incentives change again.

What about the nursing home's incentives? If Tamarack is operating in a fee-for-service environment and Mrs. Erickson is paying privately, she is billed according to the services she receives. If Mrs. Erickson is one of the more than 50 percent of nursing home residents whose nursing home care is partly or completely paid by Medicaid, it will be reimbursed according to the rate system established in the particular state. Likely, given her advanced age, dementia, and length of stay (she came from another nursing home and has already been at Tamarack for fifteen months), Mrs. Erickson has exhausted her resources and has "spent down" to Medicaid. Probably too, the nursing home receives a high rate of reimbursement for her care because of what appear to be her high functional needs and her use of intensive nursing care for her elaborate skin treatments. If the state is one of the many using so-called case-mix-adjusted reimbursement, Tamarack may appeal for higher levels based on her acuity, but eventually it will reach the maximum amount. Like all nursing homes, Tamarack has incentives to minimize its payroll expenses, maximize its revenues, and minimize turnover of residents and empty beds.

The case ponders whether Tamarack should cancel its contract with Opti-Health. Yet, unless *Medicaid* capitation is involved, the nursing home probably has no such contract. OptiHealth and *Medicare* are in a contractual arrangement. Under different facts, Dr. Wilson could be employed by a program like EverCare, a national multisite demonstration program that serves long-stay nursing home residents only. EverCare undertakes to offer medical care to nursing home residents on a capitated basis, and to be efficient it recruits physicians who serve multiple patients in particular nursing homes. Thus, economies of scale can be achieved while giving exemplary medical and health-related care in those facilities. What is in it for the nursing homes may be the extra attention received by patients from EverCare doctors and the nurse practitioners who assist EverCare patients and doctors, additional training for staff, and the marketing advantages of the affiliation. Ordinarily, a nursing home's contacts with physicians are limited to arrangements with a medical director (who may have patients at the home and who has an overall quality-assurance function). Although here doctor and nurses are at loggerheads, up to now Mrs. Erickson may well have received more conscientious medical attention than many of her counterparts at Tamarack.

The Case Revisited

Whether the bed will be helpful is a prediction; clearly, it will not be helpful in all cases. The bed rental and maintenance can easily exceed $100 a day, and it may be needed for months. Fiscal intermediaries for the regular Medicare program are often leery of authorizing such equipment.

The key point is that the costs of the intervention will be borne by OptiHealth and the benefits will accrue to Tamarack. If, over several months, the decubitus ulcers are cured, Mrs. Erickson too will benefit. But even if the decubitus ulcers are *not* cured, the nursing home stands to gain. Nursing care will be easier and require less attention because of the bed. Instead of painstakingly turning and positioning Mrs. Erickson at intervals, the magic bed will do the work. Being in favor of expenditures that come out of someone else's budget, that may help the patient and cannot hurt, and that reduce one's own staffing burden is a no-brainer. Support of this plan is hardly a reason for Tamarack to boast about its superior organizational values.

More than marketing slogans are needed to understand and evaluate Tamarack's values-based care. Of great interest is how Tamarack actually operationalizes these much-vaunted values. Has it taken steps to protect privacy as much as possible? Has it instructed its staff to individualize the times and nature of care routines? Has Tamarack staff been encouraged to adhere to these values despite increases in its own costs or declines in its profits? If Tamarack has an ethics committee, does that group largely deliberate on issues that concern end-of-life treatments and the responsibilities of others, or does it carefully consider policies, routines, and costs that are within its own discretion?

Suppose Dr. Wilson had recommended that Mrs. Erickson receive daily evaluations by a registered nurse and twice-daily (rather than the usual twice weekly) showers to promote comfort and better skin care. On average, nursing home residents receive about seventy minutes a day of care from all nursing staff including the nurse's aides and an average of five minutes of daily attention from a registered nurse. Dr. Wilson's recommendations would translate into increased expenditures for the nursing home. Do the nursing home's values require these expenditures? If the nursing home refuses to follow through, should Dr. Wilson request an ethics consult?

Neither OptiHealth nor Tamarack are philanthropists. Both compete in the "medical marketplace." They depend on government programs, though Opti-Health receives more of its proportional revenue from Medicare, and Tamarack from Medicaid. They both bear some responsibility for Mrs. Erickson's care, but each is responsible for grooming a different part of the elephant.

Back to the bed, one of three scenarios may be true: (1) it is not medically justified based on current knowledge; (2) it is medically justified, but Dr. Wilson is unaware of the latest data; or (3) it is medically justified but out of greed, fear, or some other bad motive, Dr. Wilson is denying it to the patient. Given that Dr. Wilson has spent substantial time planning Mrs. Erickson's care and OptiHealth has already paid for extensive physical therapy, their motivation merits the benefit of the doubt. The whole group must be regarded as a care team, even though not all team members are employed by the same organization, an increasingly common circumstance in health care. What might any of them do to resolve the problem?

The first tack should surely be to bring data to bear. If the nurses have any evidence to support the bed's benefits, they should bring that to Dr. Wilson's attention. They should also arm themselves with information about the price of renting various types of beds and the likely duration of the need. They might ask for a second opinion, especially if they are still convinced of the bed's efficacy. Tamarack might also enlist the involvement of its own medical director, first to elicit an opinion and then to speak with Dr. Wilson. If consultants are needed, perhaps Tamarack should employ a technical consultant to get at the facts before rushing to an ethics consult.

Certainly Mrs. Erickson's agent can disenroll her from OptiHealth. Tamarack has the right (and some would say, the obligation) to advise the agent of this possibility if facts bear out that OptiHealth is withholding a valuable treatment that would be available to her under fee-for-service or some other HMO. However, Tamarack should also inform the agent if Mrs. Erickson is likely to receive less medical attention under fee-for-service. Before giving advice, Tamarack also needs to explore whether Medicare intermediaries in its area routinely allow such beds for beneficiaries like Mrs. Erickson. Finally, Tamarack should scrutinize its own potential conflict of interest. It may even bring in a disinterested party, such as the nursing home ombudsperson, who has a statutory obligation to act as a mediator and advocate for nursing home residents.

Long-Term Care and Managed Care

Assuming Mrs. Erickson is a Medicaid recipient, the Medicaid program is responsible not only for some or all of her nursing home costs (or personal care at home) but also for the deductibles, coinsurance, and premiums related to her Medicare coverage, as well as outpatient drugs and other allowable expenses under Medicaid that are not covered under Medicare. Mrs. Erickson is one of the so-called dually eligible, a term used to describe people eligible for Medicare because of age or permanent disability status and eligible for Medicaid because of poverty. Dually eligible people are under intensive policy scrutiny.

Federal and state authorities are well aware that the Medicaid and Medicare programs are poorly articulated. When not preoccupied with cost-shifting to the other program, officials in both programs have sought to better coordinate and provide improved care at a lower cost by combining the programs under a capitated model. In such a scheme, most notably now being tested in Minnesota under the Minnesota Senior Care Organization demonstration, managed care organizations will receive capitation fees from *both* Medicare and Medicaid and be responsible for meeting the obligations of *both* programs. Would this be good for the Mrs. Ericksons of the world? How would it help Tamarack and other long-term care providers?

The financial advantages to Tamarack would depend on the deal it cut and the incentives established. Managed care organizations can form partnerships with long-term care organizations where the latter are at financial risk or can pay these providers on a fee-for-service basis (perhaps with discounted fees). They might, as in the Ever-Care example, offer additional services and coverage to enrollees, provide nurse practitioners who visit the nursing homes as representatives of the HMO, train nursing home staff, and offer other advantages to long-term care providers.

From a consumer perspective, the issue is more complicated. The face of long-term care is changing. More consumers are choosing assisted living and other congregate settings where they can get care without the high social and psychological price paid for the hour or so per day of care received in nursing homes. Home care arrangements are also becoming more common, and state Medicaid programs have begun to finance unorthodox nonagency arrangements for so-called consumer-directed home care. Some consumer advocates are afraid that if acute care and long-term care are combined in a single capitation, lifestyle decisions such as where people live and get long-term care will be made by a managed care organization that has neither expertise nor motivation to encourage individualized choices. The consolidation of power and the medicalization of everyday life inherent in such integration are off-putting. Yet, failing full integration of acute care and long-term care, the need to bring about better articulated and coordinated services for people who need both acute care and long-term care will remain pressing.

Old Battles in New Arenas?

This commentary warns against a simplistic formulation of the ethical issues at stake and warns against blaming managed care for every problem. Medicare and Medicaid may be enthralled with managed care for three reasons: (1) it seemingly caps their financial liability (though if providers have favorable selection, the presumed savings are chimerical), (2) it distances governments from rationing decisions, and

(3) for some, it is compatible with a preference for private markets, competition, and a dislike of government programs. The distancing motivation is probably the most important, yet governments make rationing decisions when they set capitation rates that determine whether a managed care organization will begrudge care to Mrs. Erickson.

More than anyone, people with multiple illnesses and disabilities who need both long-term care and acute care should be prime candidates to benefit from better management of care. Care management is needed whether acute care is capitated, long-term care is capitated, neither is capitated, or both are capitated. And under all four variants, relatively few models of good coordination exist. But it is also clear that managed care, OptiHealth style, fails to inspire trust. However pure Dr. Wilson's motivations as he strives to provide good care for a particular patient and an enrolled population within available resources, he is subject to criticisms because of the incentives inherent in capitated managed care. Many incentives operate within the plethora of managed care arrangements available under Medicare, Medicaid, or combined programs, and sometimes the providers themselves do not even know what incentives affect them. Whatever the real incentives and however selfless and scientific the motivations, the lack of trust attendant on the whiff of an HMO may be too high a price to pay.

If Mrs. Erickson's bed is a good bet in terms of predicted efficacy, ethical questions still remain. What is the right amount to spend for this anticipated benefit? Suppose that pain and discomfort are not at stake but infections from the bedsores might hasten Mrs. Erickson's death? Should her dementia be a factor, or should the same decision be made were she to be lucid, articulate, eager to try the bed, and reproachful about its being withheld? These questions are value-laden, and one would expect different answers to emerge in societies with different levels of affluence. They are not specific to managed care. With or without managed care, communities in the United States need to decide what is a just and proper allocation of acute health care and what is a decent quality of life offered through the more socially oriented programs we call long-term care.

COMMENTARY _____

Robert M. Veatch, Ph.D.

It may seem obvious that Dr. Wilson is treating Mrs. Erickson unfairly and that the task of Tamarack's nurses is to try to get testing that will eventually get her the bed they think she needs, but the case may turn out to be more ambiguous. The case states that Dr. Wilson believed the special bed was of only marginal benefit and that he will not order laboratory tests to determine her albumin level. On the other hand, the nurses believe this will require them to pursue other "more painful and less successful interventions." Are they disagreeing about the diagnostic facts or about whether the bed is worth the extra cost? The first task is to identify the disagreement exactly.

Is This a Dispute About the Diagnostic Facts?

It appears that Dr. Wilson and the nurses are disputing technical, medical facts. Dr. Wilson believes the bed will be only marginally beneficial; the nurses believe it will be of great help. Of course, if Dr. Wilson already knows the bed's benefit, it would be irresponsible to do the albumin test.

On the other hand, the nurses believe different facts. They believe, prior to testing, that, lacking the bed, Mrs. Erickson will have to undergo more painful, less successful treatment. Of course, if that could be known without testing, it would also be irresponsible. Let us assume that the nurses really believe that they cannot know whether the bed is needed without testing, but that it is possible that the bed could be of great benefit. With this assumption the picture is still rather strange. The nurses seem to be claiming that Dr. Wilson has reached an erroneous conclusion. They are, in essence, accusing him of incompetence.

Traditionally, when nurses disagreed with physicians on technical matters of whether a treatment, such as a bed, will affect the patient's condition, the assumption was that the physicians were more expert. But in this case, even as a technical matter, the situation seems more complex. Nurses and physicians are increasingly viewed as professionals with separate spheres of competence. These nurses may well know as much about decubiti as Dr. Wilson. We need to know whether the questions at stake should be viewed as matters of nursing or physician expertise.

Each party claims to know in advance the extent of the bed's effect. At least one of them must be wrong. Traditional channels of peer review and, if necessary, collegial correction might help resolve matters. More likely, however, each has overstated his or her own position.

Is This a Dispute About Whether a Potential Benefit Is Worth the Cost?

It seems likely that neither party can be sure in advance how effective the bed will be. Uncertainty also exists over how valuable the effect will be if one occurs. The patient is not described as terminal, but, given her age, she probably will not survive terribly long. In order to evaluate this case, we must estimate how bad it is for patients in this compromised condition to have decubiti as well as how long they will live and how likely it is they will improve with and without the bed. Neither Dr. Wilson nor the nurses can claim definitive expertise on these judgments. Knowledge of decubiti or their treatment cannot tell clinicians how important it is to change Mrs. Erickson's condition or whether it would be morally right to do so. It seems likely that they disagree about these value judgments rather than over more technical questions.

Should Physicians or Nurses Make These Value Judgments?

It might at first seem that physicians should make these judgments, but we shall see that would be irrational. Physicians traditionally were committed to Hippocratic ethics, according to which their duty was always to benefit patients and protect them from harm, according to the physician's ability and judgment. But in recent decades it has become clear that that principle is wrong for two reasons.

First, physicians are in no position to know what will benefit their patients. Deciding what is best is a matter of determining what fits patients' values. This involves trade-offs between medical and nonmedical goods about which physicians cannot be expert. Even within the medical sphere many competing goods can conflict. No physician can know what patients want without asking them or their surrogates. In this situation, claiming the bed is "not medically necessary" can convey no meaning. It is a deceptive term used to imply medical science can determine a nonscientific value judgment: whether a particular benefit is worth pursuing.

Second, doing what is best for patients may be terribly costly. It may be burdensome to their families, health professionals, or other patients. Using Opti-Health's resources for a bed that may have only a modest chance of even short-term benefit will come at the expense of either other patients or of other stakeholders in OptiHealth.

Let us assume for the moment that the resources, if not used for Mrs. Erickson, will go to other HMO patients. The bedside physician is hardly in a position to trade off Mrs. Erickson's interests with other patients. Many of them he has never met, and he cannot know the strength of their moral claims on resources, nor can he know either the relative amount of good that could be done or whether the moral goal is to maximize that good. Is the morally correct principle to use OptiHealth's resources to produce the most good in aggregate or to use them on the sickest, most miserable patients, even though doing so is inefficient?

Perhaps Dr. Wilson has decided that morally he is bound to use OptiHealth's resources efficiently, conserving them for patients who would benefit more.

Some ethics analysts accept this utilitarian view. Others who favor a more egalitarian principle of justice claim that it is morally preferable to benefit the worst off, even if it is less efficient. Neither position is clearly foolish; neither is obviously correct.

How can a bedside clinician claim to have the insight not only to know what Mrs. Erickson would most prefer and what the relative benefits would be of the bed but also whether utilitarianism or egalitarianism should prevail? Physicians are in no position to make these judgments. Neither are nurses. Because clinicians cannot know what is best for patients and cannot know which principle is decisive, many now insist that bedside clinicians, whether physicians or nurses, should be exempt from any social ethical duties in allocating resources. They are not supposed to be making comparative cost estimates and value trade-offs; they are supposed to serve patients.

But if clinicians should not make these judgments, then who should? Should Tamarack's values or OptiHealth's prevail? Is there a basis for concluding that Tamarack's should win out?

The HMO and the Nursing Home as Sources of Value

At first, one might be tempted to accept that Hippocrates was right, that the morally correct course is to determine what is best for Mrs. Erickson and do it. But doing what is literally best for patients is not the morally correct course—not for physicians or nurses, and not for nursing homes or HMOs.

THE IRRATIONALITY OF DOING WHAT IS BEST FOR THE PATIENT

It is even hard to imagine what would be best for Mrs. Erickson. She is in bad shape and her decubiti are likely to respond, at least somewhat, to careful management of diet and positioning. This could include assigning nurses to spoon-feed and turn her regularly as well as providing the special bed. But how much nursing and physician attention would it take to literally do what was best? Would an around-the-clock private duty nurse be better than intermittent attention? Would two constant private nurses be better? Would a private team of dietitians, dermatologists, and other specialists assigned exclusively to her offer any incremental advantage?

Clearly, no health system in a finite world would do literally everything that could help every patient, even if we could figure out what that would be; such an approach would come at the expense of other patients or societal concerns. It is irrational to strive to structure health systems to maximize patient benefit. It is likely that Dr. Wilson and the nurses disagree over exactly how to draw the lines between what is reasonable and what is marginal. There is surely some prognosis for which a critically ill, ninety-year-old demented patient should not receive certain potentially beneficial treatments because they are too marginal. If, for example, she had less than twenty-four hours to live, would testing be in order? What about a three-day or a three-week prognosis? What if she were sufficiently demented that she could not perceive the pain of the sores?

This is not an argument that Dr. Wilson was justified and the nurses wrong. Rather it suggests some lines must be drawn and that values will necessarily come into play in drawing them. Is there some reason to believe that either Tamarack's values or OptiHealth's should prevail?

THE MORAL LEGITIMACY OF INSTITUTIONAL VALUES

Both Tamarack and OptiHealth will institutionalize certain values in making these judgments. If either is a profit-making institution, those values will include some judgment about what is a fair and reasonable profit for shareholders. Even if they are nonprofit, they will not have enough resources to do every last thing that could possibly benefit every patient. In fact, if they were that well endowed, then their funders have overcommitted resources that could be doing more good some other place.

The real issue is whether either institution's values can claim legitimacy in making decisions about Mrs. Erickson's care. Tamarack or OptiHealth may be sponsored by nonprofit institutions that perhaps are religious groups. They are good at making their values explicit. If the system is Catholic, for example, it will probably be committed to good care for the poor. This could require making sure resources were not used for marginal benefits in order to have some left for basic care of the poor. If it were Orthodox Jewish, it might be uniquely committed to preserving life, even at the expense of riding roughshod over patient autonomy. If one of them reflected zealous commitment to the "religion" of libertarian free enterprise, it might manifest values ensuring that all parties including shareholders received what they bargained for. It is from this value perspective that we can consider the possibility that Dr. Wilson's agenda is not benefits for other patients but rather benefits for owners or shareholders. Some in our society believe that the free market generates efficiencies so valuable that pursuit of profit can be considered moral. They also claim that if too much is diverted to profits at the expense of patient services, subscribers will defect to other providers.

It is here that nonprofits may object, in principle, claiming that it is morally obligatory in health care to provide a decent level of patient care. But even these nonprofits would recognize that some compensation to employees and owners is legitimate and that no managed care organization—charitable or profit making—can set its rates high enough and pay its stakeholders poorly enough to be able to do everything that it possibly could for patients. Deciding which of these value sets is the right one will be more complicated than it may appear.

It can be argued that Tamarack should have the right to run its system based on its freely chosen values. But that might also be said for OptiHealth. No charitable health system will necessarily hold value commitments that will always mesh with each subscriber's; no managed care organization will manifest values inherently at odds with all enrollees' values.

THE IDEAL WAY OF SETTING LIMITS ON HEALTH CARE

One approach is to ask the question from the patient's point of view. Are Mrs. Erickson's values adequately reflected in one of the institutions? From the patient's perspective, it would be important to know whether she has in any way endorsed or subscribed to the values being used by Dr. Wilson or the nurses and their respective organizations. Once we recognize that it would be wrong morally for OptiHealth to do literally everything that it could do to benefit every one of its patients, the critical question is whether Mrs. Erickson knowingly committed to OptiHealth's values in rationing marginal care.

In a perfectly free market, Mrs. Erickson could choose from a wide range of health systems reflecting different values. She could choose one reflecting Catholic values, Jewish values, libertarian values, do-marginal-things-for-decubiti values, etc. She could choose one formally committed to allocating subscriber premiums to those uses that will produce the most good per dollar invested, regardless of who benefits. She could choose a system committed to spending on its sickest patients, rather than better-off, more-efficient-to-treat patients. She could even commit to a profit-making HMO that admitted that it structured these decisions according to the principle of maximizing profits for investors. If she had a range of HMO value systems from which to choose, it would seem morally justified that she receive care according to her chosen values. Ideally, managed care systems could make it easier, not harder, for patients to receive health care services based on their own values.

In the real world of HMOs, however, no free market in value systems exists. Many people live in areas and work for employers where at best they have one or two managed care plans from which to choose. In the even more restricted world of Medicare HMOs, how could the values of OptiHealth be considered a legitimate basis upon which to allocate scarce resources in Mrs. Erickson's case?

In the world of limited choices, a morally responsible, wise HMO would involve subscribers in making value choices for allocating health care. Certain basic allocational decisions could actually be put to subscriber vote. (Bone marrow transplant for breast cancer or life support for anencephalics could probably be handled this way.) OptiHealth could even offer a supplemental insurance rider permitting those who particularly valued some service excluded by the majority to buy the desired coverage.

Many value decisions, such as Mrs. Erickson's, will be too specific and ad hoc to lend themselves to subscriber votes. An elected council of subscribers could set policy for some allocations. It could review the practice guideline on which Dr. Wilson based his position, assessing the values necessarily incorporated in them. Other decisions could be left to professional gatekeepers accountable to subscribers and guided by value commitments actively chosen by subscribers. These would not, however, be bedside clinicians; they would be gatekeepers employed by the collective subscribers and accountable to them, rather than clinicians accountable to individual patients or managers accountable to HMO administration.

This is not to suggest that Mrs. Erickson had anything resembling this level of participation in choosing the values of OptiHealth. But, in theory, it could happen that plan subscribers were that active in choosing the values for allocating inevitably scarce resources. If, and only if, the values on which limits are based have been actively chosen by members would HMOs be justified in instructing their clinicians to exclude marginally beneficial services. In such cases OptiHealth's employees would be justified in using those values to limit beneficial services.

This position should be distinguished from the idea that patients should be asked to consent in advance to being kept ignorant of when rationing is occurring. This approach would in effect authorize OptiHealth to ration Mrs. Erickson's bed without telling her and without any assurance that she accepts the values used. By contrast if Mrs. Erickson explicitly endorsed the values, Dr. Wilson would merely carry out the policies so endorsed. He would in effect be exempted from making any bedside rationing choices himself. That seems the ideal way to allocate resources.

Implications for the Nursing Home

If, in theory, Mrs. Erickson endorsed the OptiHealth values upon which the practice guideline was based, does this mean that Tamarack must permit any managed care organization to send its physicians into its facilities, even though they will act on values that are radically different from Tamarack's? Specifically, does Tamarack have to play by OptiHealth's values when OptiHealth physicians are treating its patients at Tamarack? Clearly, at least if other providers are available, Tamarack should have the moral right to refuse to contract with OptiHealth. But if it accepts a contract with OptiHealth that makes OptiHealth's subscriber-endorsed values explicit, then it seems that Tamarack must permit Dr. Wilson to follow the orders of OptiHealth's subscribers. The alternative is to refuse to sign the contract.

One implication of this conclusion is that it is not morally necessary for a health facility to treat all its medically identical patients equally. If a hospital receives two medically identical patients with insurance based on different sets of values, assuming both insurance policies provided a basic, decent minimum, it would actually be wrong for it to treat the patients identically. If Mrs. Erickson's plan legitimately excluded the special bed and her medically identical roommate's included it, then once Tamarack agreed to serve both plans, it must treat the two patients differently.

Implications for the Nurses

This may leave the nurses in an awkward position. Their values may require providing services nearer to what is best for Mrs. Erickson than either OptiHealth or Tamarack supports. They have a right to those beliefs but surely cannot impose them on these organizations or on patients who have chosen different values. In a perfect health care world, there would be a health care system that matched their values, and they should seek employment there. In a less than perfect world, if they choose to work within Tamarack's system, they must recognize the importance of committing to its values. That will mean they cannot always deliver all the services they would like.

What If the HMO's Values Are Not Legitimate?

It seems probable that either OptiHealth's principles were not endorsed by Mrs. Erickson or its actions are contrary to its announced principles. In fact, Mrs. Erickson might well prefer Tamarack's values, which seem to commit to spending resources on patients who are very poorly off, even if it is inefficient to do so.

If that is the case, Tamarack and its employees have a duty to Mrs. Erickson. They need to take steps to alert her or her surrogates that choices are being made that seem contrary to her interest and have not received her approval. The nurses might (1) warn her and her surrogates of the inadequacies in her care and the values Dr. Wilson is using, (2) ask Tamarack's medical director to intervene to see if Dr. Wilson's mind can be changed, (3) ask for a consultation with Tamarack's and OptiHealth's ethics committees to see if the conflict can be resolved, (4) have Tamarack's risk manager alert OptiHealth's risk manager of potential liability if the nurses' belief is sustained, (5) assist Mrs. Erickson in changing HMOs or bringing charges of malpractice, (6) lobby Tamarack to sever OptiHealth's contract, and (7) lead a public relations campaign against OptiHealth so that subscribers and the public know the values upon which care is being rationed.

These actions should be pursued in order.

18

Managing Care for Seriously and Chronically Ill Children

CASE STUDY

CompleteCare Health System is a nonprofit integrated delivery system in a large East Coast city. Anne Lewis, the manager of Peerless Home Care, an operational division of CompleteCare Health System, has been told—as have all managers—to cut costs in her division, due to CompleteCare Health System's large financial losses during the last year. When a division manager is told to cut costs, the customary strategy is to identify and eliminate product lines that are losing money. Evaluating the cost-effectiveness of various home care product lines, Ms. Lewis's attention focused on the Pediatric High-Tech Home Care Program. This program offers skilled nursing care for pediatric home care clients with complex care needs, such as long-term tube-feeding and use of a ventilator. Most of these clients receive health care coverage through Medicaid. Their care often averages over eight hours a day and sometimes extends to twenty-four hours a day. Medicaid does not meet the full costs of caring for these clients. Consequently, in agreeing to service this special population, Peerless Home Care has been subsidizing some of the care given. While the costs associated with caring for these children continue to rise, there have been no commensurate increases in the level of reimbursement for services from Medicaid. The disparity between reimbursement rates and costs has continued to rise each year, vastly exceeding projected losses.

Ms. Lewis had a quality concern with this program as well: because it serviced a relatively small caseload, and the nursing care required was of such a specialized nature, Peerless Home Care could not continue to provide the quality of care required by this group of special needs clients without new financial outlays for nursing staff education. From the standpoint of improving her division's operating margin, Ms. Lewis was clear that she ought to terminate this expensive service line.

But Ms. Lewis was deeply troubled over this conclusion. Other providers in the area had already dropped pediatric high-tech home care, also for financial reasons, leaving highly vulnerable and needy clients without access to a sufficient contingent of providers. She worried that cutting the Pediatric High-Tech Home Care Program would constitute a kind of abandonment of these clients and their families. Moreover, some of CompleteCare Health System's health plan products included coverage for this specialized home care, and Peerless Home Care held contracts with other health plans to provide this service. If she decided to discontinue the program, the plan could well be selling coverage for specialized care that was not only unavailable through CompleteCare Health System's delivery system but possibly unavailable in the service area. This seemed to her to be a failure to live up to CompleteCare Health System's advertising slogan, "Quality health care services across the continuum of care."

Nevertheless, Ms. Lewis had her instructions: cut costs. From the system's perspective, her division could not continue to take such a hefty loss in one of its service lines. After being purchased by CompleteCare Health System and renamed, Peerless Home Care had become a significant locus of cost-shifting for the system. The care of expensive clients was often transferred to her division, and this led to increases in Peerless Home Care's expenses in other areas—for example, in educating nursing staff to service the more medically complex cases that were now being managed in home care rather than in the hospital. This disturbed Ms. Lewis because she had managed this home care organization as a freestanding operational unit very successfully for many years. The costs of operating this service line had always been successfully offset by gains in other service lines.

So from a system perspective, Peerless Home Care was saving CompleteCare Health System money. When the system evaluated the division's balance sheets, however, the division became a unit of analysis in isolation from its role in the system. The system asked simply: Is the division operating at an acceptable margin? How can the division cut costs so that it costs the system less? She felt the system could not have it both ways. Caught in the crossfire of two incompatible system objectives, Ms. Lewis felt compelled to decide that Peerless Home Care would get out of the business of pediatric high-tech home care so that it could meet the budget targets CompleteCare Health System had set for it. But how should Peerless Home Care deal with its twenty-one current clients?

Peerless Home Care could phase out the program by the relatively invisible strategy of not taking on new clients without discontinuing its existing clients; or it could continue to serve both existing and future clients through special time-limited contractual arrangements; or it could continue to provide services only for CompleteCare Health System's enrollees. Ms. Lewis felt CompleteCare Health System had an obligation to have pediatric high-tech home care services available for contracted enrollees of CompleteCare Health System, but not in perpetuity, given the financial losses it generated. She reasoned that Peerless Home Care could announce a new policy allowing the provision of these services for a maximum of six months, during which time Peerless Home Care would actively assist families in locating an appropriate provider. She hoped such alternative providers could be found.

Especially concerned about the families presently receiving pediatric high-tech home care services from Peerless Home Care, Ms. Lewis, members of her staff, and Peerless Home Care's ethics committee developed and implemented a complex, respectful approach to informing and eventually terminating families currently in the program. Within the constraints of her position and responsibility to the system, the approach ensured the continuation of quality services, the nonabandonment of these families, and the elimination of an overly costly program.

Each of the twenty-one families enrolled in the program was called about a certified letter they would receive that afternoon. The letter (1) informed them of the decision to terminate the Pediatric High-Tech Home Care Program within six months, (2) contained a list of other home care providers, (3) identified a staff person at Peerless Home Care who would work with them during their transition to another care provider, and (4) identified a management person they could contact with any questions. Letters were also sent, as appropriate, to the physicians, case managers, county social workers, and department heads serving affected clients/families. Also notified by letter were the CEOs, social workers, and case-workers of the three children's hospitals, which were the normal referral sources for these cases. Peerless Home Care also addressed its own employee issues, including the option of transferring its nurses to another home care agency so that they could continue with their established clients.

Despite the attention given to the process surrounding the transition of current families from the program, the decision generated such negative publicity for CompleteCare Health System in the news media that a high-level system executive reversed the manager's decision and called for a six-month moratorium and a thorough review of the matter. He subsequently announced that the program would be continued, because this exceedingly vulnerable group of clients and their families "should not be abandoned." He expressed the view that as a system, CompleteCare Health System had an obligation to serve them, despite the financial loss it incurred in doing so.

Questions for Consideration

➤ Does CompleteCare Health System have an ethical obligation to either current or future families to continue to provide these services despite its financial losses? Why?

➤ At what level of an integrated delivery system should decisions involving conflicts between care delivery obligations and business goals be made? By whom and by what process should they be made?

➤ Should CompleteCare Health System plan members be consulted for their views on using enrollment premiums to subsidize the Pediatric High-Tech Home Care Program? Why?

➤ How, ideally, might the needs of this vulnerable population be met? Is it realistic to think that our health care system as it is presently constituted can construct a provider arrangement that can manage the cost/quality issues effectively?

➤ Would it be equitable for a health care system to provide this expensive service to its own enrollees but to refuse to sell the service to other health plans for their enrollees?

➤ What obligation, if any, does CompleteCare Health System have to seek a solution to the unique needs of vulnerable populations not currently receiving cost-effective care?

COMMENTARY _____

Donald J. Brunnquell, Ph.D.

The case of Peerless Home Care's Pediatric High-Tech Home Care Program and the plight of children in our medical-industrial complex bring the deficiencies of the entire system into sharp relief. CompleteCare Health System and its subsidiary Peerless Home Care have reached decisions that betray their basic obligations to their members. The betrayal is doubly bitter because, in this case, those affected by such budget cuts are children, a group without direct political franchise, a group that has had no role in choosing a relationship with CompleteCare Health System and no direct voice in shaping that relationship.

The justice issues that lie at the core of this case and at the center of CompleteCare Health System's obligations are obscured by the organization's refusal to address them openly. They are hidden in cost-containment efforts and budget goals; no systematic effort is made to identify those who suffer harms or receive benefits. Questions of justice are pushed down to the level of an individual program and manager and, more poignantly, to the level of the individual child and family struggling to keep an intensive care unit running in their living room. The organization's inattention to the inherent conflicts of interest in its roles as insurer and provider cloud the picture further. Penetrating these layers of social and business ethics to get to the core justice questions is a complex but essential task.

Who Are These Children and Families?

To understand the decisions faced by Peerless Home Care, it is important to understand who is affected by the decisions. These are children with congenital and chronic conditions who require extensive but predictable nursing services that can, with considerable effort, be provided in their home. The children may be on a ventilator or require oxygen delivered in other ways. Many have tracheostomies or gastrostomies. Some receive total parenteral nutrition, that is, total intravenous feedings that are given through a central line, a catheter placed in a vessel near the heart. They frequently suffer from seizures or some degree of autonomic instability. They range from permanently comatose to profoundly delayed to developmentally normal, although many experience some developmental problems. Their problems often result from prematurity but may also stem from neurologic disease, cancer, or congenital heart disease.

Their families may be poor or affluent, chaotic or intact, unemployed or overworked, and isolated or well supported in their communities. No matter where the family begins, they are under extreme stress as a result of the intrusion of this service into their homes and lives. These families are frequently told by others, "I couldn't do what you are doing," and they often respond, "I'm just like you, and you would do this if you had to: there is no choice."

Children as a Special Population

That these patients are children undoubtedly affects the emotional response of many involved in the decision to drop this home care program. The CompleteCare Health System administrator's reversal of the decision, and the media's attention to the decision, reflect the immediate emotional response to denying resources to a vulnerable, dependent child. However, the legitimate moral weight the status of childhood should bear in decisions is much less clear.

The principle of respect for persons offers no reason to assign different moral status to children than to adults. However, while their status as children does not per se affect their moral worth, children are categorically vulnerable and dependent. One aspect of this vulnerability is their inability to understand, protect, and promote their own interests. This creates a special moral obligation on adults to protect children from decisions that compromise their interests.

A utilitarian approach that assesses aggregated harms and benefits may view children as categorically different, either because the length of time they may suffer harm or enjoy benefit is generally longer than in the case of adults or because they represent the continuation of human society. While such arguments may seem to give the advantage to children as compared to adults, the practical and political realities of childhood suggest otherwise. Children do not vote, have no clear voice in decisions, do not sign contracts, do not contribute to the bottom line of employers who mediate health insurance, and cannot independently access the appeals mechanisms of managed care organizations or the courts. These factors contribute to the likelihood that children's needs will be unrecognized or under-valued compared to the needs of those with political and practical power. For these reasons children deserve special protection in all systems, including the health insurance system.

Justice Issues

At every turn, questions of justice haunt the decisions about Peerless Home Care's Pediatric High-Tech Home Care Program. CompleteCare Health System allows a market-driven vision of distributive justice and a business analysis framework to determine its decisions concerning whether to subsidize this program. This analysis holds that the costs of the pediatric high-tech home care patients are unfairly borne by the other enrollees, whose premium costs are increased to pay for these patients. But this simplistic formulation misleads by ignoring many other distributive and procedural justice issues.

Political and regulatory policies support CompleteCare Health System's narrow vision of justice. CompleteCare Health System is allowed to hide distributive justice questions by targeting for contracts populations that typically have low health care costs. Regulatory decisions about the insurance industry allow health plans to shift home care costs to Medicaid before the patient reaches the contract's lifetime maximum benefit. That same political machinery then sets Medicaid reimbursement rates at levels that cannot support the necessary care, forcing CompleteCare Health System to either shift costs to other patients or not provide the service. Although families may believe that their insurance is in place to spread the cost of catastrophic medical care across the population, the political system allows insurers to ration care simply by declaring that they do not provide a service. In the end, policies shift the monetary and human costs of care to the siblings and parents of these catastrophically ill children.

The actions of CompleteCare Health System in this case also violate proce-dural justice. No mechanism exists to consider the claim of these children to resources against the claims of other groups. Asking a division manager who controls only a small part of the organization to decide eliminates fair consideration of alternatives. In short, both distributive and procedural justice questions are ignored by a health care system that supports high technology and acute interven-tions in the hospital setting such as the intensive care unit but does not recognize the obligation to do the same outside the hospital.

Any organization charged with providing health care faces these justice ques-tions or variants of them. They are not unique to managed care organizations.

Managed care organizations, however, have a greater potential to address them. If current regulatory avenues were closed to insurers—if, for example, they were not allowed to use scope-of-service definitions or targeted contracting to limit their populations or responses to health care needs—and if insurers were required to provide all care for all members up to the maximum of the contract, insurers would have to address these issues.

Health Care Organizations in a Competitive Environment

Market competition provides one account of justice. In a truly free and competitive market in which informed consumers have free choice, it may be possible to achieve this version of justice. The current competitive environment fails in many ways to meet the conditions necessary for market justice in relation to health care access and coverage. Because of historic disadvantages of certain groups, there is not equal opportunity to access health care. Given the specialized nature of the product, there is not even the possibility of full access to relevant information (Moreno 1996). Most consumers have no genuine choice of health plan or covered benefits. Managed care organizations achieve cost efficiency, in part, by restricting choice. Such compromises of consumer autonomy mean that the health insurance market operates imperfectly and therefore unjustly. Correctives to the market definition of justice are required to redress the failure of the market to promote an adequate health care environment.

The mixture of for-profit and nonprofit organizations and the lack of community dialogue or consensus on the goods to be pursued in health care reduce all of health care to a "bottom-line," cost-based competition in which neither the quality of services nor any goal beyond minimizing expenditure carries significant weight. Business unit analysis on a cost basis comes to drive decision making.

Such a business unit analysis of costly services stands in stark contrast to the stated goals of nonprofit systems like CompleteCare Health System and to the service provision portion of a for-profit company's mission. The service provision goals lose when confronted with cost-based goals of organizations struggling to compete with each other. When profits are thin for for-profit companies or when deficits accrue for nonprofits, business unit analysis of costly services emerges. High-tech home care is just one example of an expensive service that is part of the continuum of health care; treated as an individual business unit, it is likely to lose money.

Responsibilities of Integrated Delivery Systems

Nonprofit health care corporations rarely are clear about how to manage their dual roles of beneficent provider of a needed service and business competitor. Rather than being perceived as a necessary business expense or an obligation accepted by

Peerless Home Care as a cost of doing business, the financial loss in the Pediatric High-Tech Home Care Program is immediately understood to be siphoning resources away from other deserving patients. The accessibility and quality of services become secondary concerns as the nonprofit struggles to survive.

According to the case, Anne Lewis's division "became a unit of analysis in isolation from its role in the system." This situation reflects a common lack of clarity about priorities in health care. The organization has not articulated its stance regarding the core conflict within the supposedly integrated delivery system: an insurance function based on contractual obligations is asked to coexist with (and in fact given control over) a service function based on fiduciary obligations. Previously incompatible business and medical obligations (Mariner 1995) must now coexist in one organization.

The obligation of CompleteCare Health System to deliver what it explicitly agreed to in the contract with the purchaser conflicts with the obligation of Peerless Home Care to deliver what it and the families understand as a matter of duty and caring. This conflict of priorities is at the heart of the manager's dilemma. Instead of facing or resolving its organizational conflict, CompleteCare Health System has passed it to a manager. Ms. Lewis is asked to choose between her obligations to patients to provide a needed service and her obligations to the managed care organization to take part in an overall fiscal calculus to meet contractual obligations. The system shifts costs from the inpatient setting to her division by transferring patients whom she must accept, but her division is still required to maintain a positive bottom line.

Responsible Business Practices in Health Care

CompleteCare Health System has inappropriately asked an individual manager to take responsibility for an unresolved core organizational issue—not an unusual state of affairs when an organization finds itself caught in the conflict between its role as a competitor and its role as a provider. When top organizational leadership does not explicitly identify and deal with core issues, affected patients and families live through confusion, disarray, and reversals of decisions. In this scenario Ms. Lewis accepted or was forced to accept a task that should have been shouldered by the board of directors. That she involved her staff and ethics committee is in one sense admirable; in another, it only lends the appearance of legitimacy to a process that is misplaced. The highest level of any organization should make basic policy decisions that are open to public scrutiny regarding the balancing of business and care obligations. Especially in a nonprofit organization, problems like this one, which has implications for an entire class of patients, should at least be reported to the board before a final decision is made.

Such decisions are best located at the board level because, at least theoretically, it comprises members representing the community. Nonprofit organizations have tended increasingly to be dominated by business sector representatives, presumably because they bring business acumen and represent the purchasers of health care. This trend calls into question the degree to which the community is truly represented on such boards and, therefore, the moral legitimacy of the decisions reached "on behalf of the community."

Boards of directors should not be shielded from the human consequences of their decisions. Affected patients or families should be involved in the decision-making process, at least to provide the human face for the consequences of the decision. The presentation by a family affected by a decision to close the Pediatric High-Tech Home Care Program is information crucial to making a responsible decision. Without such information, which is often withheld from boards to promote their thinking as a business, a board or administrative team is not fully informed about the decision under consideration.

Justice and Decisions About Relative Benefit

Members expect that CompleteCare Health System will try to maximize benefit to those it serves, while society sanctions this expectation by conferring nonprofit status. Yet society continues to insist that allocation and justice must be addressed, while persistently avoiding the issue of how to do so. Decisions pass furtively to insurers; insurers quietly pass them to providers.

The logistic and ethical complexities of services such as home care suggest that a regular mechanism to address resource allocation issues is necessary (Arras 1995), especially given the emotional and proxy decision-making issues involved in a pediatric program. A user-provider-community advisory group can be carefully constructed to represent the many levels of information needed to reach valid decisions. Peerless Home Care apparently has an ethics committee, one model for such a mechanism, whose composition, authority, and voice within the organization are unclear but important.

Such a group would have both the knowledge and the moral legitimacy to contribute its analysis and recommendations concerning a system resource allocation issue to decision makers such as a board of directors, if a decision about terminating a program were under consideration.

A Process to Assess Justice Issues

Of course CompleteCare Health System must attend to fiscal issues; it must assess services in terms of resource use, benefit provided, and just allocation. Even without clear societal guidance, CompleteCare Health System must take action. In addition to the financial information typically used in program planning, it must gather information about the individual and aggregate impact of any decision and weigh it against its decision about alternative uses of its resources.

While in the end the CompleteCare Health System board of directors should affirm, if not make, the decision, many interim steps would add validity to the process. These steps might include:

1. The user-provider-community advisory group should obtain and consider information and make a recommendation. The group should identify the real impact of the decisions and what other options may exist besides closing the program altogether. Such a group will have greater credibility if it includes consensus leaders among those who oppose a decision to discontinue services.
2. The decision makers should discuss and agree in advance on the guidelines on which the decision will be based.
3. The decision must be made in the context of other resources available in the community, not limited to an examination of its impact on CompleteCare Health System. A decision to close the service would have a different practical impact and moral weight if there were an alternative provider available than if the community had no alternative. It must consider developing resources if none exist and involve the community in understanding what will happen if the resources are not made available.
4. Those affected must be given timely notice of impending decisions. The amount of time needed to find alternative services will vary with the situation and community, but implementing a plan within the few months that usually occur between an organization approving and implementing its budget is unreasonable.
5. CompleteCare Health System should articulate to the families involved in this decision who will make the decision and on what basis; it should also answer the question of how resource use is taken into account in other decisions about clinical care and business operations. This should be done in a public and open forum with key decision makers present. Complete honesty about the resource-based nature of the decision is required. CompleteCare Health System should not hide behind a facade of clinical criteria or force clinical providers to make decisions that are not clinical in nature. The decisions and the reasons for them should be transparent.

We Ignore Justice Issues at Our Own Peril

Bioethicists often contend that issues of resource allocation should not be decided at the bedside or in reference to an individual patient. At the same time our silence about resource allocation as a factor in decisions robs patients and their families of knowledge of the role it plays in their care. Since resource allocation is frequently a background issue influencing a patient's care, it should be raised explicitly by the provider in every case. This is ethically preferable as it will make the discussion clearer, if also more uncomfortable.

The case of Peerless Home Care's decision to terminate the Pediatric High-Tech Home Care Program demonstrates both the mechanisms and the risks of ignoring justice issues. The larger organization, CompleteCare Health System, ignored the justice issues at the administrative and board levels, as well as the question of how to balance the duties of meeting contracts and providing care. CompleteCare Health System identified only a fiscal issue and asked a midlevel manager to resolve it. The manager accepted or was forced to accept this role but was not empowered to raise and make a decision in light of the larger questions of justice involved. The members of the system and society at large were complicit in this arrangement—perhaps because of lack of understanding, perhaps because most of their own needs were currently met, perhaps because of their discomfort, perhaps because they feared that raising an explicit justice question would eventually affect their own care.

The irony of this silence lies in its hidden and unpredictable effects. Because none of us knows what health service we will need next, the injustice and irrationality of silence may affect us next. The courage to speak clearly about the needs and interests of ventilator-dependent, medically fragile children lying on their couches at home will in the end benefit us all.

References

Arras, J. D., ed. 1995. *Bringing the Hospital Home: Ethical and Social Implications of High-Tech Home Care.* Baltimore, Md.: Johns Hopkins University Press.
Mariner, W. K. 1995. "Business vs. Medical Ethics: Conflicting Standards for Managed Care." *Journal of Law, Medicine, and Ethics* 23, no. 3:236–46.
Moreno, J. D. 1996. "Recapturing Justice in the Managed Care Era." *Cambridge Quarterly of Healthcare Ethics* 5, no. 4:493–99.

COMMENTARY

Susan B. Rubin, Ph.D.
Laurie Zoloth-Dorfman, Ph.D.

To responsibly evaluate managed care, it is necessary to offer a balanced nuanced analysis, taking into account managed care's goals and intentions, the extent to which it is an ethically defensible model for the distribution of health care services, the extent to which it succeeds or fails in responding to fundamental concerns compared to alternative models of health care, and, finally, the *realpolitik* of existing managed care systems. Managed care can offer an important corrective to the excesses of fee-for-service medicine and a legitimate response to justice concerns (Zoloth-Dorfman and Rubin 1995). But in practice managed care is not without its problems.

The challenge when presented with cases of ethical dilemmas in managed care is to ascertain whether the concerns they represent are created by managed care per se or whether they would inevitably arise in any system of health care. Ethical dilemmas abound in health care today regarding real issues of justice, accessibility, accountability, safety, and quality.

For example, all systems of health care must face questions about the fair prioritization and allocation of aggregate resources. And underlying every allocation decision is a presumption about what we owe one another when we cannot all have what we might want or need. In evaluating any resultant allocation decision, the issue is not that limitations are set, or that difficult choices have to be made about how to allocate collective resources. The issue rather is what processes are in place to guide such decision making, what mechanisms are established to ensure that those most impacted by such decisions have a voice in the process, and what criteria are established prospectively to evaluate and weigh competing claims. When a managed care case involving such decisions is presented, it is necessary to consider the extent to which the particularities of managed care prompt a different response to these traditional concerns.

The Mandate to Cut Costs: A Case in Point and a Familiar Dilemma

Anne Lewis, the manager of Peerless Home Care, faces a challenge familiar to managers in a variety of health care systems across the country: how can her budget be fairly allocated while taking into account the needs of specific patient populations and important commitments to justice, duty, and fidelity. We can explore Ms. Lewis's dilemma from at least three key vantage points. First, questions of the nature and scope of our collective responsibility to care for one another and broad macrosocietal issues of justice need to be addressed. Second, at the more microsystem level, the distinctive justice concerns that arise in the distribution of a single system's aggregate internal resources must be addressed. What is owed to specific patient populations, particularly in light of promises that have been made, benefits packages that have been agreed to, and stewardship responsibilities that have been accepted? Third, the need for developing a credible and sustainable process of ethical reflection and decision making at the organizational level must be addressed. Consideration should be given to the organization's mission, core values, and fiduciary obligations, as well as the parameters within which the potentially conflicting imperatives of business and ethics will be pursued. And questions should be raised about those empowered to make difficult decisions, specifically the possibility and necessity of exercising independent moral agency within the constraints of a staff, managerial, or executive role.

Facing the Justice Question at the Societal Level

Most families with high-level home care needs ultimately need outside assistance. With the average hourly rates for caregivers beginning at $15 per hour, and care needs ranging from eight to twenty-four hours per day, the minimum cost of just receiving such care at home ranges from $43,800 to $131,400 per year. And of course as the level of skilled care needs rises, so does the cost.

The system as currently constructed is not designed to provide comprehensive care to all who need it under a system of universal coverage. Rather, we have acknowledged instead a much more modest societal obligation. As a society we fund care only when financial resources fall below a certain threshold and medical need exceeds a certain level.

Patients with long-term medical needs are put at risk when the level of services we are collectively willing to subsidize falls short of their actual needs, particularly when we have contracted with individual health plans to provide care that they can just as easily decide to discontinue. At this level, the situation CompleteCare Health System faces is of our own collective creation. Peerless Home Care's clients presumably had an initial choice of vendors for their care. And at a certain point CompleteCare Health System probably competed for its share of Medicaid clients, attracted by the stable and guaranteed reimbursement source. But as so often is the case, care costs increased faster than reimbursement and CompleteCare Health System found itself subsidizing the care of patients in the home care program. This raises significant questions of justice that are only potentiated by the fact that CompleteCare Health System's competitors have discontinued high-tech pediatric home care because it is too costly.

Rather than letting marketplace considerations exclusively drive such decisions, a more just solution would be to identify the kinds of services particularly vulnerable patient populations such as chronically ill children are likely to need and to fashion a communitywide response that would be reflective of our shared values and goals. So, for example, rather than forcing individual health plans to disproportionately shoulder the burden of providing high-cost needed care, all plans could be required to contribute to a common pool of funds that the community could earmark for such care. This would be fairer to each health plan, and it would prompt us to engage in necessary prospective conversations about our shared values and priorities.

The reality of uncovered need, the problem of reliance on private industry to subsidize care, and the question of our collective responsibility to care for the most vulnerable raise significant questions from the perspective of ethics. Even in an expansive health care system in which every citizen is guaranteed universal access to a basic decent minimum of health care, priorities have to be set and choices have to be made. The dilemma faced by managers struggling to operate within ever-tighter budgetary constraints is a microcosm of this larger and unavoidable problem.

In general, we have been woefully unwilling to develop a coherent, systematic approach to the societal problem of justice. We have settled instead for incremental, piecemeal adjustments that fail to address the larger questions. Managed care becomes an easy target in this context because it refocuses our attention on this ubiquitous challenge; but it is a challenge we would face in any system.

Facing the Justice Question at the Health Plan Level

When individual health plans like CompleteCare Health System react to the financial constraints by simply mandating cost-cutting, it is reasonable to question the necessity and legitimacy of their response. We might begin by considering what factors contributed to CompleteCare Health System's financial losses. We might seek a careful assessment of the system's expenditures on patient care, bureaucratic infrastructure, corporate offices, and compensation of top executives. Excesses or waste, once corrected, can potentially lead to better balanced costs and expenditures and make it possible to avoid dramatic cuts in services. We would want to ensure that the full range of options was considered. Rather than focusing exclusively on cost reduction, we wonder whether CompleteCare Health System has considered increasing its revenue base by instituting or raising copayments, raising premium rates, seeking to negotiate higher rates of reimbursement, or recruiting new members.

In some instances, even if such questions and alternatives are pursued, there may still be a need to cut costs. In this case, a host of questions can be raised about how a responsible organization should proceed and how it should direct its managers to proceed. Often, as in this case, the unfortunate decision is made to decentralize the deliberative process, charging managers with the entire responsibility of fixing an organization's financial problems. A far more defensible approach would be to determine at the outset what the system's overall goals, priorities, and obligations are and what potential changes in its services would be acceptable to the membership it serves. If health care organizations addressed the challenge of reducing their costs in a comprehensive rather than fragmented fashion, they would arrive at far more coherent and defensible solutions. If they also involved their membership in the process, organizations would reaffirm their sense of commitment and accountability to those they serve.

One popular approach to cost-cutting in large health care systems is to mandate an across-the-board percentage budget decrease of say 10 percent. Each department is treated equally without regard to the services it provides or the patients it serves and must adjust its budget accordingly. Some favor this approach because it treats all departments equally. But such an approach is flawed because it fails to take into account the range of services provided, the actual needs and priorities of the membership, and the needs of the most vulnerable patients. A more defensible approach would address the system's and membership's priorities directly, considering the relative weight that should be given to different services and different patient populations.

Across-the-board budget reduction proposals also fail to take into account the roles various divisions serve in an integrated system. If there is significant cost-shifting between departments, mandating an equal budgetary reduction across all departments would unfairly penalize those that absorb the cost of providing care for the most expensive clients while rewarding those that successfully avoid such costly clients.

Once the decision is made to reduce costs, questions about how to identify and select cost-cutting criteria must be addressed. When difficult decisions must be made, especially in large systems that serve a diverse membership, it is often suggested that providing the greatest number of needed services to the greatest number of people might be the fairest solution. It is a familiar utilitarian tactic to compare the good that could be accomplished by providing prenatal care to all pregnant women, for example, to providing other kinds of treatments such as organ transplants or ongoing care to patients in a persistent vegetative state. It is typical as well to rely on a cost-benefit analysis for guidance about the best course of action.

In any utilitarian scenario, however, eliminating programs on the grounds that they fail to provide the greatest good to the greatest number of people, or that their cost does not justify their benefit, raises the persistent problem of how to protect the interests of the minority. In the final analysis, maintaining programs that operate at a financial loss might nonetheless be the right thing to do. On what grounds? Often it is a matter of fidelity and the simple obligation to fulfill contractual obligations. When health plans sell products with coverage for specialized care, they have an obligation to make it available. Contractual agreements do not typically include a provision that needed care can be discontinued when necessary to save the organization money. And there might be moral obligations beyond those articulated in the contract.

Health systems should be judged by how they treat their most vulnerable and needy members. Apart from the specific claims of fidelity and contractual obligations, health care organizations assume fiduciary obligations that set them apart from other commercial businesses. At the very least, they have a distinctive obligation to consider the health and well-being of their constituents and to protect the neediest among them.

Developing a Process for Ethical Reflection at the Organizational Level

Finally, any health care system can be evaluated by examining the decision-making processes it has in place. At this level many organizations fail dismally. Despite greater emphasis in recent years on ethics at the levels of both patient care and organizational operation, much remains to be done to better integrate ethics throughout the operations of health care organizations. Health care organizations should understand the importance of articulating their underlying mission and core values, be in the practice of evaluating their options in that context, and have in place a meaningful organizational process of ethical reflection and decision making. By decentralizing decision making and failing to frame the challenge of cost-cutting as an ethical dilemma in need of collective discussion and reflection, CompleteCare Health System not only neglected to give its managers a broader frame of reference within which to operate, it also obviated the possibility of developing a comprehensive approach to the problem of fairly distributing limited resources across a varied client base. A far better approach would have been to engage the membership in a dialogue with staff and managers about their shared goals and priorities.

CompleteCare Health System has responsibilities of stewardship to its membership to use their collective resources wisely and fairly. But ultimately it is the members themselves whose lives and care will be most affected by the organization's allocation decisions, and their voice and perspective should be represented in the process. Decisions might still be made to eliminate certain programs, but different approaches to cost-cutting might be suggested, or other options might be identified. In any event, ensuring the membership a voice in the process would affirm the organization's accountability and add credence to whatever solutions were ultimately endorsed.

Health care organizations have a responsibility to set up viable processes for such ongoing discussion and decision making. One option is to expand the role of ethics committees to encompass issues of organizational and business ethics. Just as ethics committees can be available for consultation on a dilemma in the context of patient care, so too could they be available when managers, executives, or systems at large face dilemmas of cost-cutting and the fair allocation of funds. But rather than consulting the ethics committee as Ms. Lewis did to endorse and help implement a decision that had already been made, consultations should be sought earlier by key decision makers and stakeholders.

The Role of Independent Moral Agency

It is striking that managers frequently choose to substantially reduce services or eliminate programs against their better judgment. This raises significant questions about the role of independent moral agency. On the one hand, it is easy to sympathize with the plight of thoughtful managers facing difficult dilemmas. While they might like to continue providing maximal care to all clients in need, they know that might not be either viable or responsible from a financial perspective. From an ethical perspective, managers should be judged not only by the ultimate decision they make but also by the process by which they arrive at their decisions. Do managers feel they can let themselves be informed or guided by their own independent sense of what is morally right? Or do they feel compelled simply to perform their managerial duties and follow orders?

Remarkably few managers lobby for any genuine alternatives to cutbacks. Most struggle internally with their reservations but fail to voice their concerns either to those in power or to those who will be imminently affected. Do they not think there are any real viable options, or do they feel powerless to effect such changes? Given that managers could fight harder to ensure protection for vulnerable patient populations, that they could resist cost-cutting mandates, that they could attempt to mobilize the patient populations at risk, that they could leak threats of cutbacks to the press, or that they could even quit rather than be in a position to deny care to patients who they feel clearly need and deserve it, we must wonder what impact these cost-cutting decisions actually have on managers in similar situations across the country. The pressures to respond to the needs of organizations struggling to stay afloat in this competitive health care marketplace have posed serious challenges to personal and professional integrity. It is a reality that must be addressed at both the system and individual level if individuals are to remain engaged and committed to doing this important work.

Ironically, managers often lack the ultimate authority to implement their decisions. Once Ms. Lewis made her decision, for example, a top executive intervened and reinstated the program in response to public outcry. We cannot know what motivates such executives—the power of a publicity backlash or the sincere conclusion that despite financial concerns they have an obligation to continue serving a vulnerable patient population. We do know that every time a manager's decision is overturned in response to pressure, we get a glimpse once again into how fragmented and incoherent an organization's approach to cost-cutting can be.

It is a familiar phenomenon in health care policy that we tend to be more captivated and motivated by the particular patients or populations that make their needs loudly or forcefully known than by our knowledge of the aggregate but less immediately visible need that surrounds us everyday. This has advantaged more politically active and savvy patients but disadvantaged others, leading to concern about patients who may be profoundly affected by cost-cutting but are unable to effectively make their case, or about those who lack insurance and are outside the system altogether. Surely the reinstatement of a single program in response to negative publicity does not stand as the best example of how we ought to address concerns of justice at the individual, system, or national level.

What is needed in cases like these is more direct consideration of the essential questions of justice and a more responsible, comprehensive, meaningful process within which the moral issues at stake can be identified and addressed. We need to face squarely questions of what we owe one another and how we can make good decisions about distributing our inevitably limited resources. And we need to acknowledge that these are questions not about managed care as such but about how to live well together.

References

Zoloth-Dorfman, L., and Rubin, S. 1995. "The Patient as Commodity: Managed Care and the Question of Ethics." *The Journal of Clinical Ethics* 6, no. 4:339–57.

PART SIX

Responsibilities to the Community

19

Health Plan Responsibilities for Public Health Activities

CASE STUDY

The 1994 MinnesotaCare Act, building on the state's comprehensive health reform legislation of the previous two years, requires health plan companies (that is, HMOs and other managed care organizations) to contribute to the achievement of public health goals for their respective service areas. The act further requires health plan companies to collaborate with local public health units and other community organizations providing health services in the same geographic area. These requirements are designed to reinforce the renewed emphasis in Minnesota's health care system on protecting and advancing the health of populations.

After a series of meetings that brought together key leaders from managed care organizations and public health organizations in Minnesota to explore opportunities for collaboration, the West Metro Workgroup, one of the three groups that emerged from these meetings, sought in 1995 to identify and design interventions for a public health issue on the west side of the Twin Cities metro area. From the outset, Workgroup members raised a number of issues (which have yet to be resolved) regarding the state-mandated public health initiatives. For example, many sought a clearer definition of the target population, noting that while public health organizations focus on communities defined by geographic boundaries, managed care organizations focus on their enrolled population, and at times on a broader but still indeterminate "community." In addition, the managed care representatives voiced concern that the state's requirement for collaborative public health initiatives did not apply to indemnity insurers or to the self-insured segment of the market.

By applying the criteria the Workgroup had itself established for selecting an initial collaborative project (for example, suitability for joint private-public initiative; effectiveness of proposed intervention; measurability), the Workgroup agreed on a pilot project to increase hepatitis B immunizations for adolescents in selected sites in the west metro area. To further the collaborative reach of this pilot, the Workgroup contacted schools in the area. Ultimately, five schools participated. The stated objective was that at its completion, the pilot project "will have improved the accessibility to appropriate primary and preventive health services, and providers will [have been] adequately reimbursed for their services."

School administrators and staff actively supported the project and helped publicize it, and they educated their students on the risks of hepatitis B and the benefits of the vaccine. Immunizations were given at the participating schools by nurses from a local hospital who volunteered their time, since school nurses did not have the time to give the immunizations themselves. Nearly five hundred students completed the three-dose vaccination series, and the Workgroup notified the student's primary care provider, if known, after the series was completed.

The managed care organizations participating in this project (three managed care plans, representing over 80 percent of the local managed care market) provided funding for the pilot. A formula that reflected roughly each plan's market share in the west metro area was used to set the plans' respective contributions. The funding covered the cost of the vaccine and related services for insured and uninsured students alike, but it did not pay for the time of the nurses, Workgroup participants, and school staff, all of which was provided without charge. Representatives from the managed care organizations noted, however, that by paying for the immunizations for students who were already covered through capitated arrangements (which are meant to cover the cost of all care provided to enrollees), the organizations were in effect paying for the services twice. Workgroup members agreed that appropriate funding for similar joint public-private projects in the future is a major unresolved issue. They also agreed not to pursue any additional projects until this and other unresolved issues are addressed.

Questions for Consideration

➤ To what extent, if any, should managed care organizations contribute to traditional public health goals?

➤ To what extent, if any, should managed care organizations address the (public) health needs of nonenrollee populations, such as the uninsured? Do managed care organizations inherit the obligation historically recognized by physicians and hospitals to provide charity care?

➤ What "community" should managed care organizations serve?

➤ When, if ever, is collaboration between private and public health organizations an appropriate strategy for addressing public health goals? What does "collaboration" mean in this context? What should each side bring to the table?

➤ How should public-private initiatives to promote public health goals be financed?

COMMENTARY

Mila Ann Aroskar, R.N., Ed.D., F.A.A.N.

Funding for joint public-private projects is an unresolved issue in this case. No further collaborative projects will be pursued until funding and other issues are addressed: a seeming impasse. The situation in this case offers an opportunity to reflect on the distribution of responsibilities for meeting public health goals in the context of an existing legal mandate in states such as Minnesota (MinnesotaCare Act of 1994). Health plan companies, including HMOs and other managed care organizations, must submit a plan showing how they will assist in achieving public health goals. The legislation also requires collaboration among managed care organizations, local public health units, and other community health service organizations in the same geographic area.

The legal mandate and experience with this case provide an opportunity for public and private sector decision makers to think more proactively about the background issues and challenges presented by required collaborative efforts. This commentary points to ethical underpinnings for the legal mandate and reviews four background considerations that require attention in order to ensure future collaboration and sharing of responsibilities between the public and private sectors to achieve public health goals.

Three sources provide ethical support for public-private collaboration to meet society's health goals. Conclusions drawn by the President's Commission for the Study of Ethical Problems in Medicine and Biomedical and Behavioral Research (1983) in the report entitled *Securing Access to Health Care* serve as one source. These conclusions were cast in the language of ethical obligations rather than rights—the language used in the 1952 report by the President's Commission on the Health Needs of the Nation. The earlier commission viewed access to the means of attaining and preserving health as a basic human right. Over thirty years later a newly constituted president's commission concluded instead that "society has an ethical obligation to ensure equitable access to health care for all." Further, the commission concluded that "the ultimate responsibility for ensuring that society's obligation is met, through a combination of public and private sector arrangements, rests with the federal government." Private health care providers and insurers, charitable organizations, and local and state governments were all viewed as having a role in meeting this ethical obligation. The commission further concluded that efforts to contain health care costs are important, but that it would be morally unacceptable to expect the least well served or the most vulnerable populations, such as children, to suffer the negative consequences of these efforts.

A second source of ethical support for collaborative efforts and responsibilities may be drawn from the ethical principle of respect for persons. This principle emphasizes both respect for individual autonomy and self-determination *and* respect for persons as interconnected members of the human community. The distinction between the public and private sectors may serve some social purposes, but dividing them from each other and treating them separately runs roughshod over the interrelatedness and interdependence of human beings and the complex social as well as individual variables that influence health.

A third source is the ethical theory known as communitarianism. Communitarian theory holds that what makes something "right" derives from communal values, the common good, cooperation, and social goals (Beauchamp and Childress 1994). Social solidarity is central to this theoretical perspective; it is another way to talk about the interconnectedness and interdependence of individuals and organizations. Ethical commitments to cooperative values, to equitable access to health care, and to health care as a unifying rather than a divisive social force contrast sharply with a focus on individual autonomy, rights, and economic goals. Communitarian views may transform public-private sector discussions of obligations and responsibilities, including funding distributions, when decision makers deliberate about collaborative projects.

The Minnesota legislation provides a legal mandate to launch the public-private discussions necessary to develop collaborative health projects and policies that reflect society's ethical obligations. This case also points to background considerations in which intertwined ethical, legal, economic, and political factors require new social arrangements and structures as means to reach public health goals.

Background Considerations

Clarification and resolution of the issue of funding for joint public-private health initiatives require (1) engaging in ethics and politics, that is, paying explicit attention to the conflicting interests and values of both individuals and organizations, (2) establishing an operational definition of community by affected decision makers and stakeholders, (3) agreeing on overall goals and funding mechanisms for public-private initiatives prior to embarking on collaborative projects, and (4) establishing a more inclusive process for making major decisions about collaborative projects that incorporates attention to ethical values and concerns. Failure to reach some level of resolution, or at least recognition of the importance of these four background considerations, may lead to continued frustration and failure to provide important services to vulnerable populations, among them the uninsured.

Consideration I: Engaging in Ethics and Politics

Ordinarily ethics and politics are considered two separate domains. In real-life situations such as this case, however, ethics and politics share common elements for decision makers and policy developers striving to do the right thing in the midst of institutional power struggles and a highly competitive health care environment. The situation presented in this case can be described as ethical by virtue of the following characteristics. First, there is conflict or confusion about the public and private sectors' duties, obligations, and interests; second, ethical principles or values are at stake, among them, fairness and prevention of harm; and finally, a broad-based discussion is needed in order to develop a way to fund joint health projects and respond to other issues.

While medical ethical issues tend to focus on individuals, the work of developing institutional policy or public policy, such as engaging in ethics on behalf of populations or the public, is quite different. Politics, understood here as "doing public ethics," is involved because the situation concerns conflicting interests/values and power issues beyond individual interests (Aroskar 1993). These are interests and conflicts that affect the welfare of the public and public-private sector organizations themselves. Furthermore, the situation deals with ethical relations among, and the respective powers and duties of, governmental bodies and private health care systems. A response must include attention to the complex and conflicting relationships between these two sectors.

Thus, the issue of public-private funding involves paying attention to ethical concerns *and* to politics for the sake of doing what is right for individuals, for organizations, and for the public as one aspect of negotiation and compromise in decision making and policy development. This requires reflection, use of moral imagination, and a socially oriented vision of what is possible. The successful effort, in this case, to develop a public-private venture to immunize adolescents reflects a transformed vision of what can be done to achieve measurable health goals in the interests of individuals and the public good, even though issues such as funding remain.

Consideration II: Operational Definition of Community Served

The language of community needs further discussion as part of determining funding responsibilities. The case indicates that the identification of what constitutes a "community" is somewhat indeterminate; it probably means something more than a "geographic area." A brief exploration of the concept of community clarifies why managed care organizations (and others) may have difficulty in determining exactly what is meant when the language of community is invoked. The need to clarify this term becomes more urgent when the mission of the organization includes language about meeting the needs of its members *and* the community, and the organization must establish priorities and fund specific activities.

Attention must be paid to the function or purpose the language of community is expected to serve when both managed care organizations and public health agencies use it. Managed care may use it only to recognize that individual members come from and return to a community that the organization acknowledges as its relevant "service area." However, the organization should be concerned about the wider community and its environment, since they influence the health of plan members.

Public health agencies also become involved in situations where the community for which the agency is responsible is not easy to define solely in terms of geographic boundaries; this becomes clear when an outbreak of disease crosses city, county, or state lines. However, a public health agency's funding sources often dictate the community or geopolitical area to be served; this is not the case for managed care organizations.

Clues as to how the community of concern for a public-private collaborative project might be defined operationally are found in concepts of community that go beyond the idea of a geographic community. Managed care organizations may select one or more different components in constructing their definition of community. Decision makers should also realize that the language of community could, and possibly should, shift for different purposes. Thus, creation of an operational definition of community may help resolve some of the quandaries related to equitable funding distributions for public-private projects.

A general concept of community denotes a group of individuals organized into some type of unit, sharing a unifying trait, or linked by common interests and goals (Aroskar 1995a). The "west metro area" of this case could constitute a community linked by common interests and goals for a specific purpose, that is, to increase hepatitis B immunizations and preventive health services for adolescents. This way of defining community operationally provides a rationale, with identified objectives and criteria, for a specific decision—at the same time, recognizing that not all would agree with this conceptualization of a community for all purposes or under different circumstances.

The concept of "community of solution" is sometimes used to develop responses to health problems that cross the geopolitical boundaries of a single town, city, or state (Institute of Medicine 1988). Professional experience and available data dictate that often, more than one type of organization and level of government must "own" a problem and work cooperatively to achieve resolution through comprehensive programming and funding. Developing an adequate response to the risk of hepatitis B infection is only one example among others, such as prevention of HIV infection, treatment of an unsafe drinking water supply, or dealing with dangerous air pollutants. Adopting the view of "community of solution" emphasizes inclusion of a variety of different types of organizations or levels of government in order to achieve health goals and provides a "fit" with the legal and ethical mandates for public-private collaboration.

Consideration III: Goals and Priorities

Despite agreement to pursue a specific project, the differing goals of public health and managed care may have played a role in the funding issue that developed in the hepatitis B project. The conflict in this situation points to the need for a more proactive or preventive approach by addressing overlapping and differing goals of the public and private sectors as part of program development, rather than waiting until the program has been implemented. The achievement of public health goals, undergirded by ethical values of personal and collective responsibility and social justice concerns, has generally been associated with public, that is, government, support. That is now changing, as evidenced by this case.

Public health goals overlap but also go beyond those of managed care organizations. They focus on the public good and include protection and promotion of health and prevention of disease and premature death. The overall mission of public health is to fulfill society's interest in ensuring the conditions in which people can be healthy through organized community efforts that include private individuals and organizations and public (governmental) agencies (Institute of Medicine 1988). This mission includes both personal health and environmental health, which is concerned with health-related issues such as air quality, safe food supplies, safe drinking water, and safety in the workplace. While current health policy development focuses on provision of personal health services, environmental health services must also be attended to in health policy development and funding. Both influence human health and compete for societal resources with other institutions, such as education, corrections, and defense.

Managed care goals of cost control and efficiency sometimes seem to upstage other stated goals, such as provision of quality care for members and concerns for the health of populations and communities. In short, public and private sector decision makers are often focused on different goals when they sit down to discuss funding collaborative projects. This may become an unrecognized source of conflict.

Another ethical concern has to do with who is at the decision-making table when health goals and priorities are established (for example, representatives of public health agencies and managed care organizations) and who is absent from the table (for example, the self-insured segment of the market or members of minority groups). More inclusive processes to identify goals and priorities in health programming are urgently needed. More inclusive public-private collaboration to achieve society's health goals is supported by the president's commission and by ethical theory and values. All organizations involved in or even concerned about achieving public health goals have ethical obligations to work more cooperatively to provide resources toward that end.

Consideration IV: Comprehensive Decision-Making Process

A decision-making process that incorporates consideration of ethical values and principles can be used prospectively, as an explicit part of deciding, for example, how to fund collaborative efforts. It can also be used retrospectively, to evaluate an existing policy or program for its attention to or neglect of ethical concerns. Both uses might be viewed as the practice of preventive ethics at different points in the development and evaluation of collaborative policies.

The case indicates that a "formula" was developed for pilot funding by the participating plans. What we do not know is what went into development of this formula. The process presented here suggests areas that need to be addressed in developing a more comprehensive, ethically reasoned "formula" for making decisions about collaborative public-private funding (Aroskar 1995b). Elements that require attention include: (1) What are the "facts" of the situation (for example, community- or population-based needs to be addressed, legal requirements, and required resources, such as professional expertise and funding)? (2) Who are the affected parties (including individuals, populations at risk, public and private organizations, or defined communities) and how are they included in decision making? (3) What are the relevant ethical issues or conflicts (such as respect for organizational integrity and goals vis-à-vis fairness in distribution of funding for collaborative projects, or maintaining privacy of data to enhance competitive advantage vis-à-vis access to the data required for collaborative health projects)? (4) What are possible options for action and their ethical justification? (5) What are the foreseeable political, social, and economic consequences of options for action? (6) What recommendation or set of recommendations can be developed for implementation? Once these questions have been responded to, (7) action can be taken. Finally, (8) outcomes must be evaluated for use in future decision-making situations.

While consideration of these elements in a decision-making process does not guarantee a single correct or "right" response, it may rule out sometimes regrettable decisions or policies that might (and sometimes do) occur without such reflection. Paying attention to these decision-making elements enhances the possibilities for developing collaborative public-private health projects, including funding decisions, that respect affected parties and stakeholders, prevent identifiable harms, and spread costs more fairly.

In summary, it may be possible to overcome the current funding impasse in collaborative public-private efforts by paying explicit attention to community-oriented ethical values and key background considerations: the need to take into account ethical as well as political concerns for individuals and organizations, populations, and the public; the challenges of defining community; the requirement to clarify goals and priorities; and the need to develop more comprehensive and inclusive decision-making processes. Public-private efforts to move together toward achieving public health goals are not an impossible dream—not if we can develop transformed visions of what is possible and find the will to do so. One positive outcome of this case is that people of goodwill from the public and private sectors have identified important issues that need further work in order to share responsibilities for meeting public health goals—an ethical and legal mandate.

References

Aroskar, M. A. 1993. "Ethical Issues: Politics, Power, and Policy." In *Policy and Politics for Nurses*, 2d ed., pp. 200–207. Edited by D. J. Mason, S. W. Talbott, and J. K. Leavitt. Philadelphia: W.B. Saunders.

———. 1995a. "Envisioning Nursing as a Moral Community." *Nursing Outlook* 43, no. 3:134–38.

———. 1995b. "Exploring Ethical Terrain In Public Health." *Journal of Public Health Management and Practice* 1, no. 3:16–22.

Beauchamp, T. L., and Childress, J. F. 1994. *Principles of Biomedical Ethics*, 4th ed. New York: Oxford University Press, pp. 77–85.

Institute of Medicine. 1988. *The Future of Public Health*. Washington, D.C.: National Academy Press.

President's Commission for the Study of Ethical Problems in Medicine and Biomedical and Behavioral Research. March 1983. *Securing Access to Health Care*. Volume One: Report. Washington, D.C.: U.S. Government Printing Office, pp. 4–5.

COMMENTARY

Gayle Hallin, R.N., M.P.H.

This case explores the ethical responsibility of managed care organizations to society, with particular attention to their responsibility to address public health issues. How this public health responsibility is defined is affected by the prevailing health care ethic, which values individual good over common good. Health care ethics should expand its individualistic orientation to incorporate a public health perspective with its orientation of promoting the well-being of the whole population. Infusing health into health care reform requires combining the principles and goals of public health with the traditional health care reform elements of quality, access, and financing. The current trend to achieve reform through managed care models affords an opportunity to link public health goals with those of the health care delivery system.

It is often stated that if one wants to truly understand values, one should look at budgets. They are the concrete reflection of values. In the United States, the disparity between the investment in health care and the investment in public health is huge. In 1993, the "total national expenditures for population-based public health activities were estimated to be less than 1 percent of aggregate health care spending in the United States" (U.S. Department of Health and Human Services 1993). Adding the estimated allocation for preventive health care brings the collective national investment for prevention and public health to 3 percent of our total health expenditures. Something is very wrong with these proportions when we take into account that 70 percent of our health care expenditures are estimated to be related to preventable conditions (Fries et al. 1993).

The fee-for-service health care system has contributed to this disparity between resources directed to the treatment of individuals and those directed to the health of the population. The United States continues to spend more on health care than any other nation, yet it has both a growing number of uninsured citizens and a widening disparity in health status. This becomes clear in a state like Minnesota, where health status and life expectancy *averages* rank Minnesotans number one in the nation. Yet, Minnesota ranks poorly on many indicators of health status of populations of color (Minnesota Department of Health 1997). It is clear that a marketplace driven by short-term financial incentives will not lead us to social responsibility in caring for the health of the whole population.

The prevailing perspective of public health is varied governmental health services for the poor combined with protection from infectious disease and environmental hazards. The 1988 Institute of Medicine report, *The Future of Public Health*, defines public health as "what we, as a society, do collectively to assure the conditions for people to be healthy." Here public health is understood as a shared responsibility, requiring both strength in the governmental public health system and a contribution by the entire community. Such a "shared contribution" model of public health, where both public and private sectors have important roles, suggests that the expertise and resources of the private health care system can be leveraged in making progress on public health goals. At the same time, core governmental functions and funding remain essential. The shared contribution model requires a healthy governmental public health system to provide effective leadership with respect to public health priorities. While the Minnesota legislative requirement for managed care organizations to contribute to public health goals is a significant policy mechanism for engaging partnership between these organizations and the public health system, it does not define their specific priorities, responsibilities, or financial expectations.

This case highlights a variety of conditions that affect the contribution of managed care organizations when working collaboratively on public health goals and the needs of special populations. It presents a clear intersection of interests between the public and private health sectors, lifting up basic issues of justice, access to health care, and beneficence; giving specificity to the challenges of defining goals, responsibilities, and economics in the collaboration of the public and private sectors regarding shared population-based health interests; and providing insight into the elements necessary to create systemic change in the best interests of the health of the community.

Three Central Ethical Issues

Beneficence is a dominant ethical issue. Hepatitis B among adolescents is both spreading and preventable. As a communicable disease, it is of significance to the individual, public, providers, and payers. From a public health perspective, individual health care that contributes to the good of many has a higher priority than health care that has value for only one. Hepatitis B immunizations are clearly a shared common good to be achieved by protecting adolescents from this disease through a vaccination program combined with education for personal responsibility. As a communicable disease, protection of the individual also achieves a higher public good by reducing the incidence of disease in the whole population and the cost of treatment incurred by both the public and private sectors.

Access to health care is a second relevant ethical issue. Selecting adolescents as the focus for this project is in itself significant, as adolescent health care has fallen through the cracks in our health care system. It has not had the profitability of areas dominated by high technology. Adolescents are often alienated from traditional medical practice, which expects patients to meet practitioners on their turf, at their time, and on their terms. Adolescent health services consist primarily of acute care, sports physicals, and community-based reproductive health clinics. Schools and community clinics fill the void left by a health care system that recognizes little obligation toward those whom it does not see. While managed care organizations have begun to measure success in delivering preventive services, such as immunizations, annual changes in enrollment often make it difficult for providers to monitor their success in reaching an adolescent population with three separate vaccines over a six-month period.

In this scenario, justice, a third relevant ethical issue, has two dimensions. Consider first the subpopulation of adolescents. The marketplace rather than the principle of distributive justice currently determines how health care premium dollars are allocated. Until adolescents or their advocates raise their voices, resources are not likely to be directed toward their needs. This case describes alternative means to offset the failure of the current health care system to deal effectively with population-based health needs of adolescents.

The second dimension of the ethical issue of justice arises with the question of who has ongoing responsibility to pay for care provided outside the medical delivery system. It is relatively easy to get financial contributions from multiple partners for a demonstration project; it is far more difficult to put in place a systemic change for funding health services for all adolescents.

What Can Be Learned from the Case?

When the project began, the fact that there were no state guidelines meant that public and private health organizations had to establish their own framework and to learn about each other's worlds. Using agreed-upon criteria to guide selection of a common project was key. The hepatitis B immunization project has value both in and of itself and as a means to understand how to improve adolescent health care and public-private collaboration.

The project developed collaborative means to remove barriers specifically for improving hepatitis B immunization levels among adolescents through a short-term project. The project also served to identify a variety of systems issues that require attention for achieving long-term solutions, including ways to build future collaboration around public health priorities. The remainder of this commentary will focus on what can be learned that is specific to the role of managed care organizations.

PUBLIC HEALTH RESPONSIBILITIES OF MANAGED CARE IN PRACTICE

Managed care organizations have a responsibility to address public health priorities in several ways. First, they should be expected to use a significant portion of health care premium dollars for preventive health care. This would include establishing internal operational standards to ensure that enrollees are reached and receive timely and appropriate preventive health care specific to their age, sex, and culture. Achieving completed hepatitis B immunization series among adolescent enrollees would be one such example.

Second, managed care organizations have a responsibility to be corporate good citizens. Whether for-profit or nonprofit, health organizations engaged in the business of health should make corporate decisions that contribute to the well-being of their enrollees, their own employees, and the communities in which they operate. They should be expected to take the lead among their business colleagues to identify and put in place corporate best practice that integrates employee health programs, as well as corporate policy on conditions that affect the health of their environment and community. Managed care organizations should direct a portion of their philanthropy to local public health priorities. Their public affairs and legislative lobby agendas should include public health issues. This serves a greater public good and may also benefit the organization by improving the health of their employees, as well as reducing preventable health care costs among present and future enrollees. This type of benefit is exemplified through collaborative initiatives such as the adolescent hepatitis B project in the case.

Given that a substantial portion of managed care organizations' funds comes from public sources, it is reasonable to expect public accountability for contributing to the public good. The public, through its governmental representatives, has the responsibility to define, characterize, and quantify the financial aspects of managed care organizations' contribution to public health priorities. Government then has a fundamental responsibility to ensure that public resources are used in the public's best interest; fulfilling that responsibility would include private sector financial reporting of public health contributions. This would have some parallel in the hospital arena, where community benefit expectations have been developed and expected in annual reports.

As the largest single purchaser of health care, government can also use its leverage through contracts, which could justifiably include outcome measurements for specific public health goals, such as adolescent immunizations, in government service contracts. Despite limitations due to changing enrollment, this would enhance public accountability for measuring success in meeting specific public health goals.

THE INFLUENCE OF THE CHARACTER AND CONTEXT OF MANAGED CARE PRACTICE ON COLLABORATION

Experts in the field of managed care will say, "If you have seen one health plan, you have seen one health plan." Variations in managed care plans influence the nature of managed care's contribution to public health initiatives. The most significant characteristics affecting public health collaboration are the plan's organizational values, provider relationships, corporate structure, and payer mix.

Values reflected by the CEO, board, and mission statement are barometers for a managed care organization's interest in and commitment to public health priorities. Variations in organizational structure create logistic complexities, since the alignment of public health responsibilities in the departments of marketing, public affairs, operations, and foundations creates substantially different perspectives in collaborative work. The organization's payer mix also influences health plan interest and participation in public health activities. Health plans with a high governmental payer mix are more likely to participate in partnerships on public health issues than those with a high private payer mix. Finally, the health plan's provider linkages are a significant factor. In this case, health plans that prepay clinics through a loosely connected provider network have issues with double payment for hepatitis B, but they also have difficulty accounting for the extent to which their capitated adolescent population was immunized. Managed care organizations that use variations of a fee-for-service approach or own their clinics have an easier time paying "their fair share" for community-based projects, since funds are held in the corporate account until members receive services.

The environment of the managed care organizations also influences its responsibility and ability to address public health issues, particularly in three areas: regulatory conditions, business climate, and social expectations. Minnesota is the only state in the country that prohibits for-profit managed care organizations. These tax-exempt organizations have two statutory obligations: (1) collaborative plans with public health and (2) serving high-risk special needs populations. Minnesota's legislation, which provides authority to set aside antitrust issues in working together around public health issues, applies only to state-licensed managed care plans; indemnity insurers and the self-insured companies are exempt from the two obligations. The growing trend for employers to bypass health plans entirely and purchase directly from provider networks further erodes the strength of collaborative public health efforts. For the partnership to be strong, the playing field needs to be level. Business interest must be engaged through alternative incentives and corporate interests.

The business community has a strong impact on expectations of managed care to address public health issues. Business leadership commonly opposes embedding any public health or social measures in health insurance premiums. Businesses usually expect public health to be funded through their tax dollars in the general fund. Employers want their premium dollars to purchase services only for their employees. Accountability is at the individual employee service level. This narrow perspective of accountability for health challenges managed care organizations to differentiate the source of funds used for public health efforts from employer premiums. Businesses expect to express any social responsibility they acknowledge for health through the work of their foundations or their participation in United Way-type funding efforts. These mechanisms may offer a significant opportunity for linkage between managed care organizations, public health, and the business community regarding public health goals.

In a for-profit health system environment, managed care organizations would closely mirror the rest of the business community in their corporate philosophy of public health responsibility. Obligations to contribute to public health goals would need to take into account that these organizations are already paying into the tax base for funding public health measures. It is the responsibility of elected officials to establish policy that equitably redirects dollars raised from taxable health entities back into health measures for the common good.

Whether managed care organizations are for-profit or nonprofit, a large portion of their revenues come from public sources. It is therefore reasonable for the public to expect that these companies will contribute to community health and well-being and that a portion of this publicly supported health dollar will go beyond selling the public goods to selling the public good. The pilot project in this case presents a model with potential to maximize public health benefit through coordinated effort focused on a defined public health priority.

FUNDAMENTAL QUALITIES NECESSARY FOR SUCCESSFUL COLLABORATION

Successful partnerships depend on engagement, clarity, equity, and accountability. Since the government has primary social responsibility for public health, it should take the lead in building the foundation for collaboration. Engagement centers on incentives matched with environmental conditions, incentives that may take the form of public policy, economic benefit, and social marketing. In the case, the Minnesota legislature included exemptions from some spending limits as an incentive. Another incentive was statutory authority offsetting potential antitrust issues. Engagement also requires common ownership and recognition of the value of a collaborative initiative, exemplified in this case scenario in the use of selection criteria by the Workgroup.

Clarity is a second quality essential to enhance a managed care organization's contribution to public health. As part of the fundamental responsibility of government, the public health sector should be clear about public health goals, objectives, priorities, strategies, accountabilities, and financing. Clarity, or simplicity, also needs to characterize the design of public health collaboration. The fee-for-service system is not a cost-effective way to implement community-based initiatives. The case applied a model of financing simplicity through a market-share formula. The formula calls attention to a third quality needed for successful collaboration: equity. As the case description recounts, the participating managed care organizations voiced concern that the state's requirement for collaborative public health initiatives did not apply to indemnity insurers or to the self-insured segment of the market. One outcome of the project could be to begin to expect other health care organizations to contribute to public health by appealing to their various ways of contributing to community well-being.

Accountability is another characteristic essential for collaboration. The case points to two levels of accountability: for the project itself and for broader community health systems improvement. At the first level, it would be important to learn what difference the project made in getting hepatitis B immunizations completed in an efficient and effective manner for the population of adolescents. At the second level, the systems questions that are raised must be responded to with appropriate recommendations for improving adolescent health. Accountability is essential for broadening community investment in public health.

Conclusion

Managed care organizations cannot solve fundamental social policy problems. Given their large volume of public funding and orientation to enrolled populations, however, they do have corporate social responsibility to ensure that their prepaid enrolled population receives timely and appropriate health services. These organizations ought also contribute corporate resources to improve conditions affecting the health of enrollees, employees, and their communities. The good of the community at large and the good of the individual should be viewed as complementary goals.

The more we can promote health as a shared responsibility, the greater the progress we will make in improving the health of the whole community. In this shared contribution model of health, managed care has significant responsibility for promoting public health. Bringing together the responsibilities of managed care organizations to society with the priorities of public health expands our potential for achieving local and national goals for healthy people in healthy communities.

References

Fries, J. F.; Koop, C. E.; Beadle, C. E.; Cooper, P. P.; England, M. J.; Greaves, R. F.; Sokolov, J. J.; and Wright, D. 1993. "Reducing Health Care Costs by Reducing Demand for Medical Services: the Health Policy Consortium," *New England Journal of Medicine* 329, no. 5:321–25.

Institute of Medicine. 1988. *The Future of Public Health*. Washington, D.C.: National Academy Press.

Minnesota Department of Health. 1997. *Populations of Color in Minnesota: Health Status Report*. St. Paul, Minn.: Minnesota Department of Health Office of Minority Health.

U.S. Department of Health and Human Services. 1993. *For a Healthy Nation: Returns on Investment in Public Health*. Washington, D.C.: Public Health Service Office of Disease Prevention and Health Promotion.

20

Health Plan Responsibilities for Medical Education and Research

CASE STUDY

Parkview Hospital is a 550-bed tertiary care facility in the urban core of a major metropolitan area. Only the University Health Care Center, on the opposite side of downtown, is larger, with 750 beds. Consolidation in the local hospital market during the past decade, including a flurry of mergers, acquisitions, and closures, has left Parkview and University as the metro area's only independent hospitals.

Parkview is one of five teaching hospitals in the state. It has long had a mutually beneficial relationship with University, part of the state's large land-grant university system. Over half of Parkview physicians have clinical appointments at University's medical school. Parkview's physicians often collaborate with University's physicians on clinical research projects, some of which are conducted on-site at Parkview. Each year, Parkview trains approximately seventy-five full-time equivalent residents from a variety of primary and specialty programs at University. In addition, Parkview sponsors its own residency programs in pediatrics, pathology, and obstetrics-gynecology. These three programs combined train an additional fifty-five full-time equivalent residents per year. Parkview's OB-GYN program is the largest in the state and the only such program not located at an academic medical center. By being able to offer teaching and research opportunities, Parkview has been able to recruit and retain top-notch clinicians. Parkview has also used its status as a teaching hospital and its close relationship with University in its marketing efforts to attract patients.

In the past few years, Parkview has felt the same cost pressures that have affected teaching hospitals throughout the United States. In its local health care market, in which managed care is now the dominant model of health care delivery and finance, the hospital's linchpin for survival as a teaching hospital—an adequate supply of patients willing to pay such hospitals' traditionally higher charges—is seriously threatened. Parkview has seen managed care organizations become increasingly unwilling to pay the higher charges at teaching hospitals, since they can often obtain services of the same quality for lower cost at other institutions. Because these organizations are able to steer their enrollees from high- to lower-cost providers, and because the incentives for such organizations is to purchase services from providers that are less expensive, the negative impact on Parkview and other teaching hospitals in the state has been significant. In response, the leadership at Parkview is exploring a variety of strategies that would permit the hospital to continue its teaching and research programs as well as all other services that it presently provides to its patients and the community.

Six months ago, administrators at Coastal Health Plan indicated to their counterparts at Parkview their interest in acquiring the hospital. Coastal is the oldest of four managed care plans in the state and, with a total enrollment of over 825,000 in its various managed care products, is now also the state's largest nonprofit managed care company.

In the past two years, Coastal has significantly increased its support for medical education and health care research. For example, several of Coastal's clinics now participate in ambulatory training programs for medical residents (though the total number of full-time equivalent residents trained in Coastal's clinics remains below fifteen per year) and Coastal is actively seeking to engage in outcomes, epidemiologic, and other population-based research that is of particular concern to the managed care community. On the other hand, Coastal continues to have misgivings about the overall education and research enterprise. For instance, Coastal's executives have often complained that medical residents trained in this country, and especially those trained abroad, are inadequately prepared to practice in a managed care environment and that their organization, as a result, has had to "retrain" physicians who join their plan.

Two years ago, the state passed health reform legislation that has fueled further consolidation in the hospital market and has prompted the state's managed care plans to pursue aggressively a variety of expansion strategies. Coastal has so far concentrated on acquiring only physician clinics, while its competitors have also acquired or merged with one or more hospitals. Last month, however, Coastal publicly announced plans to acquire Parkview. If the purchase is completed, it would mark the first time in the state that a managed care plan bought or joined with a teaching hospital.

Questions for Consideration

➤ If Coastal purchases Parkview Hospital, should it continue the hospital's teaching and research programs? What changes to these programs would be acceptable/unacceptable? Should Coastal, for example, terminate its OB-GYN residency program? Why?

➤ What obligations, if any, do managed care organizations have to support medical education and/or health care research? Should they help fund medical education and/or health care research? If so, how? Should they provide settings for training tomorrow's practitioners?

➤ If managed care organizations help fund medical education, should they be given a say in how medical students/residents are trained? In who is trained (for example, total number or distribution between primary care physicians and specialists)?

➤ What are the incentives/disincentives for managed care organizations to support medical education and/or health care research?

➤ How should medical schools and residency programs prepare residents for managed care?

COMMENTARY

Howard Brody, M.D., Ph.D.

Consider an average American corporate executive. He gets up in the morning in his comfortable home in a rural suburb, and he shaves and makes his breakfast using electricity originally supplied to that region by the federal rural electrification program. He drives to work along a freeway constructed as part of the interstate highway program of the 1960s. While getting his education at the state university, he acquired a taste for classical music, and so he tunes his car radio to the local public radio station.

He arrives at the plant, where trucks using the taxpayer-supported road network are constantly bringing materials and taking away manufactured goods. The workforce at the factory is quite productive; most of them were taught their skills at the public schools and community colleges. Having arrived in his office, our executive remembers that he is overdue for his medical checkup and asks his secretary to call his doctor and make an appointment. He knows that his health insurance will pay for the visit—and the insurance, provided as a fringe benefit with before-tax dollars, is in effect being subsidized by U.S. taxpayers. If his physician (who also received her training at the state university) happens to prescribe a drug or recommend a medical test, it will be highly likely that it was developed by scientists supported in large part by tax funds.

At lunchtime, the executive drives to the meeting of his service club, where he gives a speech about how his success in life is due solely to individual drive and initiative, which is what has made America great.

Individual and Communal Goods

This little parable is not meant to ridicule corporate executives; all of us in America share in the same culture. Most other highly developed countries are comfortable with the idea that their success depends on some mix of private enterprise and government programs, and the precise, optimal mix can be a matter of considerable debate. By contrast, the U.S. public seems enthralled by an ideology that extols private enterprise and goes to great lengths to deny the role and value of government.

Since the United States, like its trading partners, depends greatly on government programs and regulations in many ways, this ideology has a curious effect on our political and ethical thinking. Certain features of a situation leap out at us, while others fade into the background. Perhaps the best recent example of this blind spot in American political discourse was the elderly woman who stopped her U.S. senator in an airport during the height of the debate over the Clinton health reform plan and begged him, "Don't let the government get its hands on my Medicare" (Johnson and Broder 1996). Because so many of us are like this woman, our country—in which nearly half of all health care is paid for by government, and in which even "private" insurance for employed workers is heavily subsidized by the tax system—could engage in a debate over health care reform in which it was simply taken for granted that the major objective was to "keep the government out of health care."

What does this have to do with the Parkview-Coastal case? As Americans, we can expect to have difficulty in addressing a case of this sort, which involves goods—medical research and education—that arguably ought to be seen as communal goods. We are likely to try to reduce the ethical questions to issues that can be addressed most successfully by appeals to individual rights, duties, or responsibilities. (And, of course, we tend to view corporations as large individuals, not as small communities.) But if we do this, we are unlikely to arrive at ethical wisdom.

Against Funding Research and Teaching

Suppose that Coastal's management decides that it would be healthiest in a financial sense for its plan not to engage in medical research or education. What justification might the managed care plan offer? One, of course, would be that medical research and medical education are not communal goods at all, but rather communal "bads." The case forces us to consider this possibility. For now, however, let us assume that medical research and medical education are in fact good things for all of us to have; the only question is who should pay for them and how.

If Coastal were a for-profit plan, it might join the new chorus defending this sector of the managed care industry by pointing out that it (unlike nonprofit plans) pays considerable corporate taxes (Hasan 1996). If the community thinks that medical teaching and research is good, the community is free to take those tax dollars and allocate them to that end; but it is unfair to expect the corporation to pay twice, both through taxes and internally, by supporting its own education and research. We need not assess the fairness of this position, because in the case, Coastal is a nonprofit managed care plan and therefore pays no taxes. In exchange for its nonprofit status, Coastal is supposed to supply some community service, and we can proceed to ask whether teaching and research fall under this category of expected community service.

And so do-gooders will reply that if Parkview's present programs were closed, the community would suffer a significant loss; therefore Coastal (were it to acquire Parkview) would have some responsibility to continue those programs. Coastal's objection would then be that this would place it at an unfair competitive disadvantage. Other managed care plans, with which Coastal competes, probably do not support much if any medical education and research. If Coastal is expected to sink money into these ventures, other plans will be able to underbid it and take away lucrative contracts with local employers.

There is merit in Coastal's objection. It shows why market forces alone will probably not be sufficient to protect communal goods like education and research (just as they generally fail, for example, to get industries to clean up the environment). Coastal should not be asked to do more than its share to support education and research; other managed care plans should shoulder a part of the burden. But if we can speak of a plan "doing its share" or "failing to do its share," then we presuppose some system of cooperative endeavor among all the plans. And the only way to organize this cooperative behavior among competing plans seems to be to levy a tax and impose regulation upon the industry. That is, government must step in at some point.

The Free-Rider Temptation

The term "free-rider problem" derives from the analogy of the city bus. If no one paid a fare, the buses would stop running. If, however, I can manage to ride without paying my fare, while the vast majority of riders do pay theirs, the bus system will survive. That means that it is rational in a narrow economic sense for me not to pay, because I then get two benefits—I get bus service and I save my own money. Of course, if everyone then does what is "rational," all of us will be worse off.

Private health care corporations often wish to be free riders, drawing on the fruits of medical education and research without footing the bill. Before blaming them, however, we must review the strange history of the funding of academic medicine in the United States. In effect, everyone, government included, has sought to be a free rider; no one has wanted to bear the true and full cost of the academic medical establishment. Some years ago, centers like Parkview received fairly generous subsidies from all levels of government, and yet they were still expected to generate considerable revenues on their own by charging for the services they provided. More recently, as tax-cutting became the national pastime, government assumed that it could decrease the subsidy it provided to academic centers, because they could "simply" charge more for services to make up the difference. That cost-shifting worked fairly well so long as there was a lot of fat in the fee-for-service system, and insurers could pass through these extra costs in the form of higher premiums. As soon as the actual payers (notably, Medicare, Medicaid, and the large employers) decided that they would not tolerate steadily increasing premiums, each party to the transaction developed strong incentives to make someone else pay the costs of medical education and research. So, if today the managed care industry seems unwilling to shoulder its fair share of the burden for these community goods, it is merely following a long if sad tradition.

If we were about to redesign the health care system for the United States, one important component of that plan would therefore be to decide how much we should pay for medical research and education, and how that sum can then be provided on a recurring basis without payers having an incentive to play cost-shifting games. But presently we seem to lack the political will to deal with large-scale health reform, which insures that the free-rider problem in research and teaching will be with us for some time to come.

What Kind of Research?

Recall that we set aside for later consideration the argument that medical research and medical teaching might *not* be a communal "good" at all, at least in the way they are presently conducted at institutions like Parkview. We must now turn to that concern.

The medical research record in the United States since World War II, though in some ways the envy of the world, has yet in other ways been terribly unbalanced. Medical research has until very recently been conducted as if costs did not matter. The goal has been to find what works or what works better. If the new treatment amounts to a 10 percent improvement over the old treatment, and costs three times as much, that goes down as a research success. This system of research did a great deal to fuel the runaway costs of the U.S. health care system—which led us, in turn, to adopt managed care as the best market mechanism to start to bring those costs somewhat under control. In fueling cost inflation, medical research was aided and abetted by medical education, which taught generations of doctors that they are bad people if they do not use the very latest and most complex (and hence the most expensive) technology.

Let's examine one form that criticism of this research agenda has taken recently. A movement with increasing support in medical education in Canada and the United States calls itself "evidence-based medicine" (Evidence-Based Medicine Working Group 1992). This title ought to seem odd. Whoever thought that "scientific" medicine as practiced up until very recently was *not* based on good evidence? The leaders of the new movement, however, emphasize that evidence comes in different varieties. The "old" scientific medicine was based heavily on the evidence of basic biological mechanisms as discovered in the laboratory and on treatment results derived from highly selected pools of subjects in academic referral centers. But it was, we now realize, seldom if ever based on evidence drawn from large-scale studies of "real-world" treatment results among relatively unselected patients in the community, who resemble the people whom most doctors treat most of the time. And many examples can be given of medical "breakthroughs" that seem to perform extremely well in the laboratory or in the referral center but have grave or even fatal flaws once applied on the large scale in community practice (Cardiac Arrhythmia Suppression Trial [CAST] Investigators 1989).

A group of primary care educators has proposed acronyms to aid their colleagues in critically appraising today's medical literature: POEMs and DOEs (Shaughnessy, Slawson, and Bennett 1994). POEMs are "patient-oriented evidence that matters"—studies, that is, that involve typical patients with conditions that occur relatively commonly in medical practice. The evidence is "patient-oriented," moreover, because the outcomes studied are things that matter to people, such as living longer, being free of pain, being more able to carry out activities of daily life, and so on. By contrast, DOEs are "disease-oriented evidence," which tell us more about where diseases come from and what can make them get better, but with much less importance for the life of the patient who has the disease. For example, a DOE study might reveal that taking a certain medication for six months produces a drop in serum cholesterol of fifteen points, but without being able to demonstrate that the fifteen-point drop has any impact on life expectancy or the chance of getting a heart attack in the future—or even whether the side effects of taking the medication over many years might not in themselves outweigh the benefits of lowering the cholesterol that much. The goals of this educational project are to teach primary care practitioners to tell POEMs from DOEs when they read the latest medical journals and to focus in on the POEMs for lessons to change their practice—which is not easy to do, since there are many more DOEs than POEMs in today's literature.

Coastal thus could have a positive role to play in assisting in the reform of the educational and research programs now being conducted at Parkview, if what it seeks to do is to increase the relative attention given to "evidence-based" investigation and teaching. Coastal might urge Parkview to do more research that helps managed care do a better job of delivering the outcomes that patients and physicians desire, while controlling costs (that is, generating more POEMs and fewer DOEs). And Coastal might urge Parkview to do a better job of training its students and residents in the skills of critical appraisal and evidence-based medicine, so that they will not uncritically adopt DOEs as a guide to good practice and will better understand the derivation and application of sound clinical practice guidelines. Over time, Coastal might exert even more influence over Parkview's training programs, affecting not only the skills taught to practitioners but also how many of which kinds of practitioners are trained—to ensure a future health care workforce consistent with the real needs of the community.

In seeking to acquire an academic medical center, Coastal could have something far less exemplary in mind. Coastal might want to do "research" that simply seeks to justify cost-cutting without much concern for the real well-being of patients; and to provide "education" that is merely brainwashing future corporate workers to be compliant pawns in managed care's drive to maximize its own bottom line. This would be unethical behavior, but it should not be confused with the real goals of evidence-based medicine as described here.

Just as it would be wrong to allow a plan to engage in brainwashing and public relations under the guise of evidence-based medicine, it is wrong to attack evidence-based medicine as merely the tool of managed care. Even if managed care were to disappear tomorrow, a decent and affordable health care system would depend ultimately on medicine's ability to develop POEMs to replace DOEs wherever possible.

Conclusion

Recently the mass media have been bashing managed care quite mercilessly. Some managed care practices and plans do indeed deserve all the bashing they get. But, whatever its flaws, managed care came to dominate the marketplace because of serious problems with American health care that no one else was solving.

Those problems will ultimately never be solved without some form of national health insurance that guarantees access to decent health care for all Americans; but even that system would still require some elements of managed care to work optimally (Brody 1992). Maybe we could make managed care go away, but that would not by itself solve the deeper systemic problems that led to managed care's rise in the first place. And, if medical education and research played a role in creating those deeper problems, academic medical centers must admit their responsibility and become part of the solution (Brody et al. 1993). They cannot expect special dispensation by claiming that medical education and medical research are such absolute goods as to be beyond criticism or reproach.

But we cannot tell the world of academic medicine both to reform itself to become more "evidence-based" and also somehow to expect its own funding to fall from heaven. The need to work toward better versions of medical research and education hardly eliminates the need to finance those enterprises as communal goods in which all of us have an important stake. No one in the health care system can be allowed to be a free rider where these goods are concerned.

References

Brody, H. 1992. *The Healer's Power.* New Haven: Yale University Press, pp. 186–207.

Brody, H.; Sparks, H. V.; Abbett, W. S.; Wood, D. L.; Wadland, W. C.; and Smith, R. C. 1993. "The Mammalian Medical Center for the 21st Century." *Journal of the American Medical Association* 270, no. 9:1097–1100.

Cardiac Arrhythmia Suppression Trial (CAST) Investigators. 1989. "Preliminary Report: Effect of Encainide and Flecainide on Mortality in a Randomized Trial of Arrhythmia Suppression After Myocardial Infarction." *New England Journal of Medicine* 321, no. 6:406–12.

Evidence-Based Medicine Working Group. 1992. "Evidence-Based Medicine: A New Approach to Teaching the Practice of Medicine." *Journal of the American Medical Association* 268, no. 17:2420–25.

Hasan, M. M. 1996. "Let's End the Nonprofit Charade." *New England Journal of Medicine* 334, no. 16:1055–57.

Johnson, H., and Broder, D. S. 1996. *The System: The American Way of Politics at the Breaking Point.* Boston: Little, Brown, p. 558.

Shaughnessy, A. F.; Slawson, D. C.; and Bennett, J. H. 1994. "Becoming an Information Master: A Guidebook to the Medical Information Jungle." *Journal of Family Practice* 39, no. 5:489–99.

COMMENTARY

Roger J. Bulger, M.D.

Coastal Health Plan's announcement of its intention to acquire Parkview Hospital was the product of careful self-analysis of organizational values and goals as well as hard-nosed financial due diligence. We can assume that Coastal's leadership has determined that its future and strategic purposes will be well served by assimilating Parkview, with its tertiary care capacity and educational environment, into its own large, well-established, and presumably successful nonprofit managed care enterprise. Presuming that organizational and cultural assimilation can be accomplished constructively, the effort in and of itself raises both exciting possibilities and daunting challenges as the new merged organization identifies its goals and establishes its strategic plan.

It is common sense to assume that Coastal is making this acquisition because it believes it will be stronger both in market position and in economic terms. Having a strong teaching hospital functioning within a care system adds value to the system if the hospital's higher costs can be dampened by the size and efficiency of the rest of the system. Thus, one could reasonably expect that Coastal would tolerate a 10 to 15 percent cost differential between Parkview and the rest of the system; but the cost-conscious drive to lower costs might dominate Coastal's managers, leading them to adopt major changes in organization and drastic reductions in staffing in an effort to reduce Parkview's expenses and add to the system's bottom line.

The management culture of Coastal can be assumed to be different from that which has dominated Parkview for many years. No matter how interested Coastal might be in sustaining a tertiary care teaching hospital in its system, it would be highly unlikely that Coastal would long sanction the kinds of cross-subsidy from service to education and clinical research to which the Parkview physician and nursing staff may have grown accustomed.

Similarly, the departmentally oriented culture of Parkview will do all it can to fight off the kinds of changes Coastal will seek to impose. So tensions and arguments over flagging morale will be regular characteristics of the merged environment for some time to come, all of which tends to depress productivity. The strategic focus for Coastal is the "bottom line" as well as market share, as measured in part by the number of covered lives in the new system.

In this scenario, the best we can reasonably hope for is the gradual acculturation of the Coastal leadership to a more balanced understanding of the impact of the managed care environment upon the clinical education and research activities of our teaching hospitals. A dramatic curtailment in the cross-subsidy, as distinct from a more sensitive strategy of phased reductions, could seriously jeopardize the academic output of Parkview, even though it might maximize Coastal's short-term profits. Parkview faculty and staff have at best a few years to find alternate funding for their academic pursuits. It is in one variation or another of this first approach that most current mergers are immersed. Trying to make ends meet or to make a big profit before selling out to another corporation are equally destructive of truly creative or forward thinking. These are the mergers where survival and/or winning is the name of the game.

Let's consider another scenario, one that several mergers currently on the table or recently consummated may eventually follow. This alternate scenario is directed towards the development of a "teaching integrated health care system," which I shall argue should be called instead a "learning integrated delivery system" (LIDS).

To make the LIDS scenario a reality, it will be necessary to find a plan whose leadership seeks to build a new and innovative organization that capitalizes on the strengths of the academic health center, the university, and the professions.

In attempting to construct a possible long-term vision for the new Coastal, we might agree at the outset that such a vision should flow from what most social observers say are the trends in our society, a vision that is also consistent with the direction of change in our almost twenty-first-century health system. If the direction of change in society overall is from industrialization to the knowledge-based society, and if the computer-driven information society is affecting and changing virtually every phase of life, then we can expect an information-based health system that will live under new financial drivers. Fiscal incentives have been completely reversed in capitated managed care, for example, changing the teaching hospital from a cash cow to a cost center operating within an integrated delivery system. Even so, some academic institutions have been building teaching care systems for some time.

For example, the Rush-Presbyterian-St. Luke's Medical Center University has been busy providing care to its area of Chicago for decades via its HMO and a vertically and horizontally integrated system of hospitals and chronic care venues. From obstetrics to geriatrics, from mental health to heart disease, Rush has sought to provide its patients with the requisite care somewhere in its system. A few years ago, Rush joined in partnership with Aetna, which purchased its HMO and now seeks an expanded patient base. Rush could lay claim to having had one of the earliest teaching care systems to be open to learners throughout.

As society pushes further and further toward the evolution of systems of coordinated care, academics will have to reconsider the tradition of using the teaching hospital as the main venue for clinical education, learning instead how to incorporate ambulatory settings more effectively into clinical education curricula.

If an academic center joins a major comprehensive system (such as Coastal's), one can expect the emergence of a learning (or teaching) health care system. If the definition of LIDS includes a population-based component, with strong preventive and caring themes, we shall witness a rather dramatic shift from the teaching hospital venue to that of the teaching system. If such a system embraces not only teaching but also research and community activity, then it could more properly be called a "learning system." In addition, the LIDS could become the vehicle for adding a health-oriented component to University's portfolio, perhaps involving University in health-related public policy dialogues, health promotion, and distance learning. The combination of an academic health center with its parent university in association with a developing system already exists in several places; all of them present opportunities for LIDS development. Some examples are the University of New Mexico, the University of Pennsylvania, Penn State Geisenger, the University of Florida, Parkland Hospital in Dallas, Washington University in St. Louis, the Mayo Clinic, the University of Cincinnati, the University of Massachusetts, and the University of Kentucky. It is possible to subclassify integrated delivery systems in various ways (for example, by requiring full risk-sharing by the providers, including hospitals, in capitated covered lives; this brings prevention and chronic care into the picture). However one defines the delivery organization, it will be important to link the entire system to the educational and research imperatives, thus emphasizing to the various players the centrality of these functions in the academic clinical enterprise.

Parkview's merger with Coastal creates the prospect of a health care system with a new learning dimension. It also creates the more intriguing, though more ambiguous, potential for establishing an LIDS, the still broader learning organization implied by the long-term association between Parkview and the state university. This second level of integrative planning and possible action would involve the new Coastal and University. What follows will explore both these levels in some detail.

Several assumptions underlie this analysis. First, the realities of the health care marketplace will likely continue to push the various players to greater integration and greater scale, and from case-by-case managed care toward patient- and population-based integrated delivery systems (IDS). With the acquisition of one of the five leading tertiary care centers in the state, Coastal may be well along the path to forging an IDS.

Second, a mature IDS will likely have identified its responsibilities to its clients in terms of prevention and chronic care as well as diagnosis and treatment. In doing so, a well-intended IDS commits itself never to abandon the patient, whether or not treatment is curative and whether or not chronic disease and disability are economically managed. The IDS also acts in its own best interests and those of its members to do all it can to deliver preventive services and encourage healthful behavior.

Third, Coastal through its partnership with Parkview has likely decided that it intends to transform itself more fully from a traditional IDS to an LIDS.

Fourth, the combination of the competitive market environment and the nonprofit nature of Coastal and Parkview can be expected to underscore an organizational value system based on patient and public well-being and service. This is a system, then, that is fundamentally concerned with quality and cost-effectiveness, with excellent clinical outcomes and an ever-improving collective health status for its enrollee population.

As previously noted, the entire nation is undergoing restructuring and reconfiguring throughout most of its major social institutions, moving from the postindustrialized to "the learning society." In keeping with these developments, we can envision in the health field the changes as encapsulated in the movement from the last era's fee-for-service mode through managed care and thence, to the LIDS.

A final assumption—or more properly, bias—is that the LIDS must learn to balance and integrate at least four different value structures into its daily activities, all of which rest upon the fundamental value of patient-centered, population-based service. The four value structures are (1) societal values undergirding health care (including justice, autonomy, hope, and mercy), (2) professional values (competence, commitment, compassion, and collaboration), (3) university values (the search for new knowledge and the transmission of knowledge and ideas), and (4) business values (integrity, organization, efficiency, and building wealth, while effectively distributing goods and services).

The excitement and the challenge of making an LIDS succeed lies in the creative balancing, mixing, and interpreting of these values in the work of the organization. The leadership of a successful LIDS must, from the beginning, encourage and participate in the effort to promote an ongoing organizational dialogue about these value structures and their implications, if there is to be a successful evolution of a new organizational culture.

Increasingly, universities are understanding that they must reach beyond the traditional campus to the community; and Parkview, which already enjoys a long-standing relationship with University, has been an entry point for the academic health center into the community. Just as University might see the new merger as an opportunity for it to reach further and deeper into the community, so the new health system might seek to involve University in its evolving LIDS and to influence University in appropriate ways, for example, with research assistance and direction and workforce development for the region and state. A university-based workforce needs analysis might bring data and informed opinion to the decision makers regarding specific residency program sizes. It would seem desirable for the new Coastal and University to begin formal and informal dialogue, consultation, and perhaps planning in mutually supportive efforts.

Some Specific Issues and Questions

Having purchased Parkview, should Coastal continue that hospital's teaching and research programs? On the assumption that the hospital's purchase signals the entry of Coastal into the learning environment, the new arrangement offers the creative opportunity neither to continue all programs as they are nor to discontinue all research and education but rather to review and reshape programs in the light of new realities. As "purchaser" or employer of the educational products, Coastal's management would have the opportunity to define educational shortfalls. It would also have the opportunity to encourage the creation of new and innovative ambulatory educational venues, thereby providing opportunities to model and evaluate effectiveness and efficiency of interdisciplinary teams in a variety of settings of interest to Coastal and other such providers.

If there were a mechanism for ongoing university dialogue, Coastal might in fact help University convene the main local and regional educational institutions with the main employers of newly graduated health professionals to begin a process of determining what the perceived workforce needs are for the locale, the region, and the state. In this way, Coastal could in effect be an ally with and a stimulant to University in making sense of the size and mix of its medical/health care educational programs.

Similarly, the intellectual resources of University, already engaged through associations with Parkview's large clinical faculty, should be encouraged to address issues raised by the attempt to elevate the health status of a population. Questions arising out of Coastal's interest in preventing disease or promoting health may stimulate collaborations with parts of University previously untouched by Parkview's clinical faculty.

If Coastal closed down Parkview's OB-GYN residency on short-term financial grounds without careful discussion of whether it fills a real need in the state and nationally, Coastal would have missed an opportunity for learning. If, on the other hand, the OB-GYN service at Parkview is redundant—because, say, the residency is one of several in a state with too many OB-GYN specialists and offers little of enduring value in the care of the urban poor—then a decision to close might make sense. Such reviews of specific programs at Parkview might offer a third option: in OB-GYN's case, for example, the new Coastal might create a new nurse midwifery program serving the urban poor, with a consequent reduction in the need for OB-GYN residents.

On the other hand, Coastal's serious engagement in the evolution of an LIDS would precipitate discussion about the nature and extent of its obligations to promote education and research. If Coastal perceives shortfalls in the educational products that come its way, then surely it can and should dedicate some of its resources, personnel, and sites to clinical education.

If a managed care organization seeks the evaluative information necessary for continuous quality improvement, it should also be willing to have independent researchers publish relevant studies that benefit clinical care elsewhere. If medical schools are committed to the patient's and the population's benefit first and the profession's perceived self-interest second, then managed care system education issues will likely be seen to involve nursing, dentistry, public health, pharmacy, physical therapy, and physician's assistants, as well as medicine.

Conclusion

The stalemate between the medical education establishment and the managed care establishment over paying the costs of education and research continues, but the chasms are being breached here and there. If the concept of a learning integrated system can be accepted, then the idea of education happening in a managed care setting will become routine. Information systems and technology will help bring service and academic interests together in an LIDS like the one that could be fashioned by Coastal and Parkview and the state university. The capital Coastal could bring to enhance the information system could be synergistic with University's human and financial resources to create new educational and research opportunities.

Even as the health care revolution has stopped excessive cross-subsidization among service, research, and educational funding streams, it will serve to enforce a market-like discipline upon both the education and research enterprises. If academic health centers can identify their costs in education and in research, and can organize and manage to reduce costs and enhance efficiency, the Coastal Health Plans of the world will be dealing with educational and research business plans. As academics move to accomplish this step, they move closer to more successful dialogue, planning, and negotiation with their partner health systems at the interface of service, research, and education. Coastal's purchase of Parkview could be a model in this effort nationwide.

At a larger level, a Coastal LIDS could provide grist for a university-based inquiry into the continuing ethical questions that will emerge not only from managed care but from advances in science and technology. Together, the plan and the academic health center could identify incentives and disincentives for socially desirable collaborations and could help change the environment in their favor.

Coastal's acquisition sets the stage for the emergence of a new learning organization to supplant the traditional teaching hospitals of days past. Although such a metamorphosis may seem gargantuan to many institutional stakeholders, the challenges of the current environment demand dramatic and creative strategies based on a new partnership forged upon common foundational values. Such an effort, therefore, requires a willingness to bring university, societal, professional, and business values together to serve the best interests of patients and of a defined population.

References

Bulger, R. J. 1998. *The Quest for Mercy—The Forgotten Ingredient in Health Care Reform.* Charlottesville, Va.: Carden Jennings Publishing.
———. "What Will Health Care Look Like in the 21st Century?" In *Nursing Today and in*

the 21st Century: Predictions for the Future. Edited by E.L. Sullivan. St. Louis: Mosby-Year Book.

Bulger, R. J.; Osterweis, M.; and Rubin, R. R. 1998. *Managing the Academic Health Center Mission: The Search for Integration.* Washington, D.C.: The Association of Academic Health Centers.

Contributors

Editors

Karen G. Gervais, Ph.D., is Director of the Minnesota Center for Health Care Ethics and formerly the Coordinator of the Minnesota Network for Institutional Ethics Committees. She has been developing an ethical framework for a vertically integrated health care system with the Allina Health System and has collaborated with several other health care systems and organizations. Gervais is the author of *Redefining Death*, coauthor of *The Use of Human Fetal Tissue: Scientific, Ethical, and Policy Concerns*, and has also published numerous articles on managed care.

Kimberly K. Otte, J.D., M.A., is the public policy attorney for Allina Health System, where she monitors, drafts, and implements legislation and participates in the design and implementation of Allina's ethics initiative. Previously, Otte practiced health care law at the law firm of Halleland, Lewis, Nilan, Sipkins, and Johnson. She is adjunct faculty at William Mitchell College of Law and Hamline University School of Law.

Reinhard Priester, J.D., is a health policy consultant in Minneapolis and Associate for Health Policy at the Minnesota Center for Health Care Ethics. Priester has worked with academic institutions, governmental agencies, and private organizations on a variety of health policy and bioethics issues. His work concentrates on technology assessment and reimbursement issues, resource allocation, and ethics and health care reform.

Mary M. Solberg, Ph.D., M.S.W., is a member of the Religion Department of Gustavus Adolphus College in St. Peter, Minnesota, and a Center Associate of the Minnesota Center for Health Care Ethics. She has also taught theology and ethics at Haverford College and the University of Pennsylvania. Solberg served as

Project Editor for the *Encyclopedia of Bioethics*, rev. ed., and is the author of *Compelling Knowledge: A Feminist Proposal for an Epistemology of the Cross.*

Dorothy E. Vawter, Ph.D., is the Associate Director of the Minnesota Center for Health Care Ethics. She coauthored the Minnesota Center's report, "Improving Coverage Decisions for Unproven Health Care Interventions," and is assisting in the design of a systemwide ethics model for a large, integrated health system. Vawter's other publications and research focus on cross-cultural health care ethics, professional integrity, organ and tissue donation, and research with human subjects.

Commentators

Mila Ann Aroskar, R.N., Ed.D., F.A.A.N., is Associate Professor, School of Public Health, and Faculty Associate, Center for Bioethics, at the University of Minnesota. She is an author, lecturer, researcher, and consultant on ethics in nursing, patient care, public health, and health care administration. Aroskar is a fellow of the American Academy of Nursing and a fellow of the Hastings Center.

Howard Brody, M.D., Ph.D., is Director of the Center for Ethics and Humanities in the Life Sciences and Professor of Family Practice and Philosophy at Michigan State University in East Lansing. Brody received his M.D. and his Ph.D. in philosophy from Michigan State University and completed a family practice residency at the University of Virginia. His family physician group currently works on contract with a number of managed care plans in Michigan.

Donald J. Brunnquell, Ph.D., is the resident ethicist and Director of the Office of Ethics at Children's Hospitals and Clinics of Minnesota in Minneapolis. He is a licensed psychologist with doctoral training and clinical experience in child clinical psychology in the health care setting. Further study in philosophy as a Bush Leadership Fellow led to Brunnquell's current role in clinical and organizational ethics.

Roger J. Bulger, M.D., has been President and CEO of the Association of Academic Health Centers in Washington, D.C., since 1988. He has been President of the University of Texas Health Science Center at Houston, Chancellor of the University of Massachusetts Medical Center at Worcester, and Executive Officer of the Institute of Medicine. Bulger's most recent book is *The Quest for Mercy.*

Arthur L. Caplan, Ph.D., is Director of the Center for Bioethics and Trustee Professor of Bioethics, Professor of Molecular and Cellular Engineering, and Professor of Philosophy at the University of Pennsylvania. He is a member of the Presidential Advisory Committee on Gulf War Veterans' Illness and Chairman of the Advisory Committee to the Department of Health and Human Services, Centers for Disease Control, and the FDA on Blood Safety and Availability.

Kate T. Christensen, M.D., F.A.C.P., is an internist with the Permanente Medical Group in Northern California. She is also Director of the Regional Ethics Department for the group and in that capacity organizes educational forums, conducts research, and provides leadership for the ethics activities for the Northern California Region of Kaiser Permanente.

Larry R. Churchill, Ph.D., is Professor and Chair, Department of Social Medicine, at the University of North Carolina at Chapel Hill. His most recent books are *Self-Interest and Universal Health Care: Why Well-Insured Americans Should Support Coverage for Everyone* and *The Social Medical Reader,* coeditor. With a grant from the National Human Genome Research Institute, Churchill is currently leading an interdisciplinary study of informed consent to gene therapy.

Ronald E. Cranford, M.D., is Assistant Chief of Neurology at the Hennepin County Medical Center and Professor of Neurology at the University of Minnesota Medical School. Cranford has served as a consultant to several national commissions on right-to-die issues and as a medical expert in landmark right-to-die cases including the Paul Brophy and Nancy Cruzan cases. He has published extensively on biomedical issues, especially institutional ethics committees, termination of treatment, and persistent vegetative state and other neurologic syndromes.

Kathleen A. Culhane-Pera, M.D., M.A., is a family practice physician at HealthPartners Institute for Medical Education's Family Practice Residency program in St. Paul, Minnesota. She has an M.A. in anthropology and since 1983 has worked with Hmong people, both in Minnesota and in Thailand. As Director of Cross-Cultural and International Family Medicine, Culhane-Pera attempts to bridge the gap between health care personnel and people of diverse cultural backgrounds.

Raymond G. DeVries, Ph.D., is Professor of Sociology at St. Olaf College in Northfield, Minnesota. His books, *Making Midwives Legal* and *Bioethics and Society: Constructing the Ethical Enterprise,* deal with the study of health care and medical professions. A Senior International Fellow of the Fogarty Center of the National Institutes of Health, DeVries spent 1994 and part of 1995 in the Netherlands studying its maternity care system. He is writing a book on the cultural foundations of Dutch health care.

Joanne M. Disch, Ph.D., R.N., F.A.A.N., is Vice-President of Patient-Family Services at Fairview University Medical Center and Adjunct Associate Professor of Nursing at the School of Nursing at the University of Minnesota in Minneapolis.

She is active in the American Association of Critical Care Nurses, the AACN Certification Corporation, the ANA's Committee on Nursing Practice Standards and Guidelines, and the University Hospital Chief Nursing Officers' Council. Disch has published on nursing administration, the economics of health care, and standards of practice.

Daniel O. Dugan, Ph.D., is Director of the Central Valley Institute of Ethics Education, Consultation, and Research in Modesto, California. He served as Codirector, Clinical Healthcare Ethics Support Services, at the Park Ridge Center for the Study of Health, Faith and Ethics in Chicago and is now an ethics consultant at Emanuel Medical Center, Turlock, California, and at Swedish Covenant Hospital and Covenant Retirement Communities in Chicago. His articles have appeared in leading bioethics journals.

Mary L. Durham, Ph.D., is Director of the Center for Health Research for Kaiser Permanente Northwest and Vice-President of Research for the Kaiser Foundation Hospitals and the Kaiser/Group Health in Portland, Oregon. A medical sociologist, she has focused her research on the health care of people with chronic, disabling conditions, especially those with severe mental disorders, and has designed and evaluated programs to enhance the health and functional status of older persons in HMOs.

Linda L. Emanuel, M.D., Ph.D., is Vice-President of the Ethics Standards Division for the American Medical Association and head of the Institute for Ethics. Prior to joining the AMA, Emanuel was Assistant Director, Division of Medical Ethics, and a Glessner Lee Associate Professor of Medical Ethics at Harvard Medical School. She has published and lectured extensively on clinical ethics, including accountability and professionalism.

Michael Felder, D.O., M.A., is board-certified in family practice and earned his M.A. in philosophy/bioethics. From 1991-1997, he served as the founding chairperson of what may have been the first HMO-wide ethics committee of its kind in the United States. He has been an active member of the Hastings Center Advisory Board on Value Dilemmas in Managed Care and is a member of the Rhode Island Hospital Medical Foundation.

Leonard M. Fleck, Ph.D., is Professor of Philosophy and Medical Ethics at the Center for Ethics and Humanities in the Life Sciences at Michigan State University. His book *Just Caring: The Moral and Political Challenges of Health Reform and Health Care Rationing* is forthcoming. Fleck is also coinvestigator for an NIH project, "Genome Technology and Reproduction: Values and Public Policy," which is testing a model for rational democratic deliberation about ethical and policy issues related to genetics and reproduction.

Joel E. Frader, M.D., M.A., is Associate Professor of Pediatrics and Associate Professor of Medical Ethics and Humanities at Northwestern University School of Medicine and the Children's Memorial Hospital in Chicago. Frader was a Robert Wood Johnson Clinical Scholar at the University of Pennsylvania, where he received an M.A. in sociology. He is active in many national organizations concerned with pediatrics and bioethics.

Karen G. Gervais, Ph.D., is Director of the Minnesota Center for Health Care Ethics and formerly the Coordinator of the Minnesota Network for Institutional Ethics Committees. She has been developing an ethical framework for a vertically integrated health care system with the Allina Health System and has collaborated with several other health care systems and organizations. Gervais is the author of *Redefining Death*, coauthor of *The Use of Human Fetal Tissue: Scientific, Ethical, and Policy Concerns*, and has also published numerous articles on managed care.

Bradford H. Gray, Ph.D., is Director of the Division of Health and Science Policy at the New York Academy of Medicine. Previously, he was Adjunct Professor of Research in Public Health and Director of the Institute for Social and Policy Studies and the Program on Non-Profit Organizations at Yale University and was a senior staff member and study director at the Institute of Medicine. Gray has published extensively on the changing conditions of medical professionalism.

Martin Gunderson, Ph.D., J.D., is Associate Professor of Philosophy at Macalester College in St. Paul, Minnesota. His primary areas of interest are bioethics and the philosophy of law. His publications have dealt with such topics as AIDS, informed consent, assisted suicide, and managed care.

Gwen Wagstrom Halaas, M.D., M.B.A., is Associate Medical Director of HealthPartners, a regional health plan and health care delivery system, and Assistant Professor in Family Practice at the University of Minnesota. She is board-certified in family medicine and received her MBA in Medical Group Management.

Mark A. Hall, J.D., is Professor of Law and Public Health at Wake Forest University School of Law and Bowman Gray School of Medicine and Associate Professor at the Babcock School of Management in Winston-Salem, North Carolina. He completed a Robert Wood Johnson Foundation Health Finance Fellowship and taught at Arizona State University and the University of Pennsylvania. Hall is the author or editor of ten books, including the four-volume series *Health Care Corporate Law*, *Making Medical Spending Decisions*, and *Health Care Law and Ethics*.

Gayle Hallin, R.N., M.P.H., is Public Health Administrator for the City of Bloomington, Minnesota. She is currently Cochair of the Center for Population Health and past Vice-Chair of the Minnesota Health Care Commission.

David A. Hyman, M.D., J.D., is Associate Professor of Law at the University of Maryland School of Law in Baltimore. He teaches and writes on health care financing and regulation, procedure, professional ethics, and tax.

Karen A. Jordan, J.D., is Associate Professor at the Brandeis School of Law at the University of Louisville School of Law in Louisville, Kentucky. She has also been a visiting professor of law at Seton Hall University School of Law, teaching courses offered through Seton Hall's Health Law and Policy Program.

Rosalie A. Kane, D.S.W., is Professor of Health Services Research and Policy at the School of Public Health, a graduate faculty member of the School of Social Work, and a Faculty Associate at the Center for Bioethics at the University of Minnesota. For three decades, she has conducted research and policy analyses and provided technical assistance directed toward improving long-term care practices and policies.

William T. McGivney, Ph.D., is CEO of the National Comprehensive Cancer Network, an alliance of fifteen of the world's leading cancer centers, in Rockledge, Pennsylvania. He is a nationally recognized expert in the area of drug and device regulation, technology assessment and guideline development, and coverage and reimbursement policy. In 1989 McGivney received the FDA Commissioner's Medal of Appreciation. He has served on numerous national committees, including the board of directors of the United Network for Organ Sharing.

David Mechanic, Ph.D., is Director of the Institute for Health, Health Care Policy, and Aging Research and the René Dubos University Professor of Behavioral Sciences at Rutgers University. His research focuses on social aspects of health care. In 1997, Mechanic received the Health Services Research Prize, awarded by the Association of University Programs in Health Administration and the Baxter Allegiance Foundation.

Ruth A. Mickelsen, J.D., is Vice-President and Associate General Counsel for Allina Health System in Minnetonka, Minnesota, and Adjunct Professor of Health Law at William Mitchell College of Law. In 1994, she was named a leading health law lawyer by the *Minnesota Business Guidebook to Law and Leading Attorneys*. Mickelsen frequently lectures for the Minnesota Institute of Legal Education, the National Health Lawyers Association, and the American Association of Health Plans. She is a former Director of Legal and Policy Affairs for the Minnesota Department of Health.

E. Haavi Morreim, Ph.D., is Professor in the College of Medicine, University of Tennessee, in the Department of Human Values and Ethics. For the past eighteen years, she has done clinical teaching and consulting in medical ethics at the University of Tennessee and the University of Virginia School of Medicine. Her research focuses on medicine's changing economics. Morreim has over seventy publications in leading professional journals and is the author of *Balancing Act: The New Medical Ethics of Medicine's New Economics*.

James Lindemann Nelson, Ph.D., is Professor of Philosophy at the University of Tennessee at Knoxville, Clinical Associate in Medical Ethics at the University of Tennessee Medical Center at Knoxville, and Chair of the committee coordinating UT's Graduate Concentration in Medical Ethics. With Hilde Lindemann Nelson, he is the editor of Routledge's Reflective Bioethics series and author of *The Patient in the Family* and *Alzheimer's: Answers to Hard Questions for Families*.

Genevieve Noone Parsons, M.D., is a pediatric resident at Johns Hopkins University in Baltimore. During her medical school training at the University of Pennsylvania, she spent a year at the Center for Bioethics, where she conducted a series of studies of the moral development of medical students and residents.

Gail J. Povar, M.D., M.P.H., is Clinical Professor of Health Care Sciences and Medicine at George Washington University School of Medicine and Health Sciences and practices general internal medicine. She has served as a consultant to the Institute of Medicine and is a fellow of the Kennedy Institute of Bioethics. Povar continues to publish on ethics and managed care.

Lisa J. Raiola, M.P.H., is Director of the Ethics Program for Harvard Pilgrim Health Care (HPHC) in Providence, Rhode Island. She was formerly HPHC's Director of Human Resource Development, as well as Director for Administration for the Rhode Island Group Health Association (an HPHC affiliate). Raiola was previously a principal at HRI, Inc., a management consulting firm, where she was responsible for the health care practice.

Susan B. Rubin, Ph.D., is a clinical ethicist and cofounder of The Ethics Practice, a firm devoted to providing bioethics education, research, and clinical consultation on a national basis and in a variety of health care settings. Her forthcoming book, *When Doctors Say No: The Battleground of Medical Futility*, is a critique of the concept of and the debate about medical futility. Rubin is also coeditor of a forthcoming book, *Margin of Error: The Necessity, Inevitability, and Ethics of Mistakes in Medicine and Bioethics Consultation*.

James E. Sabin, M.D., is Codirector of the Center for Ethics in Managed Care, which is sponsored by Harvard Pilgrim Health Care and Harvard Medical School. He is also Associate Clinical Professor of Psychiatry at Harvard Medical School and a practicing psychiatrist in the prepaid group practice, Harvard Vanguard Medical Associates.

Judith Shindul-Rothschild, Ph.D., R.N.C., N.A.P., is Associate Professor at Boston College School of Nursing, where she teaches health policy and health economics. She is a certified psychiatric nurse clinical specialist and has practiced in a variety of mental health care settings. Shindul-Rothschild's research and writings have focused on the relationships between health care financing, nurses' working conditions, and nursing practice. She is coauthor of *Aging and Public Policy: Social Control or Social Justice?*

Mitchell Sugarman, M.B.A., is Director of Medical Technology Assessment for the Permanente Federation in Oakland, California. He manages the process used by Kaiser Permanente to evaluate new medical technologies, including procedures, devices, and drugs. Sugarman also manages the Interregional New Technologies Committee, an interdisciplinary group of physician and nonphysician senior managers who review new medical technologies and make policy recommendations concerning them.

Peter A. Ubel, M.D., is a general internist at the Philadelphia Veterans Affairs Medical Center and a faculty member at the Center for Bioethics at the University of Pennsylvania. His primary research interests are health care allocation and decision making and the moral development of medical students and residents.

Robert M. Veatch, Ph.D., is Professor of Medical Ethics and former Director of the Kennedy Institute of Ethics, Georgetown University, in Washington, D.C. His research focuses on the role of patients in medical decisions, including the rationing of medical care. Veatch is the author of *A Theory of Medical Ethics* and *The Foundations of Justice.*

Susan M. Wolf, J.D., is Associate Professor of Law and Medicine and an Opperman Research Scholar at the University of Minnesota Law School and a faculty member in the university's Center for Bioethics. She is a past National Endowment of the Humanities Fellow and Associate for Law at The Hastings Center and a past fellow in Harvard University's Program in Ethics and the Professions. Wolf has published widely on managed care and other topics in bioethics and health law and was editor of *Feminism & Bioethics: Beyond Reproduction.*

Matthew K. Wynia, M.D., M.P.H., is Section Director for Managed Care in the Institute for Ethics at the American Medical Association. He practices in Internal Medicine and Infectious Diseases at the University of Chicago Hospitals, where he is Clinical Associate Professor of Medicine.

Laurie Zoloth-Dorfman, Ph.D., is a clinical ethicist and cofounder of The Ethics Practice, a firm devoted to providing bioethics education, research, and clinical consultation on a national basis and in a variety of health care settings. Her forthcoming book, entitled *Ethics of Encounter,* is about justice and health care reform. Zoloth-Dorfman is also coeditor of a forthcoming book, *Margin of Error: The Necessity, Inevitability, and Ethics of Mistakes in Medicine and Bioethics Consultation.*

Index

academic health centers, 348, 350,
   352, 354
access, 5, 6, 145-46, 151-67
accountability
   of health plans, for quality, 186
   of managed care organizations, in
      Medicaid contracting, 271,
      281-82
   of managed care organizations, for
      public good, 335
   of managed care organizations, in
      self-funded arrangement,
      205
   of multiple players, 9, 12
   of nurses, 188-89
   of state, in Medicaid purchasing,
      271, 275
   for vulnerable patients, 143-44
administrative pass-through for claims,
   203, 210
advocacy
   for enrollees, by health plan, 2,
      69-70
   for enrollees, by physicians, 19
   for patients, by facility, 240, 241
   for patients, by health care
      professionals, 10-11
   for patients, by physical therapists,
      233-48
   for patients, by physicians, 2, 10,

11, 20, 57, 69, 71-72, 75-76, 91,
   217-32, 241
   for patients, by nurses, 181-98,
   for patients, by social worker, 137
American Medical Association's
   Council on Ethical and Judicial
   Affairs, 222, 224
American Physical Therapy
   Association, 236, 245-46
American Physical Therapy
   Association's guide for Professional
   Conduct, 234
appeals process, 2, 51, 57, 84-85, 93,
   94, 108, 125, 138, 143, 225, 228,
   231, 246, 251, 262, 308
"assignment-despite-objection" (ADO),
   192-93
autonomy
   of patient, 25.
   See also choice

bedside rationing, 227-30, 300
behavioral health care coverage. See
   mental health care coverage
beneficence, principle of, 9-10
benefit design, 86
   responsibility for, between purchaser
      and plan, 201-16
business ethics, 225, 248, 306, 318

CEO compensation, in for-profit and
    nonprofit plans, 168-80
capitation, 2, 70, 101-17, 121, 130,
    135, 139, 147, 172, 218, 223,
    277-79, 293, 324
    emergency care and, 39
    hospitals and, 186
    impact in medically complex cases,
        127
    impact on physician, 25-26, 106,
        111, 122-23
    in nonprofit health plans, 113
    rehabilitation medicine and, 146
    risk-sharing and, 104
    systemic problems caused by, 105
carve-out of mental health programs,
    207, 274-75, 279
case management, 10, 70, 119-20,
    123, 129-31, 136, 147, 273, 282
choice, 146, 154, 207-8
    employee, of health plan, 309
    enrollee, of covered benefits, 238,
        309
    patient, of provider, 157-58, 165
    patient, of venue and provider,
        134-48
chronic illness. *See* vulnerable
    populations
clinical outcomes data. *See* outcomes
    data
clinical research. *See* medical research
Code of Ethics and Guide for
    Professional Responsibility, 236
Code for Nurses, 191
collective decision making, 21, 24-25
communal goods, 343, 344
community
    definition of, 326-29. *See also*
        managed care organizations,
    responsibilities to the community
complementary health care, coverage
    of, 66-82
confidentiality, 202, 208-9

conflicts of interest
    end of life care and, 131
    for-profit facilities and, 240
    integrated health system and, 306,
        309-10
    nursing home and, 292
    physicians and, 8, 111, 220
    organizations and, 133, 206, 310
    reimbursement arrangements and,
        109-10
continuity of care, 15, 125, 132, 135,
    146, 156, 206-7, 208
contracts
    benefits defined in, 94, 119
    language of, 59
    exceptions to, 61, 96
    exclusions in, 6, 87, 95
    interpretations of, 91
contractual arrangements, 1, 18
coordination of care, 102, 126, 127,
    135, 208
cost-containment, 2, 4, 11, 258
cost-effectiveness, 6, 18, 21, 63-65, 263
cost-shifting, 11, 46, 132, 237, 269,
    293, 304, 317, 345
    from Medicaid to other public
        funds, 267-84
    from private to public payers, 118-33
coverage
    certificate of, 50
    criteria, for complementary
        therapies, 71-74
    decisions, 59, 60-61
    denials, 2, 51, 55-56, 62, 55, 70,
        84
    eligibility, 274
    employment-based, 90
    exceptions, 10-12, 51, 59-61, 250
    exclusions for investigational
        interventions, 11-12, 53
    for durable medical equipment, 85
    for non-medical services, 93, 267-84
    limit, 85

of contractually excluded benefits, 83-98

of investigational interventions, for life-threatening conditions, 49-65

out-of-network, 84, 250-51

policies, 6, 17-32

variations, 49-50, 60

credentialing, 2, 115-67

cross-subsidization, 349, 354

cultural difference

respect for, in managed care, 66-82, 249-64

diagnosis-related groups (DRGs), 4

direct contracting arrangement, 66-68, 70-71

disclosure

by health plan, 108-9, 113-14, 157-58

by physician, 108-9, 113

disease management programs, 40

disease-oriented evidence (DOEs), 346-47

diversity, accommodation of, 66-82, 249-64

dual eligibility, 292-93

education. *See* medical education

efficiency, 186-87, 238-39

emergency services

coverage of, 33-48

Emergency Medical Treatment and Active Labor Act (EMTALA), 36, 43

Employee Retirement Income Security Act (ERISA), 44-45, 52, 89, 114

preemption of self-funded plans, 115-16, 201-2, 205, 215

ethical framework, 9-10, 13

ethical treatment standards, 113

ethicists, 210-16

ethics committees, 71, 125, 130, 131-32, 142, 161, 287, 291, 301, 305, 310-11, 318-19

ethics consultants, 125, 128, 131, 132-33, 287, 291-92

ethics resources for managed care arrangements, 9, 12-13

Ethics Advisory Group, 204

interorganizational ethics, 133

organizational ethics, 69, 128, 131, 211, 220, 314-15, 318-19, 330

organizational values, 12-13, 206, 291, 298-99, 336, 348-49, 351-52

system ethic, 154

evidence-based medicine. *See* outcomes data

external appeals mechanism, 71, 91

external review mechanism, 57-58, 88-89, 91, 92, 95-97

fiduciary relationships, 10, 111

financial incentives. *See* conflicts of interest

formulary, 227, 268-69, 280-81

for-profit health care organizations, 118, 174-75

free-rider problem, 344-45, 348

government regulation, i, 19, 89, 146

judicial, 44-45

legislative

commercially insured products and, 201-2

coverage requirements for health plans, 84

defining minimum comprehensive benefit set, 201

disclosure of financial incentives and, 114

exemption of indemnity
  insurers, 201, 323, 336
medical education support and,
  344
medical research support and,
  344
nurses accountability for harm
  resulting from short staffing
  and, 191
obligations of nonprofit health
  care organizations and, 336
public health initiatives and, 323
reimbursement and, 30

HMO Act of 1973, 4
Health Care Financing Agency
  (HCFA), 47
Health Plan Employer Data and
  Information Set (HEDIS), 174
high tech home care, 304, 309
home care patients. *See* vulnerable
  populations

Implementing Nursing's Report Card, 193
incentives, 2, 104-5, 224, 287, 290
indemnity insurance, 3, 7, 53, 66, 88,
  89, 114-46, 237, 242
informed consent, 71, 141, 251-55,
  257
Institute of Medicine, 332
interpreters, 217-18, 223, 249, 260,
  263
investigational interventions, coverage
  of, for life-threatening conditions,
  49-65

Jehovah's Witness, 250-51, 255-58
Joint Commission on the
  Accreditation of Healthcare
  Organizations (JCAHO), 193

justice, 9-10, 240-41, 306-9, 311-13,
  315-18, 320

learning integrated delivery system
  (LIDS)
life-threatening illness. *See* rescue
loss ratio. *See* medical loss ratio

managed care
  definition of, 1
  ethical neutrality of, 8
  ethic of, 8-9
  market-based, 2, 5, 8, 11, 13, 14,
    25, 91, 159-60, 241, 270
  trade-offs inherent in, 1, 2, 3, 157-58
managed care organizations
  arrangements of,
    discounted fee-for-service, 51,
      118, 250
    horizontally-integrated provider
      system, 70
    network model HMO, 102, 135
    point-of-service option, 208
    preferred provider organization,
      237, 250
    self-funded plans, 201-16
    staff model HMO, 118, 131, 237,
      285, 337
  fiduciary obligation and, 10-11,
    115-16, 240, 318
  functional characteristics of, 1
  responsibilities to the community,
    321-56
    for medical education, 13, 340-56
    for medical research, 13, 340-56
    for public health activities, 13,
      323-39
  stewardship and, 9, 12, 13, 209-10,
    314, 318
Medicaid, 49-50, 69, 105, 129, 139,
  145, 146, 292-94, 303, 308, 315, 345

Medical Assistance. *See* Medicaid
medical education, managed care
    organizations and, 340-56
medical loss ratio, 168, 171-74, 177-80
medical necessity, 5-6, 9, 11, 19, 30,
    42, 50, 57, 74, 87, 89-90, 91, 268,
    272, 279, 286
medical research, managed care
    organizations and, 340-56
Medicare, 47, 49-50, 69, 124, 136,
    145, 193, 285-302, 345
mental health services, 267-84

National Alliance for the Mentally Ill,
    274-75
National Bioethics Advisory
    Commission (NBAC), 212
National Committee for Quality
    Assurance (NCQA), 163, 174
nonprofit health care organizations,
    66, 77, 175, 177, 182
    contrasted with for-profit, 196
nurses, 181-98
Nursing Code of Ethics, 286
nursing home patients. *See* vulnerable
    populations

obligations
    balancing of, to individuals and
        population, 17-32
    of health plans, for benefit design,
        201-16
    of purchasers, for benefit design,
        201-16; 267-84
Oregon Basic Health Care Act of
    1989, 204
outcomes data, 5-7, 39, 54, 70,
    81-82, 140-41

Patient Bill of Rights, 185

Patient Safety Act of 1997, 195
physical therapists, 134-48
physicians
    fiduciary responsibilities of, 10-11
    financial incentives and, 87, 91,
        104-7
    gatekeeping and, 10, 70, 101
    professional integrity and, 10, 74-81,
        252, 256, 257
    practice guidelines and, 7, 87
population perspective, 61, 64, 160
practice guidelines, 6-7, 50, 227, 300,
    347.
preauthorization requirements, 33-34,
    36-37, 42-44, 47-48, 59, 217-18,
    221, 224, 228
prevention, 19, 89, 91-92, 277, 334-35
product design, 201-216
program termination, 303-320
prudent layperson or reasonable person
    standard, 33, 46, 47
public health, managed care
    organizations and, 323-39
purchasers, 1, 3-4, 43, 201-16, 247-48

quality, 162-63
quality of care, 151-67
quality improvement, 2, 4, 152, 156,
    160, 185, 188, 207, 244-48
quotas, 288, 293

rationing, 2, 5-6, 9-10, 21, 22, 24, 25,
    72, 86-89, 91, 92, 112, 293-94,
    308
referrals, 35, 59, 67, 72, 79, 81, 101-3,
    104, 107,
    capitation and, 101-17
rehabilitation, 134-48
reimbursement, 1, 17, 19, 30, 111
religious difference, respect for, in
    managed care, 249-64

rescue
  of patients in dire need, 12, 51, 58
  rule of rescue, 62-64, 138
resource allocation, 2, 132, 139, 297,
  299-300, 312-13, 314, 318
respect
  for cultural difference, 70, 78-80,
    101-3, 249-64
  for religious difference, 249-64
risk-adjustment, 8, 66, 109, 238,
  278-79
risk-sharing arrangements, 7-8, 40,
  70, 87, 132, 135
rural health care, 151-167

similarly situated patients
  different benefits packages and,
    233-48
social workers, 142, 143, 146
specialists, 101-17
staffing levels, 2, 240
  of nurses, in hospitals, 181-98
stakeholder theory, 225
Standards of Clinical Nursing Practice
  (American Nurses Association,
  1985, 1991), 191
Standards for Clinical Nursing Practice
  (American Nurses Association
  1998), 189

Tax Equity and Fiscal Responsibility
  Act (TEFRA), 288
teaching hospital, 340-41, 349
technology assessment, 6, 28, 50-54,
  56, 60
trust, 96, 122-23, 140, 208, 210,
  260-63, 294

universal access, 315-16, 347
utilization review, 10, 42-43, 44, 47,
  70, 218, 222, 224-25, 227-28, 237,
  282

vulnerable populations
  chronic illness, 303-20
  Medicare, 285-302
  chronic mental illness, 267-84
  managed care and, 3, 7, 10-11, 142,
    265-320
  nursing home patients, 285-302
  pediatric home care, 118-33, 303-20
  rural Medicaid population, 151-167
  seriously ill patients, 303-20

whistle-blowing, 194-95